ELSEVIER'S INTEGRATED REVIEW
PHARMACOLOGY

ELSEVIER'S INTEGRATED REVIEW
PHARMACOLOGY
SECOND EDITION

Mark Kester, PhD
G. Thomas Passananti Professor of Pharmacology
Director, Penn State Center for NanoMedicine and Materials
Co-Leader, Experimental Therapeutics, Penn State Hershey Cancer Institute

Kelly D. Karpa, PhD
Associate Professor
Department of Pharmacology
Penn State College of Medicine

Kent E. Vrana
Professor
Elliot S. Vesell Professor and Chair of Pharmacology
College of Medicine Distinguished Educator
Penn State College of Medicine

ELSEVIER
SAUNDERS

ELSEVIER
SAUNDERS

1600 John F. Kennedy Blvd. Ste 1800
Philadelphia, PA 19103-2899

ELSEVIER'S INTEGRATED REVIEW PHARMACOLOGY,
SECOND EDITION

ISBN: 978-0-323-07445-2

Notices

Knowledge and best practice in this field are constantly changing. As new research and experience broaden our understanding, changes in research methods, professional practices, or medical treatment may become necessary.

Practitioners and researchers must always rely on their own experience and knowledge in evaluating and using any information, methods, compounds, or experiments described herein. In using such information or methods they should be mindful of their own safety and the safety of others, including parties for whom they have a professional responsibility.

With respect to any drug or pharmaceutical products identified, readers are advised to check the most current information provided (i) on procedures featured or (ii) by the manufacturer of each product to be administered, to verify the recommended dose or formula, the method and duration of administration, and contraindications. It is the responsibility of practitioners, relying on their own experience and knowledge of their patients, to make diagnoses, to determine dosages and the best treatment for each individual patient, and to take all appropriate safety precautions.

To the fullest extent of the law, neither the Publisher nor the authors, contributors, or editors, assume any liability for any injury and/or damage to persons or property as a matter of products liability, negligence or otherwise, or from any use or operation of any methods, products, instructions, or ideas contained in the material herein.

Library of Congress Cataloging-in-Publication Data

Kester, Mark.
    Elsevier's integrated review pharmacology / Mark Kester, Kelly D.
Karpa, Kent E. Vrana. – 2nd ed.
        p. ; cm.
    Integrated review pharmacology
    Rev. ed. of: Elsevier's integrated pharmacology / Mark Kester ... [et al.]. c2007.
    Includes bibliographical references and index.
    ISBN 978-0-323-07445-2 (pbk. : alk. paper)
    I. Karpa, Kelly D. II. Vrana, Kent E. III. Elsevier's integrated pharmacology. IV. Title. V. Title:
Integrated review pharmacology.
    [DNLM: 1. Pharmaceutical Preparations. 2. Drug Therapy. 3. Pharmacology–methods. QV 55]

    615'.1–dc23   2011035660

Acquisitions Editor: Madelene Hyde
Developmental Editor: Andrew Hall
Publishing Services Manager: Patricia Tannian
Team Manager: Hemamalini Rajendrababu
Project Manager: Antony Prince
Designer: Steven Stave

Printed in China

Last digit is the print number: 9 8 7 6 5 4 3 2 1

Preface

It's all about integration. In fact, integration is essential for the study of pharmacology. Practitioners must consider mechanisms of action, adverse effects, and contraindications for any given drug to ensure proper and safe use by patients. Crucial to these considerations is a thorough understanding of the biochemistry, physiology, and anatomy of the targets affected by the drug. Thus, the overarching concept of the Elsevier Integrated Review series is to consider each basic science discipline within the overall context of all the other basic sciences. The foundation of clinical medicine requires that all basic sciences be integrated across disciplines. To facilitate this important learning paradigm, we have created Integration Boxes in this second edition of the text that highlight an essential pharmacologic principle that can be dramatically reinforced with information from another basic or clinical science discipline. This mode of learning facilitates deeper understanding and more complete memory of the concept.

It's also all about forging a team. Frequently, pharmacology is taught only by basic research-based scientists. We have taken a different and more dynamic approach. The team behind Elsevier's Integrated Review Pharmacology is composed of basic science researchers and educators as well as pharmacists and clinicians. It is our concept that integration must occur not only between "-ologies," but also between practitioners who prescribe, dispense, and create drugs. In this way, basic research scientists, with one voice, can effectively describe mechanisms of action for a drug, the clinician can highlight adverse effects, and the pharmacist can discuss potential interactions with other drugs and/or alternative/complementary medicines. These coordinated interactions among PhDs, MDs, and PharmDs are now the core of Penn State College of Medicine's clinically relevant and organ-based pharmacology curriculum.

It is also about voice—one consistent voice. Each chapter reflects the input of each of the three authors, reflecting an integration of basic, clinical, and pharmaceutical sciences. Each chapter includes Top 5 Lists of important concepts and case-based learning questions that reinforce the Integration Boxes.

It is also about "new and improved." Since the first edition was published, more than 100 new drug entities have come to market. More importantly, over the last several years, we have seen a revolution in pharmacologic agents. With the advent of "biologics," or genetically engineered drugs, the promise of personalized and targeted therapies is closer at hand. The second edition of Elsevier's Integrated Review Pharmacology highlights these new pharmacologic options.

It's also about color. To facilitate reinforcement of key concepts, we use a go (green) and stop (red) strategy in all our Integration Boxes and Figures. That is, if a drug turns off (antagonist) a receptor or enzyme, it is set in a red (actually purple) oval; if a drug activates (agonist) the receptor or enzyme, it is set in a green oval. In addition, we use a large red "X" to denote specifically where a drug inhibits a signaling cascade.

In the end, it's all about the students. Elsevier's Integrated Review Pharmacology provides students a rich tapestry from which to draw conclusions about specific drug classes. Detailed information is provided for major drugs in each of the classes. More importantly, this book provides students with the tools necessary to deal with the myriad new drugs that are presently moving through pharmaceutical drug evaluation "pipelines" or are first being contemplated or discovered by academic or industrial scientists. For the student, it should be more than just memorization of every minor adverse side effect for each and every drug. It's really about applying the principles of pharmacology to evaluate and assess the usefulness and effectiveness of new drugs as they come to market. Indeed, a core competency for the health care professional of the twenty-first century is to become a lifelong learner. We hope that we have provided the pharmacologic foundation for such an educational journey.

Mark Kester, PhD
Kent E. Vrana, PhD
Kelly D. Karpa, PhD, RPh

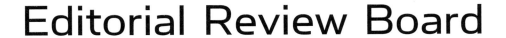

Editorial Review Board

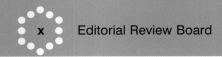

Pharmacology
Michael M. White, PhD
Professor Department of Pharmacology and Physiology
Drexel University College of Medicine
Philadelphia, Pennsylvania

Physiology
Joel Michael, PhD
Department of Molecular Biophysics and Physiology
Rush Medical College
Chicago, Illinois

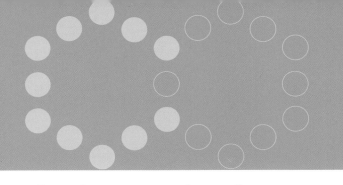

Acknowledgments

To our editors at Elsevier:

To Alex Stibbe, whose "integrative" vision is now an educational reality.

To Andrew Hall, who had to be constantly reminded that there is no such thing as a "hard and fast" deadline. Andy, more than anyone else, ensured that this labor of love came to fruition.

And to Madelene Hyde, who joined the team as we finished this project.

To our many basic, pharmaceutical, and clinical science resources: Dr. Robert Zelis, Penn State College of Medicine; Dr. Cheston Berlin, Penn State College of Medicine; Dr. Michael White, Drexel University; Dr. Kevin Mulieri, Hershey Medical Center; and Dr. Dominic Solimando Jr, Oncology Pharmacy Services, Inc.

To the hard-working Penn State College of Medicine medical students of the classes of 2007 and 2008, who provided valuable feedback concerning selected chapters and subject materials (specifically Ms. Nina Manni). For this second edition, we also wish to acknowledge Daniel Hussar, PhD (Remington Professor of Pharmacy), University of the Sciences in Philadelphia, for his excellent New Drug updates.

To Ms. Elaine Neidigh and Ms. Vicki Condran for administrative and secretarial assistance.

To all of the above, we offer our heartfelt gratitude and appreciation that you can all work so well with such difficult personalities as ours.

Contents

1   Pharmacokinetics   1

2   Pharmacodynamics and Signal Transduction   17

3   Toxicology   29

4   Treatment of Infectious Diseases   41

5   Cancer and Immunopharmacology   79

6   Autonomic Nervous System   91

7   Hematology   111

8   Cardiovascular System   125

9   Renal System   153

10 Inflammatory Disorders   161

11 Gastrointestinal Pharmacology   173

12 Endocrine Pharmacology   181

13 Central Nervous System   201

    Case Studies   227

    Case Study Answers   231

    Index   235

Series Preface

How to Use This Book

The idea for Elsevier's Integrated Series came about at a seminar on the USMLE Step 1 Exam at an American Medical Student Association (AMSA) meeting. We noticed that the discussion between faculty and students focused on how the exams were becoming increasingly integrated—with case scenarios and questions often combining two or three science disciplines. The students were clearly concerned about how they could best integrate their basic science knowledge.

One faculty member gave some interesting advice: "read through your textbook in, say, biochemistry, and every time you come across a section that mentions a concept or piece of information relating to another basic science—for example, immunology—highlight that section in the book. Then go to your immunology textbook and look up this information, and make sure you have a good understanding of it. When you have, go back to your biochemistry textbook and carry on reading."

This was a great suggestion—if only students had the time, and all of the books necessary at hand, to do it! At Elsevier we thought long and hard about a way of simplifying this process, and eventually the idea for Elsevier's Integrated Series was born.

The series centers on the concept of the integration box. These boxes occur throughout the text whenever a link to another basic science is relevant. They're easy to spot in the text—with their color-coded headings and logos. Each box contains a title for the integration topic and then a brief summary of the topic. The information is complete in itself—you probably won't have to go to any other sources—and you have the basic knowledge to use as a foundation if you want to expand your knowledge of the topic.

You can use this book in two ways. First, as a review book . . .

When you are using the book for review, the integration boxes will jog your memory on topics you have already covered. You'll be able to reassure yourself that you can identify the link, and you can quickly compare your knowledge of the topic with the summary in the box. The integration boxes might highlight gaps in your knowledge, and then you can use them to determine what topics you need to cover in more detail.

Second, the book can be used as a short text to have at hand while you are taking your course . . .

You may come across an integration box that deals with a topic you haven't covered yet, and this will ensure that you're one step ahead in identifying the links to other subjects (especially useful if you're working on a PBL exercise). On a simpler level, the links in the boxes to other sciences and to clinical medicine will help you see clearly the relevance of the basic science topic you are studying. You may already be confident in the subject matter of many of the integration boxes, so they will serve as helpful reminders.

At the back of the book we have included case study questions relating to each chapter so that you can test yourself as you work your way through the book.

Online Version

An online version of the book is available on our Student Consult site. Use of this site is free to anyone who has bought the printed book. Please see the inside front cover for full details on Student Consult and how to access the electronic version of this book.

In addition to containing USMLE test questions, fully searchable text, and an image bank, the Student Consult site offers additional integration links, both to the other books in Elsevier's Integrated Series and to other key Elsevier textbooks.

Books in Elsevier's Integrated Series

The nine books in the series cover all of the basic sciences. The more books you buy in the series, the more links that are made accessible across the series, both in print and online.

 Anatomy and Embryology

 Histology

 Neuroscience

 Biochemistry

 Physiology

 Pathology

 Immunology and Microbiology

 Pharmacology

 Genetics

Pharmacokinetics 1

CONTENTS

ABSORPTION
  Ionization
  Molecular Weight
  Dosage Form
  Routes of Administration
DISTRIBUTION
  Plasma Protein Binding
  Selective Distribution
METABOLISM
  Rates of Metabolism
  Microsomal P450 Isoenzymes
  Enzyme Induction and Inhibition
ELIMINATION
  Pharmacokinetic Changes with Aging
APPLYING THE BASIC PRINCIPLES TO CLINICAL
PRACTICE (DOING THE MATH)
  Desired Drug Level
  Drug Factors Affecting Pharmacokinetics
  Patient-Specific Variables—Determination
    of Loading Dose
  Patient-Specific Variables—Determination
    of Maintenance Dose
TOP FIVE LIST

Pharmacokinetics is all about delivery—drug delivery, that is—ensuring that an optimal concentration of drug reaches its specific target. Obstacles to drug delivery include absorption, metabolism, elimination, and distribution of drug to other body compartments. In the end, it all boils down to a dynamic equilibrium—balancing a drug's absorption and distribution with its metabolism and elimination.

A complete understanding of any drug must take into account the mechanism of action, potential side effects, and interactions with other drugs. To fully understand how drugs work, practitioners (this includes physicians, pharmacists, nurses, and physician assistants) must know the general pharmacokinetic and pharmacodynamic characteristics of the prescribed drug to maximize therapeutic benefits and avoid toxicity. Pharmacokinetic principles covering the integrated processes of drug absorption, distribution, metabolism (biotransformation), and excretion cooperatively determine the drug concentration at the receptor site. Pharmacodynamic

mechanisms determine how drug/receptor molecular interactions produce pharmacologic effects by altering intracellular signaling mechanisms (see Chapter 2).

Simply put, pharmacology is the science that studies the effects of drugs on the body (Table 1-1). A drug is any substance that alters the structure or function of living organisms. A poison is any substance that irritates, damages, or impairs the body's tissues. It is worth noting that all drugs, if given in large enough doses, have the potential to be toxic because all drugs are associated with some adverse effects. Thus the practitioner is responsible for hitting the bull's eye or, in pharmacology language, the therapeutic window—a concentration of drug at the active site that exerts a biologic response without exerting a toxic effect. The underlying principles of drug therapy can be reduced to four key statements:

- The intensity and duration of drug action depend on the time course of drug concentration at the receptor.
- Optimal steady-state drug concentration must be maintained at receptor sites to sustain the pharmacologic effect.
- Practitioners control these drug concentrations through selection of appropriate dose, dosage interval, and route of drug administration.
- The physical properties and mathematical models that determine drug absorption, distribution, metabolism, and excretion ultimately are responsible for drug/drug interactions and potential toxic side effects.

Pharmacokinetics can be reduced to mathematical equations, which determine the transit of the drug throughout the body, a net balance sheet from absorption and distribution (in) to metabolism and excretion (out). By understanding these mathematical equations, practitioners are able to determine optimal dosing for patients with impaired or altered mechanisms of absorption, metabolism, or excretion resulting from diet, genetics, environment, disease, allergy, behavior, and other drugs (prescription, nonprescription, and complementary or alternative medicines). Together, these complicating issues are known as *host factors* and represent the interface of environment, genetics, and pharmacology.

●●● ABSORPTION

Absorption is the process of delivering a drug into the bloodstream. Drugs can be administered by a variety of routes: orally (PO), intravenously (IV), intramuscularly (IM), rectally

TABLE 1-1. Pharmacology Terminology

TERM	DEFINITION
Pharmacology	The study of drugs and their effects on the body
Drug	Any substance that alters the structure or function of a living organism
Poison	Any substance that irritates, damages, or harms tissues
Pharmacokinetics	The study of the rates and movements of drugs through the body
Absorption	The process of getting a drug from its site of delivery into the bloodstream
Distribution	The process of getting a drug from the bloodstream to the tissue where its actions are needed
Biotransformation	Conversion of a drug molecule to a more water-soluble form
Elimination	The process of removing a drug from the body

(PR), topically, and via inhalation. Ultimately, to exert systemic effects, drugs must reach the vasculature. Unexpected alterations in absorption can significantly affect therapeutic goals, and certainly there are pros and cons associated with each route of administration, which will be discussed. The general physical principles that govern the rate of absorption, regardless of the route by which the drug was administered, are passive diffusion, concentration gradients, lipid solubility, drug ionization, size of the drug, and dosage form of the drug.

For a drug to be absorbed—to enter the bloodstream—the drug must cross biologic barriers. For orally administered drugs, barriers include the epithelial cells lining the gut and the endothelial cells of the vasculature. Most drugs move down their concentration gradients from an area of high concentration to an area with a lower drug concentration. This movement, called *passive diffusion*, requires no energy expenditure but does depend on the size (molecular weight) of the drug and the lipid solubility of the drug. Most drugs cross biologic barriers by passive diffusion.

On the other hand, a few drugs cross biologic barriers using active transport mechanisms. In this case, the drug moves "uphill" against its concentration gradient—from an area of low concentration to an area with higher concentration. This type of transport requires energy expenditure, typically adenosine triphosphate. Some ions, vitamins, and amino acids are absorbed in this way.

For drugs that are absorbed by passive diffusion, the lipid solubility of the drug is a key determinant for predicting how well the drug will be absorbed. Drugs that are lipid soluble easily pass through the lipid bilayer of cell walls. As a general rule, the more carbon atoms and the fewer oxygen atoms a drug has, the more lipid soluble the drug is. However, the problem with lipid solubility is that a drug must be *lipid soluble* (hydrophobic) enough to pass through cell membranes

but *water soluble* (hydrophilic) enough to dissolve in aqueous fluids (gastric juice, bloodstream). If a drug is too water soluble, it will not penetrate cell membranes. An example of an extremely water-soluble class of drugs is the aminoglycoside antibiotics. When used to treat systemic infections, aminoglycosides must be given IV because the drugs are not absorbed when administered PO. On the other hand, drugs such as phenytoin and griseofulvin are so lipid soluble that it is difficult for these agents to dissolve in aqueous media. Because of the need to be both lipid soluble and water soluble simultaneously, most drugs are administered as either weak acids or weak bases (i.e., a molecule that fluctuates between charged and uncharged states at physiologic pH).

PHYSIOLOGY

Fick's Law of Diffusion

Fick's law of diffusion states that, in a steady state of diffusion, the flux of a substance is proportional to the concentration gradient in the system. To be precise,

$$J = -DA\frac{\Delta c}{\Delta x}$$

where J is the net flux (rate of diffusion), D is the diffusion coefficient, A is the area available for diffusion, and $\Delta c/\Delta x$ is the concentration gradient. This equation concerns moving from areas of high drug concentration to areas of lower drug concentration.

Ionization

Weak acids and weak bases exist in solution as a mixture of ionized and un-ionized forms. Ionized drugs are poorly lipid soluble and do not readily cross lipid membranes, but they dissolve well in aqueous media. Un-ionized drugs, on the other hand, are highly lipid soluble and readily cross biologic membranes. Hence, the transfer of drug across a biologic barrier is proportional to the concentration gradient of the un-ionized form across the membrane; this is known as the *degree of ionization*. The ratio of ionized versus un-ionized fraction of drug depends on the pK_a (ionization constant) of the drug and the pH of the surrounding tissues or fluids. See Box 1-1 for an example.

Box 1-1.   EFFECT OF pH ON THE IONIZATION OF SALICYLIC ACID (pKa = 3)

When pH = 1   99% of salicylic acid is un-ionized
When pH = 2   90.9% of salicylic acid is un-ionized
When pH = 3   50% of salicylic acid is un-ionized*
When pH = 4   9.09% of salicylic acid is un-ionized
When pH = 5   0.99% of salicylic acid is un-ionized
When pH = 6   0.10% of salicylic acid is un-ionized

*By definition, the pKa of a drug is the pH at which 50% of the drug is ionized and 50% is un-ionized.

Box 1-2. EXAMPLES OF DRUGS BEST ABSORBED IN AN ACIDIC ENVIRONMENT

Aspirin	Iron
Calcium carbonate	Ketoconazole
Digoxin	Vitamin B_{12}

When the pH of the solution is below the pK_a, acids are preferentially un-ionized and bases are mostly ionized. On the other hand, when the pH of a solution is higher than the pK_a, acids are mostly ionized and bases are mostly un-ionized.

These principles may be illustrated in a different manner; in biochemistry, the following notation is often used to indicate the ionization status of weak acids:

$$HA \rightleftharpoons H^+ + A^-$$

In an acidic environment, such as the stomach, the weak acid, A^-, accepts a proton and becomes un-ionized. Therefore, in an acidic environment, an acidic drug is likely to be uncharged and thus preferentially absorbed. Alternatively, in an alkaline environment, acidic drugs are more likely to remain ionized and relative absorption is reduced. However, it should be realized that even though this generalization suggests that weak acids are preferentially absorbed at low pH, there is still relatively little, if any, absorption in the acidic environment of the stomach, an organ not suited for absorption. The stomach is mostly a storage depot for drugs rather than an organ for drug absorption. Thus the rate of gastric emptying into the intestines greatly affects the overall rate of absorption. Most drugs are absorbed in the intestines. The small intestines have the greatest capacity for absorption, because villi and microvilli markedly increase the absorptive surface area. The proximal areas of the small intestines (duodenum) primarily absorb drugs that are weak acids because of the acidic pH of stomach secretions. See Box 1-2 for examples of drugs that are best absorbed in an acidic environment.

Ammonia, NH_3, is an example of a weak base.

$$NH_3 + H^+ \rightleftharpoons NH_4^+$$

In contrast to weak acids, when a weak base is in an acidic environment and picks up a proton, the compound becomes ionized and, in this example, ammonium ion is preferentially formed. An alkaline drug is un-ionized in a high pH environment (such as in the small intestines) and thus more likely to be absorbed in this alkaline environment. The distal portions of the small intestines predominately absorb drugs that are weak bases because of the alkalinity of bile secretions. The key point to remember is that a weak acid is most likely to be absorbed when in an acidic environment, and an alkaline drug is preferentially absorbed in an alkaline environment. Even though weak acids are preferentially absorbed in acidic environments, they will still be absorbed, albeit to a lesser extent, in the proximal portion of the small intestines because of the large surface area designed for absorption (villi, microvilli).

BIOCHEMISTRY

The Henderson-Hasselbach Equation

The Henderson-Hasselbach equation states that there is a relationship between the pH of a solution and the relative concentrations of an acid and its conjugate base in that solution. Recall that the pKa (or ionization constant) is numerically equivalent to the pH of the solution when the molar concentrations of an acid and its conjugate base are equal.

Biochemists express this as the log ratio of protonated over unprotonated. In pharmacologic terms, this translates to:

$$\text{For acids (A): } \log \frac{A^-}{HA} \left(\frac{\text{unprotonated}}{\text{protonated}} \right) = pH - pKa$$

$$\text{For bases (B): } \log \frac{B}{BH^+} \left(\frac{\text{unprotonated}}{\text{protonated}} \right) = pH - pKa$$

For acids, the protonated form is unchanged and is the denominator. This is the more permeable chemical form. In contrast, for bases the protonated form is charged and is the denominator. However, this is the less permeable chemical form. In practical terms, this means that acids are preferentially absorbed under acidic conditions (pH below the pKa), whereas bases are preferentially absorbed at alkaline pH (higher than their pKa).

Molecular Weight

Absorption is slow for drugs that are large in size or that possess "bulky" or oxygenated side chain groups. Most drugs are 250 to 450 Da in size and can readily cross membranes.

Dosage Form

Many drugs are available in multiple dosage forms. The formulation of a drug affects the drug's absorption and onset of action. Consider, for example, an orally administered drug that is available as a tablet, a capsule, a liquid suspension, and a liquid solution. To be absorbed, the solid tablet must disintegrate into small particles, which must then dissolve into aqueous gastrointestinal fluids. On the other hand, drugs that are formulated into capsules can skip the disintegration step because capsules contain drugs that are already in small particle form. A drug suspension contains even smaller particles than capsules. With liquid formulations, the drug has already been dissolved. Hence, drugs that are available as liquid formulations are absorbed faster than drugs that are suspensions, suspensions are absorbed more rapidly than capsules, and capsules are absorbed more rapidly than tablets (Fig. 1-1).

Routes of Administration

The enteral (relating to the alimentary canal) route of administration is the safest, most economical, and most convenient way of administering drugs. Orally, sublingually, and rectally administered medications are in this category.

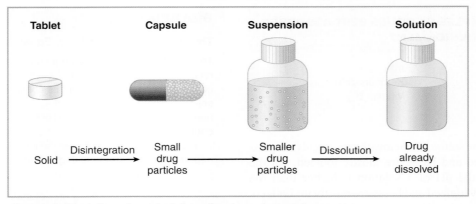

Figure 1-1. Disintegration and dissolution characteristics of various dosage forms.

ANATOMY

Drug Absorption

The first-pass effect is a major mechanism that determines the ultimate concentration of a drug in the plasma. Based solely on the anatomy of the body, drugs absorbed beyond the oral cavity are transported to the liver via the portal vein, where most drugs are metabolized to less active metabolites. After metabolism in the liver, drug metabolites are transported to the systemic circulation by the hepatic vein.

Sublingual and Oral

Medications that are administered sublingually dissolve under the tongue, without chewing or swallowing. Absorption is very quick, and higher drug levels are achieved in the bloodstream by sublingual routes than by oral routes because (1) the sublingual route avoids first-pass metabolism by the liver (Fig. 1-2), and (2) the drug avoids destruction by gastric juices or complexation with foods. Remember that drugs absorbed from the gut travel first to the liver via the portal vein. Drugs absorbed through the intestine may, thus, reach systemic circulation at a concentration significantly below the initial dose. The keys to understanding drug absorption are highlighted in Box 1-3.

Ideally, for a drug to be delivered sublingually, the drug should dissolve rapidly, produce desired therapeutic effects with small amounts of drug, and be tasteless. Examples of commonly prescribed sublingual tablets include nitroglycerin, loratadine, mirtazapine, and rizatriptan (Table 1-2).

Some diseases alter rates of drug absorption. For example if gastrointestinal motility is dramatically increased, as in inflammatory bowel diseases (Crohn disease, ulcerative colitis) or malabsorptive syndromes (celiac sprue), absorption of some drugs may be reduced (Table 1-3). On the other hand, absorption of other drugs may be increased in patients with these inflammatory gut disorders, because gastrointestinal membranes often do not remain intact as a consequence of these autoimmune diseases. Alternatively, consider situations in which gastrointestinal motility is slowed (i.e., diabetic gastroparesis). Here, drug absorption could be enhanced as a result of prolonged contact time with the absorptive areas of the intestine. Likewise, there are drugs that alter the rate of

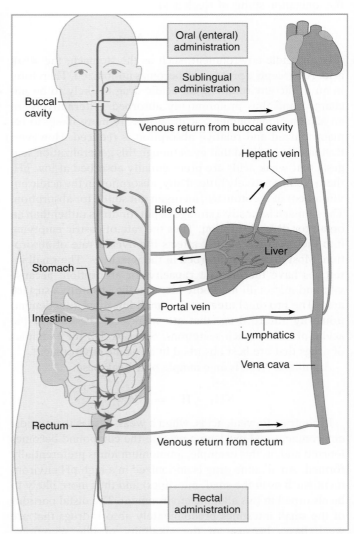

Figure 1-2. Drugs administered sublingually and rectally avoid first-pass metabolism in the liver.

absorption for other orally administered medications (Table 1-4).

Food can also affect absorption of drugs by either increasing, decreasing, or delaying the rate at which absorption occurs (Table 1-5). As a generalization, food tends to slow the

Box 1-3. KEYS TO DRUG ABSORPTION

- The biochemical properties of a drug determine the optimal route of administration.
- Optimal absorption of weak acids/bases depends on the pH of the gastrointestinal tract or surrounding environment.
- Gastrointestinal disease can affect the absorption of drugs.

TABLE 1-2. Drugs Commonly Prescribed Sublingually

DRUG	USE
Loratadine	Allergies
Mirtazapine	Anxiety
Nitroglycerin	Angina
Rizatriptan	Migraine headache

TABLE 1-3. Effect of Intestinal Disease on Drug Absorption

DISEASE	ABSORPTION INCREASED	ABSORPTION DECREASED
Celiac sprue	Aspirin Cephalexin Clindamycin Erythromycin Propranolol Sulfamethoxazole Trimethoprim	Acetaminophen Amoxicillin Penicillin V
Crohn disease	Clindamycin Propranolol Sulfamethoxazole Trimethoprim	Acetaminophen Cephalexin Methyldopa Metronidazole

TABLE 1-4. Drug Effects That Alter Absorption

EFFECT	DRUG
Changes in gastric or intestinal pH	H_2 blockers, antacids, proton pump inhibitors
Changes in gastrointestinal motility	Laxatives, anticholinergics, metoclopramide
Changes in gastrointestinal perfusion	Vasodilators
Interference with mucosal function	Neomycin, colchicine
Chelation	Tetracycline, calcium, magnesium, aluminum
Resin binding	Cholestyramine
Adsorption	Charcoal*

*Note that the final example is administered deliberately to alter drug absorption. The remainder display altered absorption as a side effect.

rate of gastric emptying. This results in slower absorption of many drugs. For this reason, drugs are often administered on an empty stomach—to increase absorption. However, if drugs are irritating to the gastrointestinal tract, a light, nonfatty meal may be recommended. There are other reasons to consider giving drugs with or without food. For example, penicillin V should be administered on an empty stomach (1 hour before meals or 2 to 3 hours after meals) because it is unstable in gastric acids. On the other hand, metoprolol and propranolol (β-blockers) should be taken with meals because food enhances their bioavailability. Although the oral route of administration is the most common, there are a few instances in which the oral route of administration should not be used (Box 1-4).

Rectal

Sometimes drugs are administered rectally via suppository or enema. Absorption from the rectum is erratic and unpredictable because the rectum contains no microvilli. In addition, most drugs irritate the rectum. However, rectal administration can be useful in patients who are unconscious or vomiting or in those with severe inflammatory bowel disease. An additional

TABLE 1-5. Effect of Food on Absorption of Selected Drugs

REDUCED ABSORPTION	DELAYED ABSORPTION	INCREASED ABSORPTION
Ampicillin Aspirin Atenolol Captopril Hydrochlorothiazide Tetracyclines Iron Levodopa Penicillamine Sotalol Warfarin	Acetaminophen Aspirin Cephalosporins Sulfonamides Diclofenac Digoxin Furosemide Valproate	Carbamazepine Diazepam Griseofulvin Labetalol Metoprolol Propranolol Nitrofurantoin

benefit of this route of administration is that the first-pass effect of the liver is avoided because a portion of the rectal blood supply (inferior and middle hemorrhoidal veins) bypasses hepatic portal circulation.

Parenteral

The parenteral routes of administration include any routes that bypass the gastrointestinal tract entirely. The IV route of administration is the quickest way to get a drug to its site of action, so IV drugs are of the greatest value during emergencies when speed is vital. Advantages and disadvantages of IV drug administration are found in Boxes 1-5 and 1-6.

IM and SC administrations are not affected by first-pass hepatic metabolism, but both routes of administration are directly affected by blood flow at the site of injection. Exercise, activity, and massage at the injection site increase blood flow,

which speeds drug absorption by allowing drug contact with vasodilated capillaries.

Relatively large volumes of solution can be administered IM with less pain or irritation than SC injections. This route is particularly useful for lipophilic substances. IM aqueous solutions are typically absorbed within 10 to 30 minutes, although depot formulations have been designed for some drugs that promote gradual absorption over a prolonged period. Drugs administered SC are absorbed slightly more slowly than drugs administered IM. Patients are more likely to be able to give themselves SC injections (e.g., insulin) than to self-administer medications by any other parenteral route.

In the event of an overdose after IM or SC injections, absorption may be reduced by immobilizing the limb, applying ice, administering a vasoconstrictive agent (e.g., epinephrine), or applying a tourniquet.

Other examples of parenteral administration options are listed in Table 1-6.

Inhalation

Anesthetic gases, metered-dose inhalers, and dry-powder inhalers all deliver drugs to the lungs. The smaller the particle size of the drug, the more likely the drug will reach the alveoli. Inhaled glucocorticoids and β-adrenergic agonists are often given to directly affect bronchial and alveolar targets, thus achieving efficacy with minimal systemic effects. However, it should be remembered that a proportion of inhaled drugs still reaches the systemic circulation.

Mucous Membranes

Several drugs are administered topically to mucous membranes of the eye, nose, throat, and vagina. Although typically only local effects are desired, some level of systemic drug absorption does occur through mucous membranes. In fact, some vaginal estrogen products are specifically formulated to provide systemic effects. Likewise, undesired systemic side effects can occur from drug administration to mucous membranes, such as when ocular β-blockers aggravate asthma or when nasally delivered corticosteroids contribute to osteoporosis, cataracts, or elevated intraocular pressure.

TABLE 1-6. Additional Parenteral Routes of Administration and Rationale for Use

SITE OF ADMINISTRATION	RATIONALE (EXAMPLE)
Intra-arterial	Local perfusion of an organ (cancer chemotherapy, radiocontrast agent)
Bone marrow (burn patients)	Other sites inaccessible
Intradermal	Allergy testing
Intracardiac	Emergency treatment of cardiac arrest
Intraperitoneal	Home dialysis; some ovarian cancer treatment protocols

Topical

In general, absorption through the skin is extremely slow. Absorption can be increased by incorporating drugs into fatty, lipid-soluble vehicles such as lanolin, by rubbing the application site to increase blood flow, or by applying a keratolytic (e.g., salicylic acid) to reduce the keratin layer. Drugs applied topically may be used either for their local effects (e.g., hydrocortisone) or for systemic effects (e.g., nitroglycerin, scopolamine, estrogen, nicotine). The latter examples are available as *transdermal* formulations and are time released.

●●● DISTRIBUTION

The process of translocating drugs from the bloodstream into the tissues is referred to as *distribution*. The apparent volume of distribution (Vd) describes the area of the body to which drugs are distributed and may be defined as the fluid volume required to contain all the drug in the body at the same concentration observed in the blood. The Vd may be calculated by dividing the total amount of drug in the body by the initial concentration of drug in the plasma (e.g., C_0 or plasma concentration at time zero). Remember, Vd assumes that the concentration of drug is the same in all locations throughout the body (which is not always true). Mathematically, Vd (in liters) is equivalent to

$$\frac{\text{Dose (mg)}}{\text{Concentration (mg/L)}}$$

Another way to think about Vd is that it is equal to the amount of space in the body that a drug needs to fill up. It should in no way be confused or associated with any particular physiologic compartment. In many cases, the volume of distribution is normalized to body weight and will then be expressed as units of liters per kilogram.

Vascularity is the most important determinant of distribution. After all, very little drug can be distributed to an area of the body that gets minute amounts of blood flow. Frankly, most drugs are not uniformly distributed. Drugs are typically distributed in several phases. In the first phase, drugs are distributed to high-flow areas such as the heart, liver, kidneys, and brain. In later phases, drugs are distributed to low-flow areas such as bones, fat, and skin.

There are many body compartments in which drugs can be distributed, and the Vd varies for each drug, depending on how widely distributed the drug is. Some drugs that circulate in the body tightly bound to albumin will remain primarily in the vasculature, a compartment with a Vd of about 5 L, the volume of plasma. Other hydrophilic drugs distribute to both the vasculature and extracellular fluid compartments, with a Vd of about 15 L. Still other agents distribute throughout all body fluids, including intracellular fluids, and possess a Vd of 40 L or more. With respect to Vd, some key points to understand are (1) when a drug has a large Vd, it means that a larger dose of drug will be needed to achieve a target drug concentration in the plasma; and (2) lipid-soluble drugs (hydrophobic) have a larger Vd than water-soluble drugs.

In fact, lipophilic drugs can dissolve in fat and can accumulate in adipose tissues, yielding Vd greater than 100 L. Note that a drug may have a high Vd and distribute to peripheral compartments, but those compartments are not necessarily the sites of drug action. However, the real value of Vd is that it allows determination of steady-state dosing regimens when a particular concentration of drug is desired in the plasma.

Plasma Protein Binding

Numerous drugs bind nonspecifically to serum proteins, especially albumin, as well as other cell constituents in the skeletal system (bones, teeth, muscle), through a process known as nonspecific protein binding. Protein-bound drugs are not bioactive (i.e., protein-bound drugs have no therapeutic efficacy while bound nonspecifically to plasma proteins). Bound drugs cannot be filtered by the glomerulus nor are they subject to metabolism by microsomal P450 enzymes. Protein-bound drug can be thought of as a *reservoir*—with drug gradually released from nonspecific binding sites when plasma concentrations of the drug decline. For sports enthusiasts, think of plasma proteins as the hockey penalty box; when bound to plasma proteins, drugs (i.e., hockey players) can no longer participate in biologic activity, free distribution, metabolism, or excretion. On the other hand, unbound (or "free") drugs are able to distribute and bind to their specific receptor targets and exert biologic effects.

When a drug is nonspecifically protein bound, the disappearance of the drug from the blood is slowed, because only free drug (1) is metabolized by hepatic enzymes and (2) is filtered by renal glomeruli and eliminated. Because albumin is the primary plasma protein to which drugs bind nonspecifically, alterations in albumin levels can affect free drug concentrations (Table 1-7). Other plasma proteins that nonspecifically bind drugs include α_1-acid glycoproteins and lipoproteins.

There is a theoretical risk of drug-drug interactions any time a drug is greater than 80% protein bound. Drugs compete with one another for binding to plasma proteins, and drugs frequently displace each other. Consider the anticoagulant drug warfarin, which is greater than 99% protein bound. This means that less than 1% of warfarin is circulating freely, and it is this small amount of free drug that is therapeutically active. If a patient has been stabilized on a dosage of warfarin and another highly protein-bound drug is

TABLE 1-7. Free Drug Levels with Albumin Alterations

ALBUMIN LEVEL	ILLNESS	FREE DRUG LEVELS
Hyperalbuminemia	Dehydration	Decreased
Hypoalbuminemia	Burns	Increased
	Renal disease	Increased
	Hepatic disease	Increased
	Malnutrition	Increased

Box 1-7. EXAMPLES OF HIGHLY PROTEIN BOUND DRUGS

Warfarin	Sulfonylureas
Sulfonamides	Nifedipine
Valproate	
Nonsteroidal antiinflammatory drugs	

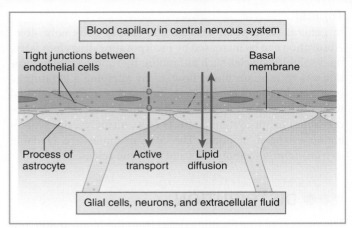

Figure 1-3. The blood-brain barrier.

administered (e.g., a sulfonylurea; Box 1-7), the second drug may compete with warfarin for binding sites and may displace some warfarin from albumin. Even if this displacement results in only 2% of warfarin circulating freely, the amount of free drug has doubled, and this may lead to toxic, potentially life-threatening consequences.

There is a growing feeling that plasma protein binding is not as important as originally thought, because drugs displaced from plasma proteins would then be subject to distribution, excretion, and metabolism. As such, concentrations of free drug in plasma may only be transiently and minimally increased. However, clear cases of toxicity have been observed following administration of highly protein-bound drugs. For example, sulfonamide antibiotics are never used in infants younger than 2 months. Sulfonamides are highly protein-bound drugs, and, in neonates, these drugs have displaced bilirubin from plasma protein-binding sites. This has resulted in hyperbilirubinemia and kernicterus (brain damage caused by bilirubin). In addition, numerous examples of drug-drug interactions involving warfarin and other highly protein-bound drugs exist in the literature.

Selective Distribution

Some molecules are preferentially taken up by specific cell membranes (e.g., iodide by thyroid). It is important to remember, however, that tissues with the highest drug concentrations are not always the sites of drug action. Digoxin, a drug used to manage heart failure, binds nonspecifically to skeletal muscle, but its desired effects are in the heart.

Just as there are reservoirs for drugs, there are also barriers. The term *blood-brain barrier* is a bit of a misnomer. There is not a true barrier that keeps all drugs from entering the central nervous system. The blood-brain barrier refers to decreased permeability of brain capillaries because of endothelial cells fitting tightly together. To enter the central nervous system, drugs must first transverse the capillary endothelium and then cross astrocyte membranes (Fig. 1-3). The blood-brain barrier is impermeable to water-soluble drugs, but Box 1-8 lists criteria for drugs that readily permeate the central nervous system.

The placental barrier protects the fetus from maternal drugs and metabolites. However, the placental barrier is also not a true barrier. In fact, the barrier becomes thinner during pregnancy, decreasing from the beginning of gestation through term. Drugs are distributed to a developing fetus if they are (1) highly lipid soluble, (2) un-ionized, and (3) small in size. Key points about drug distribution are highlighted in Box 1-9.

Box 1-8. CHARACTERISTICS OF DRUGS THAT READILY PENETRATE THE CENTRAL NERVOUS SYSTEM

- Low ionization at plasma pH
- Low binding to plasma proteins
- Highly lipophilic
- Small molecular size

Box 1-9. KEYS TO DRUG DISTRIBUTION

- Drugs are distributed into interstitial or cellular fluids after absorption or injection into the bloodstream.
- Drug distribution may be limited by drug binding to plasma proteins.
- Lipid solubility, pH gradients, and binding characteristics to intracellular or membrane components are determinants that can lead to accumulation of drug in some tissues at higher concentrations than would be expected from diffusion equilibrium alone.

●●● METABOLISM

Biotransformation is pharmacology language for metabolism and is the first step toward metabolizing a drug. The end result of metabolism is that the original drug molecule is altered in ways that make the drug more polar, hydrophilic, and water soluble (and hence excretable). Remember that free metabolites are readily filtered in the glomerulus (in contrast to those that are protein bound) and that these polar hydrophilic metabolites are preferentially excreted rather than reabsorbed across the lipid barrier of the peritubular capillary network of the nephron. Although metabolism can occur in any tissue, the liver is typically thought of as being the primary metabolic site. Without metabolism, 99.9% of all drugs filtered at the glomerulus would be reabsorbed into systemic circulation by the peritubular capillaries of the kidney.

Rates of Metabolism

In the liver, drugs are metabolized at various rates, either by zero-order kinetics or first-order kinetics. Only a few drugs (e.g., alcohol and phenytoin, an anticonvulsant drug) follow zero-order kinetics for metabolism. With zero-order kinetics, the rate of metabolism is constant and does not vary with the amount of drug present. With drugs eliminated in this manner, there is a *fixed amount* of drug that can be handled at any one time. That is because the enzymes involved with metabolism are saturable. Consider alcohol as an example. Only 10 to 14 g of alcohol can be eliminated per hour because alcohol dehydrogenase gets saturated with drug at these doses and simply cannot handle any more drug. When an amount greater than this is ingested, an individual experiences side effects (i.e., "gets drunk"). The amount of time necessary for alcohol to be metabolized increases with the amount of alcohol ingested. If 100 g of alcohol is initially ingested but only 10 g can be metabolized per hour, it will take 10 hours for that alcohol to be metabolized and eliminated. Zero-order reactions are shown in Figure 1-4.

Most drugs, however, are metabolized by first-order kinetics. In other words, a *constant fraction* of the drug is metabolized per unit of time. Another way to think about first-order kinetics is that metabolism increases proportionately as the concentration of drug in the body increases. The more drug there is in the body, the faster metabolism will occur. The enzymes involved with metabolizing most drugs are not saturable at normal drug concentrations. Graphically, first-order reactions are shown in Figure 1-5. When plotted on linear paper, the resulting graph is curvilinear. However, if the log of drug concentration versus time is plotted, the result is a straight line. This line can provide very useful information. Because a constant fraction of drug is metabolized per unit time and metabolism increases proportionately as the concentration of drug in the body increases, the time to clear the body of 50% of drug will always be constant. This is the definition of half-life ($t_{1/2}$). The $t_{1/2}$ of a drug is defined as the time necessary to remove 50% of drug from the body. With first-order reactions, the $t_{1/2}$ of a drug is constant and independent of the dosage given. For example, if 100 mg of a drug is administered and it takes 4 hours to eliminate 50 mg, the $t_{1/2}$ is 4 hours. Knowing that information, it will take 4 more hours to eliminate 25 mg, 4 additional hours to eliminate 12.5 mg, and another 4 hours to eliminate 6.25 mg. Another way to say this is that the peak plasma concentration is reduced in half every $t_{1/2}$. As a general rule of thumb, it takes five $t_{1/2}$ to effectively eliminate (more than 97%) a drug from the body.

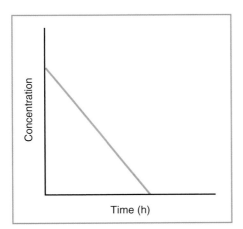

Figure 1-4. *Zero-order* reactions are linear.

BIOCHEMISTRY

Kinetics

Kinetics is the study of rates of chemical reactions; it is concerned with the detailed description of the various steps in reactions and the sequence in which they occur. Enzyme kinetics is the study of the binding affinities of substrates and inhibitors and the maximal catalytic rates that can be achieved.

Only a few drugs are metabolized by zero-order kinetics (e.g., alcohol, phenytoin), in which the enzymes that carry out the reactions are saturable, allowing a fixed amount of drug to be metabolized at any given time. Most drugs are metabolized according to first-order kinetics, in which the time necessary for half of the initial substrate to be eliminated ($t_{1/2}$) is constant and independent of the initial concentration of the substrate.

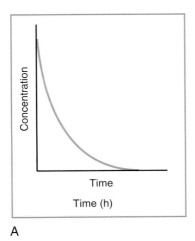

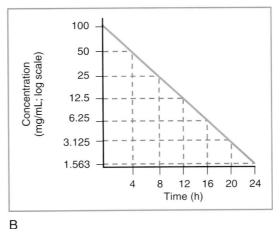

A   B

Figure 1-5. *First-order* reactions are curvilinear (**A**) unless the concentration is plotted on a logarithmic scale (**B**).

Microsomal P450 Isoenzymes

In the liver, the microsomal (endoplasmic reticulum) P450 mixed-function oxidases play a major role in drug metabolism. P450 enzymes have modest specificity for substrates and catalyze the metabolism of widely differing chemical structures. The ability of a drug to be metabolized by various enzymatic reactions depends on the drug's side chain groups and chemical structure. There are 17 families of cytochrome (CYP) P450 genes and 39 subfamilies. Three of these families preferentially metabolize drugs—CYP 1, 2, and 3. Genetic polymorphisms exist for these genes. For example, 7% to 10% of whites are deficient in CYP2D6, and CYP2C19 is completely absent in 3% of whites and 20% of Asians. Because these two genes largely determine how people break down drugs, genetic variations in these metabolism genes can have important consequences for patients. "Poor metabolizers" have a greater risk than the general population of experiencing adverse drug reactions. These P450 polymorphisms (genetic variants) are the basis for the emerging field of pharmacogenomics, a discipline in which an individual's genetic information can guide drug and dose selection.

Phase I Reactions

Also known as *nonsynthetic reactions,* phase I reactions include oxidation, hydrolysis, and reduction reactions. Cytochrome P450s are the enzymes that catalyze phase I reactions. Addition of oxygen groups or removal of methyl groups causes drugs to be more polar than the parent compounds, but even after phase I reactions, the drugs often lack the water solubility necessary for elimination. One aspect of phase I reactions is to prepare drugs for subsequent phase II conjugation reactions.

In addition to serving as a first step in normal metabolism, phase I reactions can have beneficial or negative consequences (Box 1-10). In some cases, phase I reactions activate pro-drugs. For example, the inactive enalapril is activated to enalaprilat (an angiotensin-converting enzyme inhibitor). Conversely, phase I metabolism of benzo[a]pyrene (a tobacco pyrolysis product) produces genotoxic diol epoxide metabolites.

Phase II Reactions

Phase II, or synthetic, reactions are energy-dependent reactions in which chemical structures are added to the drug to increase polarity and enhance water solubility. Such chemical modifications include glycine conjugation, glutathione conjugation, sulfate formation, acetylation, methylation, and glucuronidation (the addition of the polar sugar glucuronic acid, $C_6H_9O_6$). Phase II reactions typically cause drugs to be inactivated. In addition, phase II reactions often enhance polarity so that the molecules can be readily excreted.

Box 1-10.   RESULTS OF BIOTRANSFORMATION

Active drug → Active metabolite
Active drug → Inactive metabolite
Pro-drug → Active drug
Active drug → Toxic metabolite

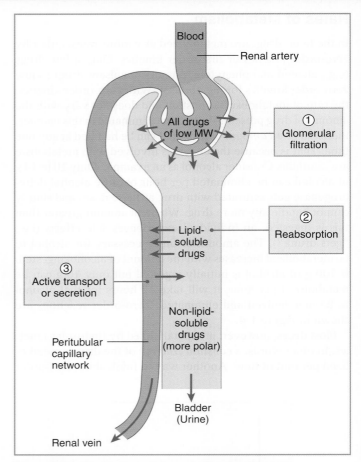

Figure 1-6. Elimination of drugs in the renal tubule.

Figure 1-6 illustrates phase I and phase II metabolism of aspirin. (An additional example of sequential phase I and II metabolism is illustrated by acetaminophen in Chapter 3).

Enzyme Induction and Inhibition

Frequent administration of certain drugs leads to increased synthesis (transcription or translation), or induction, of P450 enzymes. Enzyme induction increases metabolism of all drugs that are metabolized by that particular P450 isoenzyme. Therefore, when multiple drugs are given, drug interactions are likely at the level of P450 metabolism. *This is the major mechanism for drug-drug interactions.* For example, the antiepileptic drug phenytoin induces the CYP1A2 P450 isoenzyme. The antipsychotic drug haloperidol is metabolized by the same isoenzyme. If haloperidol is given concurrently with phenytoin, the metabolism of haloperidol will occur faster than normal as a result of enzyme induction, and the drug will be less effective. In this situation, practitioners may need to prescribe larger doses of haloperidol to achieve desired therapeutic effects. Other chronic inducers of CYP450 enzymes include the anticonvulsant drug phenobarbital and the antimycobacterial drug rifampin. As a potent P450 enzyme inducer, rifampin is associated with drug interactions of substantial clinical significance. Rifampin induces the P450 enzymes responsible for metabolizing oral contraceptives and immunosuppressant drugs. The end result of these drug interactions could be an unplanned pregnancy or immune rejection in a transplant patient. The antiseizure medication carbamazepine is a unique example of an auto-inducer. Carbamazepine induces its own metabolism via CYP3A4, meaning that the longer the drug is given, the more rapidly it is metabolized.

In contrast to enzyme induction, some drugs block, or inhibit, the CYP enzymes that metabolize other drugs. The H_2 (histamine) blocker cimetidine (used to treat acid reflux) is an example of a CYP2C9 P450 enzyme inhibitor. Because diazepam (an anxiolytic) is metabolized by the same CYP450 enzyme, when cimetidine (available as an over-the-counter medication) is administered concurrently, diazepam will not be metabolized as rapidly as normal and may accumulate in the body. This can lead to a longer $t_{1/2}$ for diazepam and associated toxic effects. Box 1-11 lists major drugs whose metabolism may be altered if they are given concurrently with P450 enzyme inhibitors or inducers. Remember, the plasma level of substrates increases with coadministration of a P450 enzyme inhibitor and decreases with coadministration of a P450 enzyme inducer, with varying degrees of clinical significance. Natural and herbal products can also alter the activities of the microsomal P450 isoenzymes and alter drug metabolism (Table 1-8). To prevent adverse drug-drug interactions that occur as a result of altered metabolism, review the key points highlighted in Box 1-12.

CLINICAL MEDICINE

Drug Interactions

Although hundreds of potential drug-drug interactions exist, a few are deemed to be exceptionally important from a clinical standpoint. Keep in mind that some drug-drug interactions warrant careful monitoring, whereas other drug combinations must be avoided entirely. This list is not intended to be exhaustive of all serious drug-drug interactions.

Drug-Drug Interactions of Significant Clinical Importance

Object Drug (or Drug Class)	Precipitant Drug (or Drug Class)	Potential Adverse Clinical Outcome
Benzodiazepines	Azole antifungal	Increased benzodiazepine toxicities
Cyclosporine	Rifampin	Decreased cyclosporine efficacy
Dextromethorphan	MAO inhibitors	Serotonin syndrome; avoid combination
Digoxin	Clarithromycin	Increased digoxin toxicities
Ergot alkaloids	Macrolide antibiotics	Increased ergotamine toxicities
Estrogen-progestin products (oral contraceptives)	Rifampin	Decreased oral contraceptive efficacy
MAO inhibitors	Anorexiants; sympathomimetics	Hypertensive crisis; avoid combination
Meperidine	MAO inhibitors	Serotonin syndrome; avoid combination
Methotrexate	Trimethoprim	Increased methotrexate toxicities
Nitrates	Phosphodiesterase-5 inhibitors	Enhanced vasodilatory effects; avoid combination
Pimozide	Macrolide antibiotics; azole antifungal agents	QT prolongation, life-threatening arrhythmias; avoid combination
Selective serotonin reuptake inhibitors	MAO inhibitors	Serotonin syndrome; avoid combination
Theophylline	Ciprofloxacin; fluvoxamine	Increased theophylline toxicities, especially seizure risk
Thiopurines (azathioprine, mercaptopurine)	Allopurinol	Increased thiopurine toxicities
Warfarin	Sulfinpyrazone, nonsteroidal anti-inflammatory drugs, cimetidine, fibrate derivatives, barbiturates thyroid hormone	Increased bleeding risk
Zidovudine	Ganciclovir	Increased zidovudine toxicities

MAO, monoamine oxidase.
From Malone DC, Abarca J, Hansten PD, et al: Identification of serious drug-drug interactions: results of the partnership to prevent drug-drug interactions, J Am Pharm Assoc 44:142–151, 2004.

ELIMINATION

Elimination is the process of excreting drugs or their metabolites from the body. The kidneys play a large role in drug removal. When glomerular filtration rates are decreased in disease, as evidenced by decreased creatinine clearance (see Chapter 9), the dose of drugs that are eliminated by the kidney must be reduced to avoid toxicity. In other words, renal disease leads to reduced drug excretion, drug accumulation, and increases the risk of drug toxicities. Physicians often need to lower drug dosages for patients with renal disease.

As blood enters the renal glomeruli, plasma is filtered of all substances that (1) are smaller than 60 Da in size and (2) are

Box 1-11. P450 ENZYME INHIBITORS AND INDUCERS*

P450 Substrates	P450 Inducers
Benzodiazepines	Carbamazepine
β-Blockers	Phenobarbital
Ca^{++} channel blockers	Phenytoin
Carbamazepine	Rifampin
Cyclosporine	**P450 Inhibitors**
Haloperidol	Cimetidine
Oral contraceptives	Erythromycin
Phenytoin	Fluoxetine
Theophylline	Isoniazid
Tricyclic antidepressants	Ketoconazole
Warfarin	Ritonavir

*This list is not exhaustive. It is merely a representation of selected drugs that have been associated with clinically significant drug interactions resulting from altered P450 metabolism.

TABLE 1-8. Examples of Natural Products That Alter P450 Isoenzyme Metabolism

P450 INDUCERS	P450 INHIBITORS
Broccoli	Black tea
Brussels sprouts	Chamomile
Cabbage	Clove
Cauliflower	Dandelion
Charbroiled meats	Ginger
Cigarette smoking	Grapefruit juice
Oregano	Kava kava
	Milk thistle
	Licorice
	St. John's wort*

This list is not exhaustive. More than 40 foods and natural products are known to alter P450 metabolism.
*Although St. John's wort appears to inhibit CYP3A4 acutely, it also seems to induce the enzyme with repeated administration.

Box 1-12. KEYS TO DRUG METABOLISM

- Most drugs undergo metabolism before being eliminated from the body.
- Drug metabolites are generally more polar than their parent compound.
- The cytochrome P450 enzymes are selective but not specific.
- Concurrent ingestion of two or more drugs can affect the rate of metabolism of one or more of them.

not protein bound. Drugs that are un-ionized and lipid soluble are readily reabsorbed into the peritubular capillaries from the renal tubules, whereas drugs that are ionized or polar tend to be retained in the renal tubule and excreted in the urine (Fig. 1-7). Changes in urine pH can alter (increase or decrease) drug elimination, just as discussed in the section on absorption. Briefly, acidifying the urine (with vitamin C or NH_4Cl) promotes reabsorption of drugs that are weakly acidic (acidic environments render weak acids un-ionized, $H^+ + A^- \rightarrow HA$). On the other hand, alkalinizing the urine ($NaHCO_3$) causes a weak acid to be ionized and thus accelerates its excretion. This is a great way to detoxify weak acids (i.e., salicylate). Equally, toxins that are weak bases can be preferentially excreted by acidifying the urine.

In addition, some drugs are actively secreted out of the bloodstream and into the proximal renal tubule via energy-dependent cationic and anionic transport pumps (Table 1-9). Drugs can compete with one another for binding sites on these transport pumps; as a result, one drug can inhibit the elimination of another. Probenecid (used for chronic gout) competes with penicillins and cephalosporins for binding to the anionic transporter, hence extending the actions of the antibiotics. Likewise, cimetidine competes with metformin (an antihyperglycemic) for the cationic transporter, causing metformin levels to increase substantially. These types of competitive interactions are another classical example of how drug-drug interactions may lead to toxicity.

Other organs also play roles in drug elimination. The mammary glands typically secrete drugs, such that drug concentrations found in breast milk approximate 1% of the total maternal dose. Because breast milk is slightly acidic, some weak bases may be preferentially concentrated (trapped) and eliminated through this "excretory" organ. Some drugs are eliminated via sweat glands, saliva, or tears. Although these are minor routes of drug elimination, they may account for skin rashes associated with use of some drugs. Substances such as alcohol and volatile anesthetics are eliminated by the lungs. The liver also plays a role in elimination because some drugs are eliminated via the bile and pass out of the body with fecal matter. This latter route of elimination is also associated with *enterohepatic recirculation* for some lipid-soluble drugs. For example, polar estrogen metabolites are excreted by the liver into the bile and are then returned to the intestines by the bile duct. Once in the intestines, normal gut flora can cleave the estrogen glucuronide, thus recycling the estrogenic parent compound. Because of the lipophilic nature of steroids, estrogen can then be reabsorbed and recycled. The end result for a drug that is recycled in this manner is a prolonged $t_{1/2}$. Note that when antibiotics are administered and the gut flora has been reduced, estrogen is less likely to be recycled and hence excreted in feces. Whenever antibiotics are administered to women using hormonal contraception, there is a possible risk of reduced efficacy of the contraceptive and a back-up barrier method of contraception should be used. The key points to remember about drug elimination are highlighted in Box 1-13.

Pharmacokinetic Changes with Aging

It is no secret that the population is living longer. Because a number of the physiologic changes that occur with aging have a direct effect on drug delivery, a brief overview is warranted. For drugs administered orally, decreased gastric acid production, delayed gastric emptying, slowed intestinal transit, and decreased gastrointestinal blood flow occur with aging. These changes can have profound effects on a drug's absorption and bioavailability. Dramatic increases in body fat and decreases

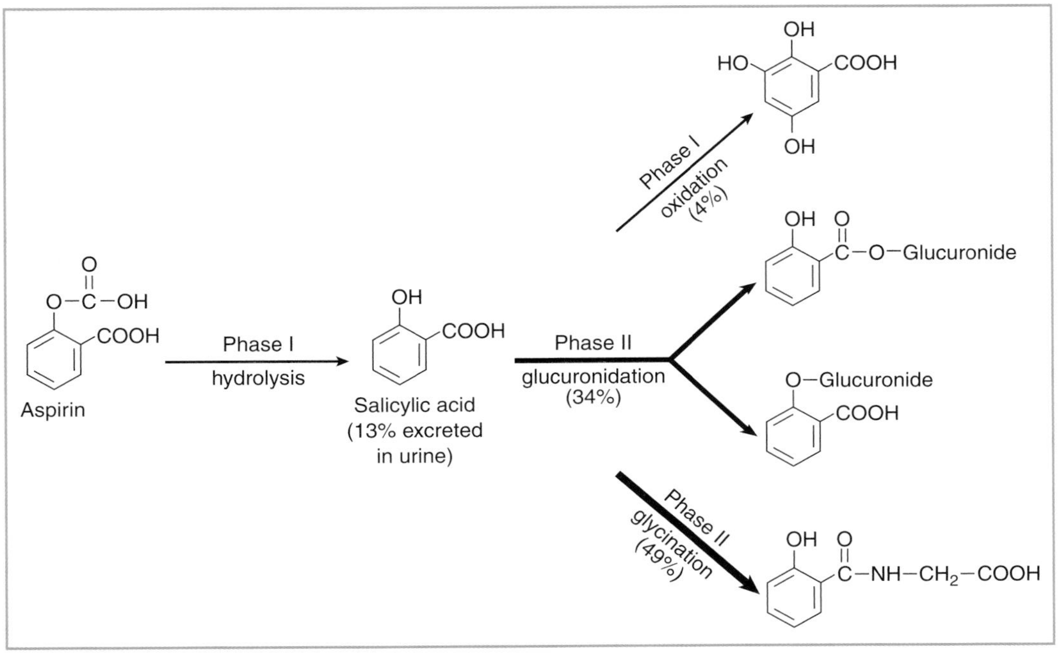

Figure 1-7. Phase I and phase II metabolism of aspirin increases drug solubility for elimination. Metabolites on the right are renally excreted.

TABLE 1-9. Drugs That Are Actively Secreted

ANIONIC TRANSPORTER	CATIONIC TRANSPORTER
Furosemide	Amiloride
Thiazides	Cimetidine
Penicillins	Digoxin
Cephalosporins	Metformin
Probenecid	Morphine
Nonsteroidal anti-	Procainamide
inflammatory drugs	Quinidine
	Ranitidine
	Triamterene
	Trimethoprim
	Vancomycin

Box 1-13.   KEYS TO DRUG ELIMINATION

- Renal and fecal excretion are the most important routes of drug elimination.
- Urine pH can be manipulated to enhance renal clearance of drugs.
- Some drug conjugates are hydrolyzed in the lower gastrointestinal tract back to the parent compound and reabsorbed in a process called enterohepatic recirculation. This process extends the duration of drug action.

in water content also occur with aging. Changes in body composition can affect a drug's Vd, dosing, and side effect profile. Aging is also associated with lower levels of albumin. This results in higher free concentrations of medications that are normally highly protein bound. Furthermore, the activity of active transporter mechanisms (including cellular efflux

pumps such as P-glycoprotein) declines with age, resulting in higher than normal levels of drug reaching certain organs, including the brain. This may partially account for the increased risk of confusion and heightened risk of falls in elderly individuals. Finally, decreased hepatic volume and declining renal function with aging are associated with decreased drug elimination and side effects that result from accumulation of drugs in the body. Because some of the parameters that change with aging can decrease the amount of drug that is absorbed, whereas other parameters such as declining hepatic and renal function can increase drug toxicity, it is important to consider pharmacokinetic factors as an underlying cause any time an expected pharmacologic response is achieved in an elderly patient.

●●● APPLYING THE BASIC PRINCIPLES TO CLINICAL PRACTICE (DOING THE MATH)

When health care professionals administer medication to patients, numerous factors need to be considered (Box 1-14). In the final sections of this chapter, basic pharmacokinetic principles and equations are applied to determine dosing regimens for patients.

Desired Drug Level

Any time a drug is given, there is a "target" level of drug in the plasma that the physician is trying to achieve. Typically, the drug concentrations should become relatively constant and stable when the amount of drug administered during each $t_{1/2}$ is equal to the amount of drug metabolized and eliminated from the body during the same time interval. Thus, it is said that the physician is trying to reach steady state (drug concentration in plasma at steady state, or Cpss).

Box 1-14. **THERAPEUTIC CONSIDERATIONS WHEN SELECTING DRUG DOSAGES**

- Dose
- Bioavailability (F)
- Route of administration (PO, IV, etc.)
- Drug interactions
- Time interval between doses (τ)
- Plasma level of drug initially (Co)
- Plasma concentration of drug reported by laboratory (Cp)
- Desired steady-state plasma concentration of drug (Cpss)
- Volume of distribution (Vd)
- Clearance (Cl)
- Half-life ($t_{1/2}$)

If a drug is given once every $t_{1/2}$, it takes 4 to 5 $t_{1/2}$ for that drug to reach Cpss. Likewise, it takes 4 to 5 $t_{1/2}$ for the drug to be eliminated from the body. When the dosage "in" equals the dosage "out" at any time after 4 to 5 $t_{1/2}$, the Cpss has been reached.

Steady-state concentrations can be achieved either by administering a continuous IV infusion or by giving a series of intermittent doses (either as IV bolus injections or orally) (Fig. 1-8). Note several key points illustrated in Figure 1-8: (1) a new dose is administered once every $t_{1/2}$, (2) 50% of the preceding peak plasma concentration is eliminated each $t_{1/2}$, and (3) Cpss is attained after 4 to 5 $t_{1/2}$, regardless of whether the drug was given by constant IV infusion or by repeated intermittent doses. It is important to realize that the steady state presented in Figure 1-8 can be achieved more quickly by administering a large loading dose early in therapy.

It is worth noting, too, that controlled-release dosage formulations have been created whose plasma levels mimic continuous IV infusions. A few advantages of controlled-release formulations include (1) reduced dosing frequency, (2) reduced fluctuations in drug levels, and (3) a more uniform pharmacologic response.

Drug Factors Affecting Pharmacokinetics

The bioavailability (F) of a drug refers to the fraction of a drug that reaches the systemic circulation. For drugs given IV, the F is 1.0. Two major factors that alter oral bioavailability are (1) the amount of drug *absorbed* from the gastrointestinal tract and (2) the amount of drug *metabolized* by the liver during the first-past effect. Note that bioavailability does not take into account metabolism subsequent to first-pass metabolism or excretion. Often, pharmacologists refer to a term known as *area under the curve*. This is a reference to the graphic representation of the systemic concentration of a drug versus time. This analysis encompasses the factors that elevate concentration (absorption, bioavailability) versus those factors that decrease concentration (metabolism, excretion). This is

illustrated in Figure 1-9. Although generic drugs must contain the same active ingredients as their trade name counterparts, inactive ingredients are permitted to vary. Sometimes, this change in inert ingredients may alter the dissolution rate of a drug, and, thus the shape of the curve may vary. Clinically, this can be important if two different products (albeit containing the same active ingredient) produce differential pharmacologic responses. Similarly, different dosage forms (tablets, gelcaps, liquid) of the same drug may not always be bioequivalent with each other.

For drugs eliminated by first-order kinetics, the $t_{1/2}$ is constant. That is to say, the time to remove 50% of drug from the body is always the same. Doubling the dosage of a drug does not alter its $t_{1/2}$.

A drug's $t_{1/2}$ provides the information that helps determine or predict (1) how often a drug should be readministered, (2) the time necessary to reach Cpss, (3) how long it will take

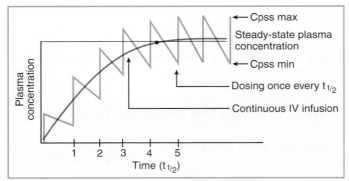

Figure 1-8. Multiple dosing regimens attain steady-state plasma concentrations. *Cpss*, drug concentration in plasma at steady state.

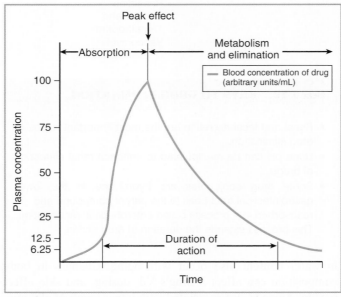

Figure 1-9. Plasma levels of drug during absorption and elimination phases. The integral of this curve represents the area under the curve.

to completely eliminate the drug, and (4) plasma levels of the drug (Cp) at various time points.

Patient-Specific Variables— Determination of Loading Dose

Briefly, Vd is the apparent volume in which a drug is at equilibrium in the body:

$$Vd = \frac{Dose}{Cp}$$

Importantly, the term Vd assumes that the body is a single compartment in which drugs are equally distributed. This apparent Vd allows us to calculate a loading dose (a higher initial dose to quickly achieve the desired Cpss).

$$Loading\ dose = \frac{(Vd)(Cpss)}{F}$$

Reduced to its simplest form, this calculation takes into account the size of the patient (Vd) multiplied by the plasma concentration desired (Cpss).

Sometimes, the desired Cpss is not being attained (e.g., impaired bioavailability because of gastrointestinal disease, enhanced metabolism because of CYP450 enzyme induction, unusual body composition), and the loading dose may need to be boosted. If a patient has already been receiving a drug but is below the desired Cpss, the loading dose can be recalculated according to

$$Loading\ dose = \frac{(Vd)(Cpss\ desired - Cp\ inital)}{F}$$

Patient-Specific Variables— Determination of Maintenance Dose

Knowing a person's rate of clearance (Cl) is especially important for calculating maintenance doses. Clearance is defined as the volume of plasma from which a drug is completely removed by the processes of excretion or metabolism per unit time. Clearance is expressed in units of flow (L/h, mL/min). When the physician wants to achieve Cpss, it is important that the amount of drug cleared from the body in a given time interval is equivalent to the next dose given (e.g., "what goes in must come out"). Clearance is the "out" component for the drug. The value of 0.693 is a mathematical constant that reflects first-order clearance (metabolism and excretion).

$$Cl = \frac{0.693(Vd)}{t_{1/2}}$$

Using this information, maintenance doses can be calculated:

$$Maintenance\ dose = \frac{(Cl)(Cpss)(\tau)}{F}$$

where τ stands for the interval of time between doses of the drug.

Additionally, for some drugs (e.g., aminoglycosides) it is useful to predict peak and trough levels. This can be estimated using the following equation, where *Cp max* stands for maximal plasma concentration (i.e., the peak) and *Cp min* represents the minimal plasma concentration (i.e., the trough).

$$Cp\ max = Cp\ min + \frac{(F)(Dose)}{Vd}$$

●●● TOP FIVE LIST

1. Pharmacokinetics comprise a collection of equations that predict drug concentrations at the target site over time.
2. Pharmacokinetic principles integrate drug *a*bsorption, *d*istribution, *m*etabolism, and *e*xcretion (ADME).
3. Practitioners often need to know mathematical terms specific for a drug ($t_{1/2}$, bioavailability) as well as for a patient (volume of distribution, clearance) to determine the steady-state concentration of drug in plasma (Cpss).
4. Because clearance and volume of distribution change in patients as a function of disease or age, practitioners often need to quantify plasma concentrations of drug directly (from laboratory measurements) to ensure that drugs reach therapeutically effective concentrations without causing toxic effects.
5. Frequently, practitioners must determine volume of distribution and clearance in selected groups of patients (i.e., in renal, gastrointestinal, or hepatic disease). This is necessary to achieve appropriate therapeutic responses.

Self-assessment questions can be accessed at www. StudentConsult.com.

Pharmacodynamics and Signal Transduction

2

CONTENTS

DOSE-RESPONSE RELATIONSHIPS
TIME-RESPONSE RELATIONSHIPS
DRUGS AS AGONISTS
DRUGS AS ANTAGONISTS
SIGNALING AND RECEPTORS
THE FUTURE IS NOW
TOP FIVE LIST

Signal transduction is all about the targets. The targets may be membrane or cytosolic receptors, ion channels, transporters, signal transduction kinases, enzymes, or specific sequences of RNA or DNA, but the pharmacodynamic principles that govern these interactions remain the same (Table 2-1). Drugs bind to specific targets, activating (stimulating) or inactivating (blocking) their functions and altering their biologic responses.

●●● DOSE-RESPONSE RELATIONSHIPS

Often, the lock-and-key concept is useful to understand the way drugs work. In this analogy, the target is the lock and the drug is the key. If the key fits the lock and is able to open it (i.e., activate it), the drug is called an *agonist*. If the key fits the lock but can't get the lock to open (i.e., just blocks the lock), the drug is called an *antagonist*.

The pharmacodynamic properties of drugs define their interactions with selective targets. Pharmaceutical companies identify and then validate, optimize, and test drugs for specific targets via rational drug design or high-throughput drug screening. Table 2-2 identifies some pharmacodynamic concepts that determine the properties of drugs.

Terms such as *affinity* and *potency* (see Table 2-2) are most appreciated in graphic form. Figure 2-1A illustrates a graded (quantitative) dose-response curve. Often, this type of curve is graphed as a semi-log plot (see Fig. 2-1B). Notice that the y-axis is depicted as a percentage of the maximal effect of the drug, and the x-axis is the dose or concentration of the

drug. Several important relationships can be appreciated through graded dose-response curves:

1. *Affinity* is a measure of binding strength that a drug has for its target.
2. Affinity can be defined in terms of the K_D (the dissociation constant of the drug for the target). In this instance, affinity is the inverse of the K_D ($1/K_D$). The smaller the K_D, the greater affinity a drug has for its receptor.
3. The dose of a drug that produces 50% of the maximal effect is known as the ED_{50} (effective dose to achieve 50% response). If concentrations are used, then the concentration to achieve 50% of the maximal effect is known as the EC_{50}.
4. When plotted on a *linear* graph, the dose-response relationship for most drugs is exponential, often assuming the shape of a rectangular hyperbola.
5. By plotting response versus *log* dose, a graded dose-response curve can be translated into more linear (sigmoidal) relationships. This facilitates comparison of the dose-response curves for drugs that work by similar mechanisms of action. Without knowing anything about the mechanisms of opioids or aspirin, Figure 2-1C shows that hydromorphone, morphine, and codeine work by the same mechanism, but aspirin works by a different mechanism. Often, the slope of the curves and the maximal effects are identical for drugs that work via the same mechanism. These curves also show that of the three opioids, hydromorphone is the most potent. That is, responses are observed at lower doses compared with the other agents. *Potency* is a comparative term that is used to compare two or more drugs that have different affinities for binding to the same target.
6. Below the *threshold* dose, there is no measurable response.
7. E_{max} is a measure of maximal response or efficacy, not a dose or concentration. After the maximal response is achieved, increasing the concentration/dose of the drug beyond the E_{max} will not produce a further therapeutic effect but can lead to toxic effects.

Does the curve depicted in Figure 2-1B look familiar? The same mathematical relationships that define how a drug (ligand) interacts with a receptor to elicit or diminish a biologic response also govern the ways in which substrates (ligands) interact with enzymes to generate metabolic end

TABLE 2-1. Examples of Drug Targets

GENERAL TARGET CLASS	SPECIFIC TARGET	DRUG EXAMPLE
Plasma membrane receptor	β-Adrenergic receptor	Isoproterenol
Cytosolic receptor	Corticosteroid receptor	Prednisone
Enzyme	Cyclooxygenase	Aspirin
Ion channel	GABA receptor	Barbiturates
Transporter	Serotonin transporter	Fluoxetine
Nucleic acid	Alkylating chemotherapeutics	Chlorambucil
Signal transduction kinases	Bcr-Abl	Imatinib
	mTOR	Sirolimus

GABA, γ-aminobutyric acid.

TABLE 2-2. Pharmacodynamic Concepts for Determining Properties of Drugs

TERM	DEFINITION
Affinity	The attraction (ability) of a drug to interact (bind) with its target. The greater the affinity, the greater the binding
Efficacy	The ability of a drug to interact with its target and elicit a biologic response
Agonist	A drug that has both affinity and efficacy
Antagonist	A drug that has affinity but not efficacy
Selectivity	Interaction of drug with receptor elicits primarily one effect or response (preferably a therapeutic response)
Specificity	Interaction of a drug with preferentially one receptor class or a single receptor subtype
Potency	Term for comparing efficacies of two or more drugs that work via the same receptor or through the same mechanism of action*

*When comparing potency between two drugs, the drug that can achieve the same biologic effect at the lower concentration/dosage is considered more potent.

products. In fact, the terms K_D and E_{max} (ceiling effect) can easily be redefined as K_m and V_{max}, as per Michaelis-Menten enzyme kinetics.

Another useful mathematical concept is quantal ("all-or-none") dose-response curves. These population-based, dose-response curves include data from multiple patients, often plotting percentages of patients who meet a predefined criterion (e.g., a 10 mm Hg reduction in systolic blood pressure, going to sleep after taking a sleep aid) on the y-axis versus the dose of drug that produced the biologic response on the x-axis (Fig. 2-2A). These curves often take the shape of a normal frequency distribution (i.e., bell shape). These all-or-none responses can easily be thought of in terms of drugs that are sleep aids. The drug either puts people to sleep or it doesn't. There is no in-between. However, the dosage that induced sleep may differ among various people. Most people will fall asleep with a medium-range dose, but there will be outliers—some will be very sensitive to the drug at low doses, whereas others will be relatively resistant to hypnotic effects until higher drug levels are achieved.

These data can be transformed into a cumulative frequency distribution (see Fig. 2-2B), where cumulative percent maximal patient responses are plotted versus dose. This type of sigmoidal curve yields useful safety information when the all-or-nothing responses are defined as therapeutic maximal

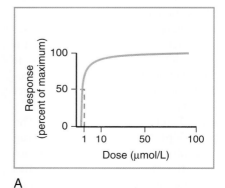

A

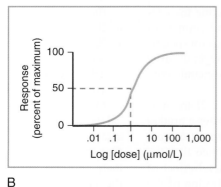

B

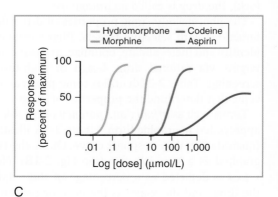

C

Figure 2-1. Graded dose-response curves, in which the K_D value is 1 μmol/L.

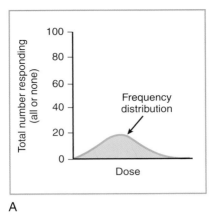
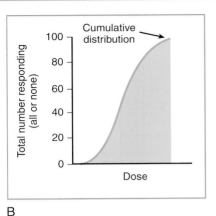
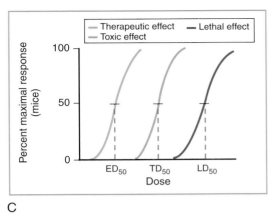

A   B   C

Figure 2-2. Quantal dose-response curves.

responses, toxic responses, or lethal responses. In this way, for a single drug, cumulative frequency distributions can be compared for therapeutic efficacy, toxicity, and lethality (see Fig. 2-2C). This type of analysis can be used to compute the therapeutic index for any drug. The therapeutic index is defined as the TD_{50} (the dose that results in toxicity in 50% of the population) divided by the ED_{50} (the dose at which 50% of the patients meet the predefined criteria). As a rule of thumb, when a drug's therapeutic index is less than 10 (meaning that less than a 10-fold increase in the therapeutic dose will lead to 50% toxicity), then the drug is defined as having a narrow therapeutic window. Examples of drugs with narrow therapeutic windows are listed in Box 2-1. Plasma concentrations are routinely assessed for drugs with narrow therapeutic windows. This is especially critical for patients whose pharmacokinetic parameters are compromised by renal or hepatic diseases.

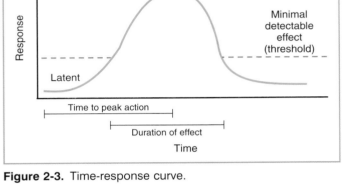

Figure 2-3. Time-response curve.

●●● TIME-RESPONSE RELATIONSHIPS

For some analyses, it is advantageous to graph time to drug action versus defined response. This time-response curve (Fig. 2-3) depicts the latent period (time to onset of action), the time to peak effect, as well as the duration of action. Often the y-axis for this type of relationship is given as the plasma concentration of the drug (because plasma concentration is directly related to response). The maximal peak response should be below the toxic dose and above the minimal effective dose. If it isn't obvious why the processes of absorption, distribution, metabolism, and excretion determine the shape of this curve, refer back to Chapter 1.

●●● DRUGS AS AGONISTS

How does a practitioner interpret two drugs that have equal affinities (binding) for a specific target but have different efficacies (degree of response) (Fig. 2-4)? In this example, even though all these drugs are agonists for the target, the drugs that elicit a maximal response are full agonists (drugs C and D), whereas those that do not elicit a maximal response are often referred to as *partial agonists* (drugs A and B in Fig. 2-4). In other words, despite occupying all of the receptors for the drug at the target site, the biologic response for partial agonists is muted or lower than that of full agonists. Often the reasons for this muted or weak biologic response at full receptor occupancy (saturation) is unknown. However, the key point is that partial agonists are often used clinically to inhibit competitively the responses of full agonists; thus they can be thought of as competitive pharmacologic antagonists. Buspirone is an example of a partial agonist; buspirone exhibits full agonist properties at presynaptic $5HT_{1A}$ serotonin receptors but very weak agonist activity at postsynaptic $5HT_{1A}$ receptors. The net result of these disparate biologic responses leads to classification of this drug as a partial agonist.

Continuing with Figure 2-4, there can be cases when partial agonists (drug A) display greater potency (greater effect at a

Box 2-1. DRUGS WITH NARROW THERAPEUTIC WINDOWS

Theophylline	Digoxin
Warfarin	Carbamazepine
Valproate	Phenytoin
Lithium	Gentamicin

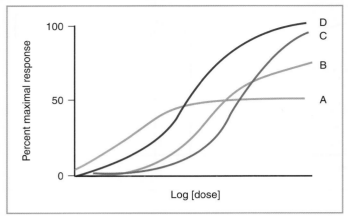

Figure 2-4. Graded dose-response curves for four drugs of the same class. Drugs C and D are full agonists, whereas drugs A and B are partial agonists. Drug A is the most potent agent, despite being a partial agonist. Drug D is more potent than C, even though both are full agonists.

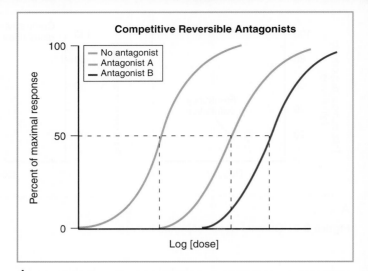

A

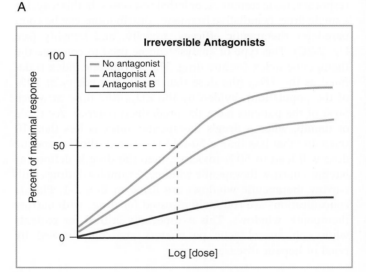

B

Figure 2-5. Antagonists shift dose-response curves of agonists. **A,** Competitive reversible antagonists. **B,** Irreversible antagonists.

lower concentration) than full agonists (drug D). Understanding these dose-response curves requires an appreciation of the two-state model for receptor activation. Receptors can be thought to undergo a dynamic conformational or structural transition between inactive and active states in the presence of ligands. This model can be useful to explain why partial agonists exhibit weak biologic responses at full saturation of receptors. In this model, full agonists preferentially bind to the active form of the target with high affinity, whereas partial agonists have affinities to both the active and the inactive conformations of the target. By extending this model, drugs can be designed to stabilize the inactive form of targets. These drugs theoretically would exhibit negative efficacy and are called *inverse agonists*. For inverse agonism to be observed, there must be some level of constitutive activity in the absence of agonist. Although these issues are frequently incorporated into test questions, there are few, if any, demonstrated examples of inverse agonism in vivo.

●●● DRUGS AS ANTAGONISTS

Often physicians prescribe a drug that blocks or competes with an endogenous metabolite or pathway or exogenous *xenobiotic* (foreign substance) or drug. These agents are antagonists in that they block (or antagonize) the natural signal. These antagonists change the shape of dose-response curves. For example, a competitive, reversible antagonist shifts the dose-response curve to the right, indicating that the agonist must now be given at a higher dose to elicit a similar response in the presence of the antagonist (Fig. 2-5A). In contrast, an irreversible antagonist shifts the dose-response curve downward, indicating that the agonist can no longer exert maximal effects at any therapeutic dose (see Fig. 2-5B). There are also allosteric interactions (binding at an alternative or "distant" site), where different drugs bind to distinct sites on one target in a reversible but not competitive manner. In these cases, the action of one drug positively or negatively affects the binding of a second drug to the target, a phenomenon known as *cooperativity*.

Antagonists, such as β-adrenergic receptor antagonists (β-blockers) have affinity, but no efficacy, for β-adrenergic receptors. These drugs compete for and block endogenous norepinephrine or epinephrine from stimulating adrenergic receptors. Because membrane receptors may be recycled after drug binding (desensitization), may be newly transcribed, or may have amplified responses through actions at multiple effectors, the actual magnitude of antagonism corresponding to a reduced biologic response may not always be linear and, in fact, may be less than expected. The term *spare receptor* is often used to describe this phenomenon.

●●● SIGNALING AND RECEPTORS

The critical concepts of signal transduction pathways are amplification, redundancy, cross-talk, and integration of biologic signals. From a pharmacologic perspective, identification of individual signal transduction elements often uncovers

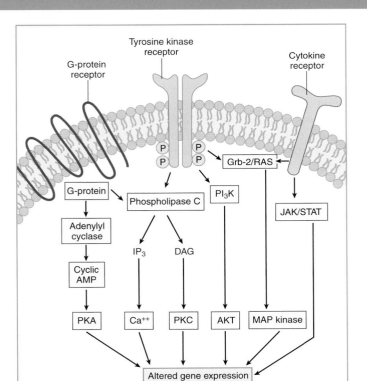

Figure 2-6. Signal transduction: it all leads to altered gene expression. *IP₃*, inositol-trisphosphate; *DAG*, diacylglycerol; *AMP*, adenosine monophosphate; *PKA*, protein kinase A; *PKC*, protein kinase C; *PI₃K*, phosphatidylinositol-3-kinase; *AKT*, a cell-survival kinase; *JAK/STAT,* dimerized proteins that couple cytokine receptors to downstream targets; *Grb-2/Ras*, scaffold network of proteins that couple tyrosine kinase receptors to downstream targets such as the MAP kinases; *MAP kinases*, mitogen-activated protein kinases.

potential targets for drugs to selectively disrupt the integrated circuits that control cell growth, survival, and differentiation. To appreciate fully the complexity of signaling networks requires an understanding of a "subway map" of interconnected receptors, effectors, targets, and scaffold proteins. The physician should understand the critical concepts of cell signaling as well as some of the therapeutic targets that can now be modified with drugs.

Figure 2-6 depicts several intracellular signals that are regulated via receptor activation. A major family of membrane receptors is the seven-transmembrane–spanning domain G-protein–coupled receptors. These receptors couple to heterotrimeric guanosine triphosphate (GTP)-binding proteins, which regulate downstream effectors, including adenylate cyclase. This is a critical element in the discussion of the autonomic (see Chapter 6) and central nervous systems (see Chapter 13).

As depicted in Figure 2-7, amplification of the signal occurs as one receptor interacts with multiple G-proteins that remain activated even after the receptors dissociate. In a cyclical fashion, activated receptors couple to the α/β/γ subunits of the inactivated G-protein (bound to guanosine diphosphate [GDP]). This interaction induces GDP dissociation, followed by GTP binding, and activation of the G-protein. The activated

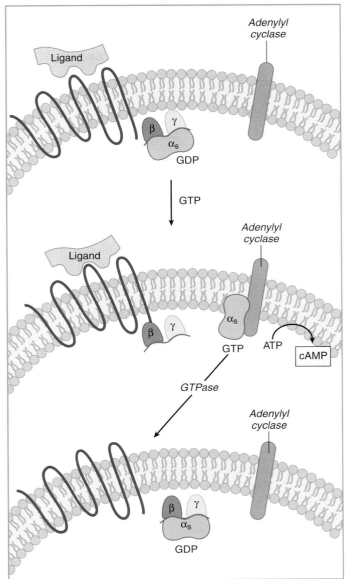

Figure 2-7. A G-protein–centric view of signaling. *GTP*, guanosine triphosphate; *GDP*, guanosine diphosphate; *ATP,* adenosine triphosphate; *cAMP,* cyclic adenosine monophosphate.

G-protein dissociates into distinct α and β/γ subunits. The α subunit interacts with adenylyl cyclase, the enzyme that produces cyclic adenosine monophosphate (cAMP), the biologic cofactor for protein kinase A. Hydrolysis of GTP to GDP dissociates the α subunit from adenylyl cyclase and permits reassociation with the β/γ subunits, resetting the cycle for subsequent activation by another receptor. Leading to further complexity is that distinct α subunits couple to different and specific effectors (Fig. 2-8) as well as the fact that β/γ subunits themselves can interact with other downstream effectors, including phospholipases.

Examples of a receptor class that couples to Gₛ ("s" stands for "stimulatory" as opposed to Gᵢ, in which the "i" stands for "inhibitory") to activate adenylate cyclase and generate cAMP are the β-adrenergic receptors. Pharmacologic intervention with a β-agonist such as isoproterenol activates β-adrenergic

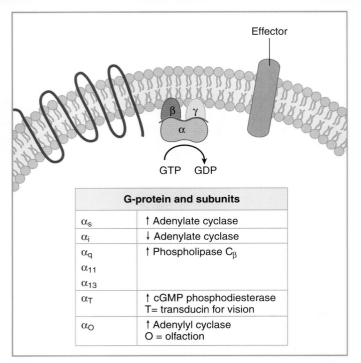

G-protein and subunits	
α_s	↑ Adenylate cyclase
α_i	↓ Adenylate cyclase
α_q	↑ Phospholipase C_β
α_{11}	
α_{13}	
α_T	↑ cGMP phosphodiesterase T= transducin for vision
α_O	↑ Adenylyl cyclase O = olfaction

Figure 2-8. G-proteins come in different flavors. The G-protein complex is composed of α, β, and γ subunits. The α-subunits are distinct proteins that subserve different functions by coupling to different effectors. *GTP*, guanosine triphosphate; *GDP*, guanosine diphosphate; *cGMP*, cyclic guanosine monophosphate.

receptors, whereas antagonists such as propranolol, a β-blocker, prevent endogenous activation of these receptors.

Understanding the mechanisms by which these receptors undergo desensitization or internalization helps explain why receptor responses dissipate over prolonged activation (Fig. 2-9). Interaction of β-adrenergic receptors with epinephrine promotes phosphorylation of the receptor by β-adrenergic

receptor kinases. The hyperphosphorylated receptors interact with arrestin, a molecule that either prevents activation of G-proteins by the receptor and/or induces receptor internalization. One of the critical concepts in signal transduction is that posttranslational modifications of targets by phosphorylation alter receptor function.

Besides coupling to adenylate cyclase, G-protein–linked receptors can regulate lipid turnover in membranes. Another critical concept in signaling is that altered lipid metabolism generates lipid-derived second messengers that amplify primary signals. Simply put, it's all about metabolism of a phosphorylated lipid that makes up less than 0.01% of the total lipid content of the membrane. G-protein–coupled receptors, such as the angiotensin II receptor, activate phospholipase C via G_q, which preferentially hydrolyzes phosphatidylinositol 4,5-bisphosphate (PIP_2) to form two distinct lipid-derived second messengers (Fig. 2-10A): inositol 1,4,5-trisphosphate and diacylglycerol. Inositol 1,4,5,-triphosphate, being hydrophilic, leaves the membrane and interacts with Ca^{++} channels on the endoplasmic reticulum, producing an increase in intracellular free Ca^{++}. Calcium-regulated kinases impact multiple systems responsible for blood clotting, neuronal function, and proton secretion in the stomach. In contrast, diacylglycerol, being hydrophobic, remains at the plasma membrane, where it is a lipid cofactor that activates protein kinase C.

To complicate matters, growth factor receptors, such as platelet-derived growth factor, which are tyrosine kinases, also couple to phospholipases to form lipid-derived second messengers (see Fig. 2-6). Another critical concept in signaling is that dimerization and resultant autophosphorylation of tyrosine kinase receptors often leads to propagation of the signal. Many of the latest therapeutic approaches work through inhibiting these tyrosine kinase receptor activation mechanisms. In addition, these tyrosine kinase receptors also activate phosphatidylinositol-3-kinase (PI_3K; Fig. 2-10B), which can

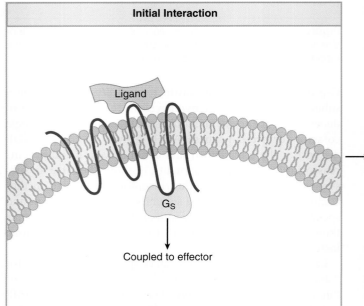

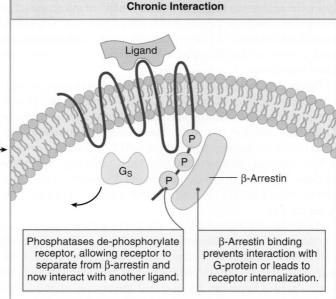

Figure 2-9. Hyperphosphorylation of G-protein receptors leads to desensitization. *S*, stimulatory.

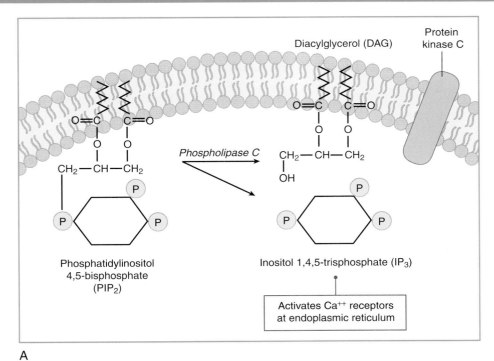

A

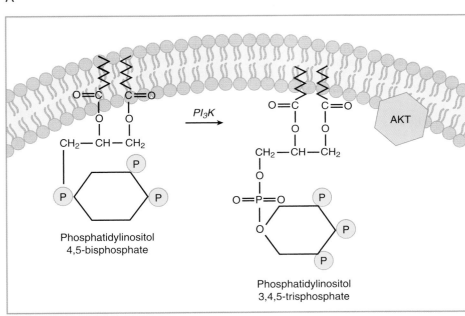

B

Figure 2-10. Phosphatidylinositol 4,5-bisphosphate, a lipid substrate for multiple enzymes. *PI₃K*, phosphatidylinositol-3-kinase; *AKT*, a cell survival kinase.

form a third messenger from phosphatidylinositol 4,5-bisphosphate. The generated phosphatidylinositol 3,4,5-trisphosphate can interact with proteins containing pleckstrin homology domains, such as AKT (a cell survival kinase), which are critical kinases for cell survival. Growth factor receptors are overexpressed in cancerous lesions. Figure 2-11 depicts several of the pro-mitogenic cascades activated by this class of receptors as well as designated targets for therapeutic intervention.

Figure 2-12 illustrates another lipid metabolite formed from hydrolysis of PIP₂. Phospholipase A₂ hydrolyzes fatty acids from lipids, such as PIP₂ or phosphatidylcholine. These fatty acids are often highly unsaturated, containing multiple double bonds. Fatty acids containing 20 carbons with 4 double bonds that occur starting 6 carbons from the carboxyl terminus are known as *arachidonic acid*. These fatty acids can be oxidized by multiple enzymes to form prostaglandins, leukotrienes, and epoxides (hydroxy-eicosatetraenoic acids) by cyclooxygenase, lipoxygenase, and epoxygenases, respectively.

The onslaught of lipid-derived messengers is referred to as *arachidonophobia*. Multiple drugs, either irreversibly (aspirin) or reversibly (nonsteroidal antiinflammatory agents) inhibit cyclooxygenase and are reviewed in Chapter 10.

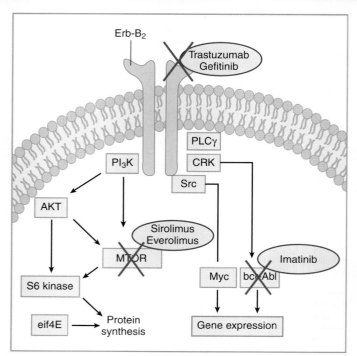

Figure 2-11. Targeted cancer therapy. *Erb-B₂*, a tyrosine kinase receptor; *PLCγ*, phospholipase C subtype that couples to tyrosine kinases; *CRK/Src*, another group of scaffold proteins that couple tyrosine kinases to downstream effectors; *cABL, Myc, mTOR, S6 kinase*, various downstream kinases and transcriptional factors that can serve as selective "targets" for drugs; *PI₃K*, phosphatidylinositol-3-kinase; *AKT*, a cell survival kinase.

Inhibitors of leukotriene synthesis, such as montelukast, are effective in asthmatic patients.

Another signaling concept is that lipid-derived second messengers such as prostaglandins can themselves activate G-protein–coupled receptors, again amplifying responses (Fig. 2-13). It should be noted that lipid-derived messengers can signal by creating structured membrane microdomains (also called *lipid rafts*), directly interacting with lipid-binding domains on proteins, or by posttranslationally modifying proteins. Examples of posttranslational modifications include proteins made hydrophobic by covalent modifications with 14-carbon (myristoylate) or 16-carbon (palmitoylate) fatty acids. A critical example of a myristoylated target protein is Ras, which is overexpressed or mutated in multiple cancers.

Signal transduction cascades can interact with and dramatically impact ion channels. In fact, ligand-gated ion channels themselves serve as targets for both intracellular signal transduction cascades as well as therapeutic drugs. Pharmacologic regulation of ion channels serves as one approach to controlling cardiac (verapamil, a Ca^{++} channel blocker), renal (furosemide, an $Na^+/K^+/Cl^-$ cotransporter antagonist), and neuronal (benzodiazepines, a Cl^- channel allosteric modulator) function. Modifying pathologic ion channel activity with therapeutics can be affected by direct interaction with the channel itself or upstream/downstream signal transduction targets of that ion channel. Ligand-gated ion channels can be regulated by Ca^{++}, cAMP, lipid mediators, and tyrosine phosphorylation signal transduction mechanisms.

A detailed example of ion channel modulation with therapeutics is γ-aminobutyric acid (GABA)–activated neuronal Cl^- channels. Benzodiazepines are examples of drugs that work via modulation of GABA-activated Cl^- channels. GABA serves as the endogenous ligand for this ligand-gated ion channel (Fig. 2-14). Benzodiazepines cannot activate GABA receptors in the absence of GABA, but benzodiazepines do facilitate the actions of GABA to alter the conformation of the receptor-ion channel, increasing the frequency of Cl^- channel opening events. The enhanced Cl^- flux hyperpolarizes the membrane, diminishing neuronal transmission and inducing sedation or cessation of anxiety (anxiolytic). The target of benzodiazepines, then, is a ligand-gated ion channel. This is also an example of positive cooperativity between the GABA neurotransmitter and a drug.

CLINICAL MEDICINE

Why Do Physicians Need to Know Signaling 101?

More and more drugs that alter signal transduction cascades are being validated, tested, approved, and marketed. These drugs offer the promise of specificity, selectivity, and reduced toxicity because signaling elements are often mutated or overexpressed in disease states, including cancer and inflammation. In this way, normal tissues may not be dramatically affected by the drug, resulting in reduced side effects. Examples of some approved designer drug targets include the following:

Target Signal	Approved Pathology
Erb-B₂ receptor	Breast cancer
Erb-B₂ receptor	Non–small-cell lung cancer
Erb-B₂ receptor	Colorectal cancer
BCR-ABL	Chronic myelogenous leukemia
mTOR	Restenosis after coronary stenting
Peroxisome proliferator activator receptors	Diabetes

The *Her2/neu* gene product, the Erb-B₂ receptor, a member of the human epidermal growth factor family of tyrosine kinases, is overexpressed in multiple cancers and is associated with a poor prognosis. Erb-B₂ forms a heterodimer with other Erb receptors that exhibit enhanced mitogenic signaling potential. Several different strategies have been used to target this receptor. Monoclonal antibodies (trastuzumab) as well as low-molecular-weight inhibitors (gefitinib) have been designed to block these actions. Additional strategies, including coupling a specific antibody to cytotoxins or ligands that activate immune cells, are being investigated.

●●● THE FUTURE IS NOW

It's no longer just about small molecules (pure, structurally defined, drugs that are produced through industrial scale chemistry) that affect receptors, ion channels, and signal transduction cascades. New strategies in biotechnology and

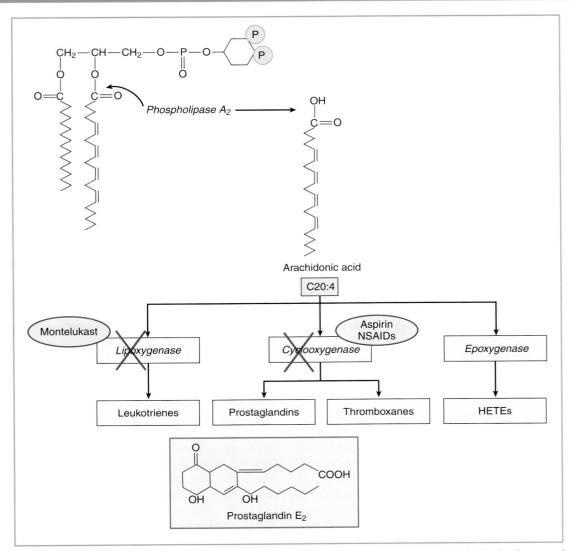

Figure 2-12. Arachidonophobia: 20 carbons, 4 double bonds, and the precursor to multiple lipid-derived second messengers (leukotrienes, prostaglandins, thromboxanes, and hydroxy-eicosatrienoic acids) that regulate myriad physiologic responses from vasoreactivity, to bronchial constriction, to labor, to protection of the gastrointestinal tract, to inflammation, and so on. The inset prostaglandin E$_2$ is an example of the types of structures that are created. *NSAIDs*, nonsteroidal antiinflammatory drugs; *HETEs*, hydroxyeicosatetraenoic acids.

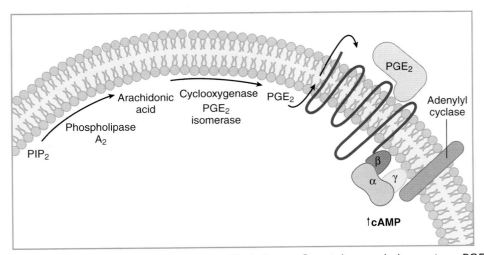

Figure 2-13. Lipid-derived second messengers can interact with their own G-protein–coupled receptors. *PGE$_2$*, prostaglandin E$_2$; *cAMP*, cyclic adenosine monophosphate. *PIP$_2$*, phosphatidylinositol 4,5 bisphosphate.

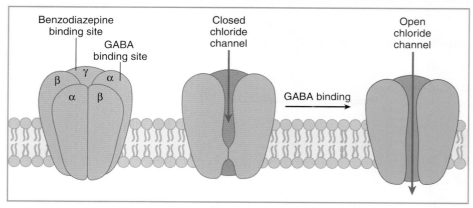

Figure 2-14. Ligand-gated channels regulate the flow of ions through plasma membrane channels. This example depicts the γ-aminobutyric acid (GABA$_A$) receptor, which modulates Cl$^-$ conductance.

molecular biology have expanded a class of drugs, known as *biologics*, that are themselves endogenous natural substances such as growth factors, receptors, enzymes, cytokines, or peptides. Biologics are often produced in living cells through recombinant DNA technologies. As examples, biologics are produced to treat endocrine disorders, rheumatoid arthritis, oral mucositis, and cancer complications (Table 2-3). These and other biologics are discussed in more detail throughout this book.

Recombinant enzyme biologics have also revolutionized the treatment of lysosomal enzyme diseases, a group of congenital defects in which enzyme deficiencies result in dysfunctional metabolism of glycosphingolipids. These sugar-conjugated lipids are major components of neuronal cells and contribute to immunogenicity and autoimmunity. Recent Food and Drug Administration (FDA)-approved examples of recombinant enzymes to treat lysosomal enzyme diseases are listed in Table 2-3. The term *enzyme replacement therapy* is often used to define therapeutic approaches that use these recombinant

enzyme biologics. An alternate strategy known as *substrate reduction therapy* has also recently been approved for Gaucher disease, in which an inhibitor (miglustat) of the rate-limiting enzyme in glycosphingolipid metabolism, glucosylceramide synthase is used to reduce total glycosphingolipid content.

The new biologics that have been approved by the FDA offer the potential of more specific and selective cell targeting. Recent examples include monoclonal antibodies that specifically target and neutralize growth factor receptors or bind up their ligands (see Table 2-3). Another use of the monoclonal antibody approach is to employ these biologics to achieve more targeted delivery of conventional small-molecule therapy. For example, gemtuzumab ozogamicin is a biologic in which the antitumor substance calicheamicin is coupled to an antibody that binds to CD33, a protein epitope preferentially expressed on acute myeloid leukemic blast cell populations. Other targeted monoclonal approaches include iodine-131 tositumomab or yttrium-90 ibritumomab tiuxetan, in which radiotherapy is coupled to a CD20 antibody, whose

TABLE 2-3. Biologics (Examples of the Revolution)	
Growth factors	Sermorelin (a recombinant form of growth hormone–releasing factor used to treat dwarfism)
	Mecasermin (a recombinant form of insulin-like growth factor [IGF] for children with IGF deficiency)
	Palifermin (a recombinant form of human keratinocyte growth factor used to treat oral mucositis)
	Filgrastim and sargramostim (recombinant forms of colony-stimulating factor used to treat cancer-therapy–induced neutropenia)
Growth factor receptors	Etanercept, a recombinant form of tumor necrosis factor receptor that binds up circulating tumor necrosis factor, used for rheumatoid arthritis
Enzymes (lysosomal storage diseases)	Agalsidase β (Fabry disease)
	Alglucosidase alpha (Pompe disease)
	Imiglucerase (Gaucher disease)
	Idursulfase, laronidase, galsulfase (mucopolysaccharidosis)
Cytokines	Denileukin diftitox (interleukin-2 coupled to diphtheria toxin)
Peptides	Synthetic insulin used to treat diabetes
Antibodies	Trastuzumab (Erb-B$_2$ receptor)
	Gefitinib (epidermal growth factor receptor)
	Bevacizumab or ranibizumab (vascular endothelial growth factor)
	Gemtuzumab ozogamicin (CD33)
	^{131}I-tositumomab or ^{90}yttrium ibritumomab tiuxetan (CD20)

receptor is preferentially expressed on B-cell non-Hodgkin lymphoma cells. A similar approach is used by the biologic denileukin diftitox, in which recombinant cytokine interleukin-2 protein sequences are coupled to diphtheria toxin to direct the toxin to cutaneous T-cell lymphomas.

The holy grail of the pharmacology revolution involves molecular-based therapeutics that have the potential to target gene products. As an example, aptamers, which are stabilized RNA sequences that bind to proteins, have now been approved as therapeutics. Pegaptanib is an aptamer-based therapeutic that targets vascular endothelial growth factor and is used for treatment of age-related macular degeneration. The upside of molecular-based therapeutics is the potential to selectively target mutated gene products. The downside of using molecular-based therapeutics, such as aptamers or small interfering RNAs, is systemic degradation by RNAases or Toll-like receptor-mediated inflammatory side effects. Thus, a new modality has been embraced to deliver and protect these labile substances. The burgeoning field of nanomedicine uses nanoscale (<100 nm) delivery systems (liposomes, colloids, dendrimers, polymers) to protect labile bioactive cargos, such as RNAs. Several nanoscale products have now been approved by the FDA, including a nanoliposome that encapsulates the cancer-agent doxorubicin, as well as a nanoscale bioconjugate between albumin and the cancer agent docetaxel. Both nano "solutions" improve the pharmacokinetic parameters of the encapsulated drug. The future for design of small molecule inhibitors, biologics, and molecular-based therapeutics can only get brighter as the "omic" revolution defines new targets in diseased tissues. Functional genomic, proteomic, transcriptomic, metabolomic, and lipidomic approaches offer the potential to define a myriad of new dysfunctional cell signaling cascades in disease.

BIOCHEMISTRY

Gene Targeting

The future of pharmacology may well be to target signaling elements at transcriptional or translational levels. Strategies being investigated to selectively silence genes include:

- Antisense oligonucleotides
- siRNAs (small interfering RNAs)
- RNAzymes (enzymes that degrade RNA)
- DNAzymes (enzymes that degrade DNA)

These strategies are presently limited by the technology needed to selectively and efficiently deliver these nucleic acids to specific tissues without inducing toxicity.

●●● TOP FIVE LIST

1. Drugs bind to targets; these targets can be receptors, ion channels, transporters, signaling molecules, enzymes, or specific nucleic acid sequences.
2. Interactions between drugs and targets can be agonistic or antagonistic.
3. Pharmacodynamic terms used to define drug-target interactions include affinity, potency, and efficacy.
4. Drugs with a narrow therapeutic window (therapeutic index equals toxic dose [TD_{50}] divided by effective dose [ED_{50}]) must be closely monitored by the practitioner.
5. The future will be defined by designer drugs applied to individuals, tailored to a specific molecular or metabolic pathology. This is the essence of personalized medicine.

Self-assessment questions can be accessed at www.StudentConsult.com.

Toxicology 3

CONTENTS

APPROACHES TO THE POISONED PATIENT
Activated Charcoal
Gastric Lavage
Ionized Diuresis
SPECIFIC ANTIDOTES
Neurally Active Drugs/Poisons
Cardiovascular Drugs/Poisons
Hepatotoxic Drugs/Poisons
Heavy Metal Poisons
Cyanide Poisoning
COMPLEMENTARY AND ALTERNATIVE MEDICINES
TOP FIVE LIST

Toxicology is all about excess—too much of a good thing can be bad. In fact, according to the ancient pharmacology proverb, "If one is good, two is not necessarily better." More than just the memorization of acronyms or mnemonics, toxicology involves the practice of life-saving modalities and therapeutic interventions that reduce levels of hazardous substances within the body. Almost any substance, if taken in large enough doses, can produce harmful effects. It is therefore critical to be able to identify common toxins and to be able to initiate appropriate measures in a timely fashion.

●●● APPROACHES TO THE POISONED PATIENT

When managing the adverse effects associated with drugs or poisons, always begin with the ABCs (*airway*, *breathing*, and *circulation*) and initiate cardiopulmonary resuscitation if necessary. That is, make sure the patient is stable before worrying about the specific treatments or antidotes.

Activated Charcoal

Activated charcoal is often used in emergency departments for suspected overdose situations when antidotes with higher specificity are not available. Activated charcoal is a highly purified adsorbent form of charcoal that binds (adsorbs) drugs in the gastrointestinal tract, preventing their absorption. However, charcoal is ineffective for treating hydrocarbon (e.g., ethanol) or metal (e.g., iron, lead, lithium) overdoses. Risks

associated with activated charcoal include emesis (vomiting) after administration, pulmonary aspiration leading to pneumonitis, and constipation or bowel obstruction.

Gastric Lavage

Another common technique used in emergency departments is gastric lavage (pumping the stomach), which is helpful only if a patient comes to the hospital within 1 hour of a toxic ingestion. Lavage decreases absorption of toxins by approximately 50% at 5 minutes, 25% at 30 minutes, and 15% at 60 minutes. Lavage may be used to speed removal of many drugs ingested orally, but it is contraindicated for ingestion of caustic substances or hydrocarbons. Complications associated with gastric lavage include aspiration pneumonitis, laryngospasm, mechanical injury to the esophagus or gastrointestinal tract, hypothermia, and fluid and electrolyte imbalances.

Ionized Diuresis

Ionized diuresis may be used to facilitate excretion of poisons that are eliminated by the kidneys. Ionized diuresis refers to the process in which excretion of weak acids or weak bases is enhanced by trapping the ionized portion of drug in the renal tubules. For example, take ammonia ($NH_3 + H^+ \rightleftharpoons NH_4^+$). Ammonia, NH_3, is a weak base that readily crosses biologic membranes because it is uncharged. If filtered from the plasma by the glomeruli, ammonia would be prone to reabsorption in the bloodstream because it is un-ionized and not particularly polar. However, the situation changes if the urine is acidified. In an acidic environment, the positively charged ammonium ion cannot easily penetrate biologic membranes and thus is not readily reabsorbed (i.e., a higher percentage of metabolite would be excreted). Historically, the ion-trapping principle was applied to hasten removal of drugs that are weak bases (amphetamines, phencyclidine). However, this practice is no longer recommended because rhabdomyolysis (muscle breakdown) is common after these overdoses and acidification of urine may increase the risk of renal failure. On rare occasions, ammonium chloride can be used to acidify urine and facilitate secretion of weak bases.

The same principle applies to weak acids. For example,

$$\text{Salicylic acid} \rightleftharpoons \text{Salicylate} + H^+ (HA \rightleftharpoons A^- + H^+)$$

In other words, to excrete toxic weak acids, alkalinize the urine. In alkalinized urine, drugs that are weak acids are ionized and excreted—not reabsorbed. To treat poisonings associated with weak acids (salicylates, phenobarbital), the urine can be alkalinized with intravenous sodium bicarbonate while the patient is monitored for alkalosis and fluid and electrolyte disturbances (Table 3-1).

PHYSIOLOGY

Anion Gap—Acids and Bases

The term *anion gap* refers to the concentration of all the unmeasured anions (negatively charged molecules) present in the plasma. It is estimated by subtracting measurable anions (chloride and bicarbonate) from the measurable cations (Na^+ and K^+). A normal anion gap is between 8 and 16 mEq/L. The resulting anion gap is then assessed as normal, high, or low. A high gap is deemed a sign of acidosis and is used in the emergency department as an indication of conditions such as ketoacidosis, lactic acidosis, or renal failure.

PHYSIOLOGY

Aspirin Toxicity Is an Acid-Base Problem

Aspirin is a commonly used drug that can potentially lead to fatalities in overdose situations. Acute intoxication causes an initial respiratory alkalosis via hyperventilation resulting from direct stimulation of the respiratory centers. High-dose salicylates also cause uncoupling of oxidative phosphorylation. Catabolism occurs secondary to the inhibition of adenosine triphosphate–dependent reactions, which leads to hyperpyrexia (markedly elevated body temperature) and metabolic acidosis from the accumulation of endogenous acids.

●●● SPECIFIC ANTIDOTES

Specific antidotes are available for only a few drugs and poisonous substances. Be aware that (1) the duration of action of most antidotes is shorter than that of the toxic agent, so antidotes may need to be given repeatedly until the effects of the poison are eliminated; and (2) antidotes should never replace good supportive care.

Neurally Active Drugs/Poisons

Organophosphates
Antidote: pralidoxime

Toxic exposure to irreversible acetylcholinesterase inhibitors such as the organophosphates usually stems from occupational hazards, given that the chemicals are used as insecticides and pesticides in the agricultural industry (parathion, malathion) and as biologic warfare agents (soman). As a result, farmers are at risk of developing life-threatening complications if crop-dusting airplanes inadvertently spray them. Military personnel are also at risk in the event that they are attacked with weapons containing nerve agents.

Organophosphates are highly lipophilic and can permeate the body via inhalation or absorption through the skin. These agents covalently bind to and inhibit acetylcholinesterases, the enzymes that usually terminate the actions of acetylcholine. The most important thing for health care providers to remember when organophosphate poisoning is suspected is to protect themselves. Because of the lipophilic nature of the drugs, health care professionals can become cross-contaminated simply from skin contact with the affected individual (Table 3-2).

Exposure to organophosphates results in widespread toxicity because acetylcholine plays key roles within the sympathetic nervous system, the parasympathetic nervous system, and the neuromuscular junction. Signs and symptoms of organophosphate overdose include *s*alivation, *l*acrimation, *u*rination, *d*efecation (known as the *SLUD syndrome*), miosis, bronchospasm, bradycardia, sweating, paralysis of respiratory muscles, convulsions, and coma. Another popular mnemonic is DUMBELS (*d*iarrhea, *u*rination, *m*iosis, *b*ronchoconstriction, *e*xcitation, *l*acrimation, *s*alivation). The most common cause of death is respiratory failure, so mechanical ventilation may be necessary.

Pharmacologic management of organophosphate poisoning includes atropine and pralidoxime. Atropine competitively blocks the actions of acetylcholine at muscarinic receptors (see Chapter 6 for more details). Thus it is palliative in nature because it does not reverse the inhibition of acetylcholinesterases caused by the organophosphates. Atropine reverses bronchorrhea but not pupil size. Pralidoxime is truly an antidote for organophosphate poisoning. Pralidoxime breaks the

---

TABLE 3-1. Presentation and Management of Salicylate Poisoning

AGENT	SIGNS/SYMPTOMS	INTERVENTIONS	ANTIDOTES
Salicylates (e.g., aspirin)	Acidosis Coma Confusion and lethargy Dehydration Hyperthermia Hyperventilation Hypokalemia Seizures Tinnitus	Manage acidosis and electrolytes Intravenous hydration Intubation and mechanical ventilation (severe cases)	Urinary alkalinization Hemodialysis (severe cases)

TABLE 3-2. Presentation and Management of AChE Inhibitor Poisoning

AGENT	SIGNS/SYMPTOMS	INTERVENTIONS	ANTIDOTES
AChE inhibitors (e.g., physostigmine, insecticides [organophosphates, carbamates])	Diarrhea Urination Miosis Bronchoconstriction Excitation (muscle twitches) Lacrimation Salivation, sweating, seizures Gastrointestinal cramps	Respiratory support Intravenous hydration	Atropine Pralidoxime

AChE, acetylcholinesterase.

covalent bond between organophosphates and acetylcholinesterases to regenerate the active enzyme. Pralidoxime is an effective antidote for organophosphate poisoning only if the antidote is administered before the "aging" process (i.e., within 24 hours of exposure), which stabilizes the organophosphate-enzyme complex (Fig. 3-1).

Anticholinergics
Antidote: physostigmine
In contrast to organophosphates, where toxicity is the result of increased concentrations of acetylcholine, numerous medications including muscarinic receptor antagonists, such as benztropine, possess anticholinergic properties. In addition, some antihistamines and phenothiazines possess anticholinergic properties, as do natural products such as Jimson weed and some mushrooms (e.g., *Amanita muscaria*). Physicians have to actively manage side effects associated with anticholinergic agents, and it may be a surprise that

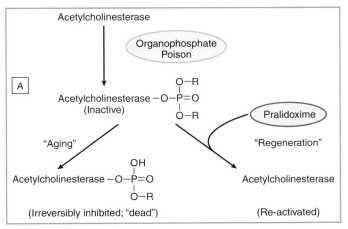

Figure 3-1. Pralidoxime is an antidote for organophosphate-inactivated acetylcholinesterase activity. The organophosphate toxin covalently modifies acetylcholinesterase. Over time, the organophosphate can be modified (aged), losing one or more of the attached "R" groups. Pralidoxime does not work effectively against these aged enzymes. Therefore, therapy should be initiated promptly.

acetylcholinesterase inhibitors may sometimes have to be administered as antidotes.

Signs and symptoms of anticholinergic syndrome are opposite those of the SLUD syndrome and include hypertension, tachycardia, fever, dry eyes/mouth, urinary retention, and ileus (decreased intestinal motility). Central nervous system side effects, including visual hallucinations, disorientation and confusion, seizures, and coma, also occur. Thus a patient with anticholinergic syndrome may generally be described as being dry as a bone, red as a beet, hot as a pistol, blind as a bat, and mad as a hatter. To alleviate excessive anticholinergic side effects, acetylcholinesterase inhibitors such as physostigmine may be administered. Physostigmine inhibits the degradation of acetylcholine in the synaptic cleft, thus enhancing the action of acetylcholine. Physostigmine is indicated if anticholinergic side effects of agitated psychosis, seizures, or supraventricular arrhythmias are occurring (Table 3-3).

Benzodiazepines
Antidote: flumazenil
Benzodiazepines have largely replaced barbiturates as sedative-hypnotic agents because of their superior safety profile. However, in benzodiazepine overdose situations, respiratory depression is still a major concern. Other signs and symptoms accompanying sedative-hypnotic syndrome include hypothermia, miosis, ileus, and bradycardia (Table 3-4).

Flumazenil competitively antagonizes the benzodiazepine binding site of the γ-aminobutyric acid receptor. If benzodiazepine toxicity is suspected, flumazenil treatment may prevent the need for subsequent intubation of the patient. Flumazenil has a relatively short half-life ($t_{1/2}$) compared with many benzodiazepines, often necessitating readministration. Caution is also necessary when using flumazenil during detoxification in patients who may be physically dependent on benzodiazepines because the antidote can induce seizures as a result of sudden benzodiazepine withdrawal.

Opioids: Heroin
Antidote: naloxone
The opioid analgesics and heroin possess a variety of depressant effects, the most dangerous of which is decreased respiratory drive. Naloxone was the first opioid receptor

TABLE 3-3. Presentation and Management of Anticholinergic Syndrome

AGENT	SIGNS/SYMPTOMS	INTERVENTIONS	ANTIDOTES
Muscarinic antagonists (e.g., atropine), mushrooms	Dry mouth, eyes Tachycardia Hypertension Hyperthermia Delirium and hallucinations Sedation Urinary retention Constipation Agitation, disorientation, confusion Seizures Coma	Manage cardiovascular symptoms and hyperthermia	Physostigmine or neostigmine

TABLE 3-4. Presentation and Management of Sedative Hypnotic Syndrome

AGENT	SIGNS/SYMPTOMS	INTERVENTIONS	ANTIDOTES
Sedative-hypnotics (e.g., benzodiazepines, barbiturates, alcohol)	Lethargy Disinhibition Ataxia Nystagmus Miosis Stupor Coma Hypothermia Hypotension Bradycardia Respiratory failure	Ventilatory support	Flumazenil for benzodiazepines only

antagonist made available to reverse toxicities associated with opioid overdoses. Use of this specific antidote may prevent both intubation and aspiration. Naloxone should be used if the patient has both respiratory depression and miosis. Because naloxone has a relatively short $t_{1/2}$ compared with the depressant effects of most opioid receptor agonists, the antidote may need to be readministered numerous times to reverse respiratory depression (Table 3-5).

Serotonin Syndrome
Antidote: benzodiazepines followed by cyproheptadine or metoclopramide

Serotonin syndrome is a hyperserotonergic state that is dangerous and potentially fatal. It is a condition that has been on the rise since the 1960s when drugs that affect serotonergic neurotransmission (e.g., lysergic acid, selective serotonin reuptake inhibitors, monoamine oxidase inhibitors) came into

TABLE 3-5. Presentation and Management of Opioid Overdose

AGENT	SIGNS/SYMPTOMS	INTERVENTIONS	ANTIDOTES
Opioid analgesics (e.g., morphine, heroin, oxycodone)	Lethargy and sedation Bradycardia Hypotension Hypoventilation Miosis Constipation Coma Respiratory failure	Ventilatory support	Naloxone

use. In addition, toxicity from excess serotonin is observed in the case of carcinoid tumors.

Signs and symptoms of serotonin syndrome include euphoria, sustained rapid eye movements, overreaction of reflexes, clumsiness, rapid muscle contractions and relaxations in ankles and jaw, dizziness, feelings of intoxication, sweating, shivering, diarrhea, loss of consciousness, and death. Treatment of serotonin syndrome first involves discontinuing any offending drugs. Second, benzodiazepines may be administered, followed by drugs that possess serotonin antagonist activity such as cyproheptadine or metoclopramide (Table 3-6).

Serotonin syndrome may occur as a consequence of inadvertent combinations of drugs that affect serotonin levels in the central nervous system. Combining drugs that act as selective serotonin reuptake inhibitors, serotonin receptor agonists, serotonin release agents, or serotonin catabolism inhibitors could result in a patient exhibiting the serotonin syndrome. Examples of agents that in combination elicit serotonin syndrome are monoamine oxidase inhibitors, clomipramine, trazodone, lithium, amphetamines, cocaine, dextromethorphan, meperidine, venlafaxine, tricyclic antidepressants, buspirone, triptans (serotonin $5HT_{1D}$ agonists), and reserpine (Table 3-7; see Chapter 13 for details). The natural supplements L-tryptophan and St. John's wort have also been implicated in serotonin syndrome, as has electroconvulsive therapy.

CLINICAL MEDICINE

Carcinoid Syndrome

Toxicologic syndromes, such as the symptoms associated with serotonin syndrome, may not always be a result of improper uses of medication. As an example, carcinoid syndrome is a constellation of symptoms that arise as a result of a carcinoid tumor. Carcinoid tumors arise from peripheral neuroendocrine cells (especially of the gut) and are generally defined by their ability to synthesize and release large amounts of serotonin. Because of the inappropriate release of this bioactive amine neurotransmitter and neurohormone (see Chapter 13), patients have a wide range of symptoms, including flushing of the neck and face, diarrhea, wheezing, and palpitations. In some patients, right-sided heart problems arise as a result of tricuspid valve stenosis.

CLINICAL MEDICINE

Serotonin Syndrome and Neuroleptic Malignant Syndrome

Physicians are required to make differential diagnoses based on a combination of symptoms and patient history. Many different clinical problems may present with similar symptoms. As an example, neuroleptic malignant syndrome (idiosyncratic toxicologic reaction to antipsychotic neuroleptic drugs; see Chapter 13) often presents with the same symptoms as serotonin syndrome. This latter condition is more predictably associated with excess serotonin activity as a result of treatments with serotonergic drugs such as the selective serotonin reuptake inhibitors antidepressants; see Chapter 13). In this case, serotonin syndrome can be distinguished from neuroleptic syndrome on the basis of a detailed medical history with particular attention devoted to recent changes in drug administration.

Methanol
Antidote: ethanol or fomepizole

Methanol is found in fuel antifreeze, windshield washer fluids, and "moonshine." Its ingestion leads to optic nerve damage and associated blindness as well as severe metabolic acidosis.

Metabolized by the same hepatic enzymes that biotransform ethanol, methanol is first converted by the enzyme

TABLE 3-6. Presentation and Management of Psychotropic Drug Overdoses

AGENTS	INTERVENTIONS	ANTIDOTES
Selective serotonin reuptake inhibitors (e.g., sertraline); serotonin receptor agonists (e.g., buspirone, sumatriptan)	Manage hyperthermia and seizures	Cyproheptadine Antipsychotics Benzodiazepines Dantrolene Metoclopramide
Tricyclic antidepressants (e.g., imipramine)	Manage seizures, hyperthermia, and acidosis	Antiarrhythmics
Central nervous system stimulants (e.g., cocaine, amphetamines)	Manage cardiovascular symptoms, hyperthermia, and seizures	Benzodiazepines Antipsychotics Antiarrhythmics
Antipsychotics (e.g., haloperidol)	Dose reduction Switch to different agent Manage seizures	Botulinum toxin for acute dystonia Bromocriptine and/or dantrolene for neuroleptic malignant syndrome Antimuscarinics and antihistamines for extrapyramidal reactions

SSRI, selective serotonin reuptake inhibitor

TABLE 3-7. Drugs That Can Cause Serotonin Syndrome When Used in Combination

SELECTIVE SEROTONIN REUPTAKE INHIBITORS	NONSELECTIVE SEROTONIN REUPTAKE INHIBITORS	SEROTONIN AGONISTS
Fluoxetine	Trazodone	Buspirone
Fluvoxamine	Nefazodone	LSD
Sertraline	Clomipramine	Mescaline
Paroxetine	Imipramine	Triptans
Citalopram	Desipramine	
Escitalopram	Amitriptyline	
	Nortriptyline	

DRUGS THAT PROMOTE SEROTONIN RELEASE	DRUGS THAT INHIBIT SEROTONIN BREAKDOWN
Cocaine	Pargyline
Amphetamines	Phenelzine
Codeine	Selegiline
Dextromethorphan	
Reserpine	

LSD, lysergic acid diethylamide.

alcohol dehydrogenase to formaldehyde, which is then converted to formic acid by aldehyde dehydrogenase (Fig. 3-2).

The formaldehyde and formic acid metabolites are responsible for the visual damage and acidosis. Surprisingly, ethanol is an effective antidote for methanol ingestion because it successfully competes with methanol for alcohol dehydrogenase and saturates the enzyme. This slows the metabolism of methanol and provides time to remove methanol by dialysis, if needed (Table 3-8). Alternatively, fomepizole, an inhibitor of alcohol dehydrogenase, can also be used for methanol and ethylene glycol poisoning.

PATHOLOGY

Causes of a High Anion Gap

Numerous toxins, metabolic syndromes, and drugs produce a high anion gap acidosis. A simple mnemonic for these conditions and poisonings is MUDPILES.

Methanol
Uremia
Diabetic acidosis
Paraldehyde or phenformin
Isoniazid or iron
Lactic acid (carbon monoxide, cyanide—inhibition of aerobic metabolism)
Ethylene glycol
Salicylates

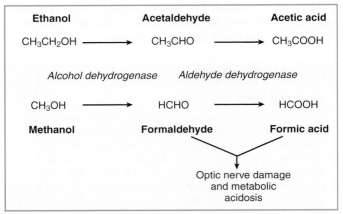

Figure 3-2. Ethanol can be used to treat methanol poisoning. Because ethanol has greater affinity for alcohol dehydrogenase than methanol, the conversion of methanol to active metabolites is slowed.

automobile exhausts. After hurricanes, CO poisoning incidence increases because of the use of generators for power. Headache often is the first symptom, followed by confusion, malaise, tachycardia, syncope, coma, convulsions, and death. Administering either 100% O_2 or hyperbaric O_2 (available at selected facilities) reverses CO poisoning (Table 3-9). Hyperbaric O_2 treatment is the most rapid means of reducing CO content.

Cardiovascular Drugs/Poisons

Carbon Monoxide
Antidote: 100% or hyperbaric oxygen

Carbon monoxide (CO) is an odorless, colorless gas that binds to hemoglobin with a more than 200-fold greater affinity than oxygen (O_2), resulting in tissue hypoxia. Most CO poisonings occur as a result of furnace or space heater malfunctions or

Hematologic and Cardiovascular Toxidromes
Antidote: protamine, vitamin K, digoxin immune Fab

Overdoses of many cardiovascular medications result in toxic syndromes, or toxidromes, for which appropriate interventions must be used (Table 3-10). For example, bleeding complications as a result of heparin or warfarin overdoses are particularly life-threatening. Protamine sulfate is a basic polypeptide that binds to and neutralizes the anticoagulant properties of

TABLE 3-8. Presentation and Management of Alcohol Poisoning

AGENT	SIGNS/SYMPTOMS	INTERVENTIONS	ANTIDOTES
Methanol, ethylene glycol	Lethargy Disinhibition Ataxia Nystagmus Miosis Stupor Coma Hypothermia Bradycardia Respiratory failure	Ventilatory support	Ethanol Fomepizole

TABLE 3-9. Presentation and Management of Carbon Monoxide Poisoning

AGENT	SIGNS/SYMPTOMS	INTERVENTIONS	ANTIDOTES
Carbon monoxide	Nausea and vomiting Dyspnea Mydriasis Vertigo or syncope Hypotension Tachycardia Arrhythmias	Decontamination	Hyperbaric O_2 (severe cases) Humidified 100% O_2 (mild to moderate cases)

O_2, oxygen

TABLE 3-10. Presentation and Management of Anticoagulant and Cardiac Glycoside Poisoning

AGENT	SIGNS/SYMPTOMS	INTERVENTIONS	ANTIDOTES
Anticoagulants (e.g., heparin)	Bleeding Osteoporosis HIT Skin necrosis Hypersensitivity	Manage medical condition (e.g., hypertension) to reduce risk of bleeding	Protamine for heparins Vitamin K for warfarin (mild to moderate cases) Fresh frozen plasma (severe cases or rapid correction)
Cardiac glycosides (e.g., digoxin)	Nausea Anorexia Shortened QT interval T-wave inversion Disorientation Visual halos Hallucinations Arrhythmias	Manage electrolytes Cardioversion for unstable cardiac arrhythmia Cardiac pacing	Digibind (Fab) Potassium (competes with digoxin for K^+ binding site on the Na^+/K^+-ATPase pump) Antiarrhythmics

HIT, heparin-induced thrombocytopenia; *ATPase*, adenosine triphosphatase.

heparin (see Chapter 7). Because warfarin reduces vitamin K–dependent coagulation factors, the antidote for warfarin toxicity is slow intravenous infusion of vitamin K with transfusion of fresh-frozen plasma, if necessary. Both protamine and vitamin K therapies have a slight risk of anaphylactic shock.

As another example of a cardiovascular toxidrome, cardiac glycosides, including digoxin, exert efficacy within a narrow therapeutic window. Despite monitoring serum digoxin concentrations, cardiac glycoside toxicity—as evidenced by delirium, fatigue, blurred vision, nausea, and life-threatening cardiac arrhythmias—may be seen in the emergency department. The initial antidote for digoxin toxicity is administration of K^+ to compete with digoxin for the Na^+/K^+-adenosine triphosphatase pump and, if toxicity is severe enough, intravenous infusion of digoxin immune Fab (Digibind), an anti-digoxin antibody.

Hepatotoxic Drugs/Poisons

Acetaminophen

Antidote: *N*-acetylcysteine

Acetaminophen is one of the most commonly used drugs in children (e.g., Tylenol) and is often used in suicide attempts by teenagers and adults. Approximately 100,000 cases of acetaminophen overdose occur annually. It is available in various oral dosage forms and is frequently found in combination with other medications including pain relievers and cough and cold preparations in both prescription as well as over-the-counter medications. Patients may not realize that acetaminophen is contained in several different products they are taking; thus acetaminophen toxicity may be unintentional.

Acute acetaminophen poisoning results in hepatotoxicity and occurs in several stages. Within the first 24 hours of an acetaminophen overdose, toxicity begins with nausea and vomiting. Hepatic necrosis is most likely in those who are malnourished, those who abuse alcohol, and patients who take other hepatotoxic medications (Table 3-11).

Acetaminophen is metabolized in the liver to glucuronide or sulfate conjugates (phase II reactions), which subsequently are excreted renally. A small fraction of acetaminophen, about 5%, is metabolized by P450 isoenzymes (phase I reactions) to a reactive metabolite *N*-acetyl-p-benzoquinone-imine (also discussed in Chapter 1). Normally, this metabolite is conjugated with glutathione, a sulfhydryl-containing compound, in the liver and would be excreted in the urine as an inactive mercapturate conjugate. However, in acetaminophen overdose situations, sulfate stores are depleted, thereby depleting glutathione stores. The reactive metabolite *N*-acetyl-p-benzoquinone-imine then reacts with other hepatocellular sulfhydryl groups in the cytosol, cell plasma membranes, and endoplasmic reticulum, forming reactive and necrotic tissue adducts and results in hepatotoxicity (Fig. 3-3).

In acetaminophen overdose situations, *N*-acetylcysteine, a sulfhydryl-containing acetaminophen-specific antidote, replenishes hepatic stores of glutathione by acting as a glutathione surrogate, combining directly with reactive acetaminophen metabolites and preventing hepatic damage. *N*-acetylcysteine should be initiated within 10 hours of acetaminophen overdose to achieve optimal results. Although *N*-acetylcysteine helps prevent liver damage by inactivating reactive acetaminophen intermediates, the antidote does not reverse hepatic injury

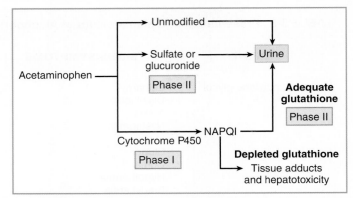

Figure 3-3. Metabolism of acetaminophen. Acetaminophen is metabolized by both phase I and phase II pathways. The phase I pathway (cytochrome P450–mediated) generates a reactive intermediate (*N*-acetyl-p-benzoquinone-imine [NAPQI]) that normally undergoes further metabolism via a phase II bioconjugation reaction with glutathione to form a metabolite that is excreted in the urine. During an acetaminophen overdose, glutathione stores are depleted, and the reactive NAPQI intermeditate forms tissue adducts leading to liver toxicity. *Administration of* N-*acetylcysteine replenishes glutathione stores, diminishing toxicology.*

once it has occurred. Unfortunately, the antidote has an unpleasant odor when administered orally, which often triggers nausea and vomiting and impairs the full course of therapy. For this reason, an injectable form of *N*-acetylcysteine was recently approved by the Food and Drug Administration (FDA) (Table 3-12).

Heavy Metal Poisons

Antidote: deferoxamine, deferasirox, dimercaprol, ethylenediaminetetraacetic acid, penicillamine, pentetate zinc trisodium, penetrare calcium trisodium, Prussian blue, succimer

Humans are exposed to heavy metals every day because these elements are used in various industrial processes from which many modern conveniences are derived. For example:

- Arsenic is found in wood preservatives, insecticides, pesticides, and poisons.

TABLE 3-11. The Four Stages of the Clinical Course of Acetaminophen Toxicity

STAGE	TIME AFTER INGESTION	CHARACTERISTICS
I	First 24 hours	Anorexia, nausea, vomiting, malaise, pallor, diaphoresis
II	24 to 48 hours	Resolution of above; right upper quadrant abdominal pain and tenderness; elevated bilirubin, prothrombin time, hepatic enzymes; oliguria
III	72 to 96 hours	Peak liver function abnormalities; anorexia, nausea, vomiting, malaise may reappear; jaundice
IV	4 days to 2 weeks	Resolution of hepatic dysfunction or complete liver failure

From Behrman RE: *Nelson Textbook of Pediatrics,* ed 16, Philadelphia: WB Saunders, 2000.

TABLE 3-12. Presentation and Management of Acetaminophen Poisoning

AGENT	SIGNS/SYMPTOMS	INTERVENTIONS	ANTIDOTES
Acetaminophen	Nausea and vomiting Abdominal pain Hepatic failure	Repeat blood levels to assess for toxicity	*N*-acetylcysteine

TABLE 3-13. Presentation and Management of Heavy Metal Poisoning

METAL	ACUTE SIGNS/SYMPTOMS	CHRONIC SIGNS/SYMPTOMS	INTERVENTIONS/ANTIDOTES
Arsenic	GI distress Garlic breath Watery stools Torsades de pointes Seizures	Pallor Skin pigmentation Alopecia Stocking/glove neuropathy Myelosuppression	Charcoal and/or dimercaprol for acute poisoning Penicillamine or succimer for chronic poisoning
Iron	Severe GI distress Hematemesis Bloody diarrhea Necrotic bowel	Dyspnea Shock Coma	Gastric aspiration and carbonate lavage Deferoxamine IV
Lead	Nausea and vomiting GI distress Abdominal pain Malaise Tremor Tinnitus Paresthesias Encephalopathy	Anemia Neuropathy Nephropathy Hepatitis Mental retardation Sterility Stillbirth	Gastric lavage and dimercaprol for severe cases EDTA or succimer Succimer PO in children
Mercury	Chest pain Dyspnea Pneumonitis GI distress GI bleeding Shock Renal failure	CNS effects Ataxia Paresthesias Auditory changes Visual changes	Succimer PO Penicillamine PO Add charcoal for orally ingested toxin

CNS, central nervous system; *EDTA*, ethylenediaminetetraacetic acid; *GI*, gastrointestinal; *IV*, intravenous; *PO*, orally.

- Iron is found in vitamin supplements.
- Lead is found in tap water, old paint chips, herbal remedies, and glazed kitchenware.
- Mercury is found in older thermometers, batteries, dyes, electroplating, photography, and dental amalgams.

Similarly to drug overdoses, continued exposure to these heavy metals has devastating toxicologic consequences. Treatment of heavy metal toxicity relies on the use of chelating agents. Chelators are organic compounds with two or more electronegative groups that form stable covalent bonds with cationic metal atoms. These stable complexes are readily excreted, thereby reducing toxicity associated with heavy metals (Table 3-13).

Arsenic

Acutely, arsenic toxicity causes gastrointestinal distress, "garlic" breath, and watery stools. Long-term exposure causes alopecia and anemia and may be carcinogenic. Dimercaprol is one chelator used to treat arsenic exposure. It is useful in lead, mercury, and cadmium poisonings as well. Dimercaprol is a chelator (forms two bonds with the metal ion) that is given parenterally as an oily liquid. It is highly lipophilic and readily enters cells throughout the body, including the central nervous system. As a result of its permeability, even at therapeutic doses this chelator is associated with a high incidence of adverse effects, including transient hypertension and tachycardia, headache, nausea, vomiting, and paresthesias.

BIOCHEMISTRY

Electron Transport Chain

The electron transport chain passes electrons from one protein (cytochrome or flavoprotein) to another in order to capture energy and pump hydrogen ions from the mitochondrion. The potential energy of this hydrogen ion gradient is harnessed to make adenosine triphosphate in oxidative (aerobic) metabolism. This is so named because the final acceptor for the electrons is molecular oxygen with the subsequent production of water. A number of toxic substances interfere with the electron transport chain (e.g., cyanide) or the transport of oxygen (e.g., carbon monoxide).

Iron

Iron is the most frequent cause of accidental overdose in children. Iron is irritating to the gastric mucosa, and acute toxicity may cause hemorrhage and gastric perforations. Once absorbed, iron is taken up by tissues, especially the liver, and acts as a mitochondrial poison by perturbing the electron transport chain and inhibiting oxidative phosphorylation. Because of the pharmacologic characteristics of iron, gastrointestinal distress is common within the first several hours after ingestion of toxic amounts. Within 24 to 36 hours of ingestion, hepatic injury, cardiovascular shock, metabolic acidosis, seizures, and coma may ensue.

Iron overdoses are also common in conditions that require frequent blood transfusions (e.g., hemophilia, thalassemia) and are treated with deferoxamine. Deferoxamine is a chelator with selective affinity for iron. Fortunately, it competes poorly with iron in hemoglobin and the cytochromes. At high doses, deferoxamine may cause visual disturbances, including cataract formation and retinal degeneration. Patients should be warned that deferoxamine may change the color of their urine to pink or orange. Unfortunately, deferoxamine must be administered via long infusions (more than 8 hours). Deferasirox is a recently FDA-approved iron chelator that can be administered orally, a clear advantage. However, as compared with deferoxamine, higher serum creatine levels and higher incidence of hepatic toxicities are observed with deferasirox.

Lead

Acute inorganic lead poisoning is not common in the United States at present but may occur in children who have ingested large amounts of lead-containing paint. Signs and symptoms of chronic inorganic lead poisoning include peripheral neuropathies, anorexia, anemia, tremor, weight loss, and gastrointestinal upset. Basophilic stippling of red blood cells is especially common after lead overdose. If encephalopathy occurs, prompt chelation is imperative. Treatment includes dimercaprol, ethylenediaminetetraacetic acid (EDTA), penicillamine, or succimer. Because EDTA also binds to calcium, EDTA is given as a calcium disodium salt to prevent hypocalcemia. Penicillamine is a water-soluble bidentate chelator that is well absorbed from the gastrointestinal tract and is excreted unchanged, although serious toxicities including aplastic anemia, lupus erythematosus, hypersensitivity reactions, and nephrotoxicity have been reported. Succimer is a polar chelator that can be administered orally and is well tolerated. It chelates extracellular but not intracellular lead and arsenic. Gastrointestinal distress, rash, and adverse central nervous system effects have been reported.

PATHOLOGY

Basophilic Stippling

Basophilic stippling is a typical sign of lead poisoning. The term refers to small, blue, dot-like structures scattered uniformly throughout the hemoglobin area of red blood cells. The stippling is derived from nuclear remnants and causes cells to resemble reticulocytes (immature red blood cells).

Mercury

Mercury poisoning usually occurs via inhalation of elemental mercury. Chest pain, shortness of breath, nausea and vomiting, kidney damage, gastrointestinal distress, and effects on the central nervous system may result. Treatment of mercury intoxication is with penicillamine or succimer. There have been public concerns that the mercury used as a preservative in pediatric vaccines has contributed to a rise in the prevalence of autism. Even though the Institute of Medicine reports no link between vaccines and autism, mercury is no longer used as a preservative in many new vaccine formulations.

Trans-Uranium Elements

Laboratory or industrial accidents as well as, unfortunately, the contents of a "dirty bomb" could expose individuals to toxic doses of plutonium, americium, or curium. Pentetate zinc trisodium and penetrare calcium trisodium are recent FDA-approved antidotes to contamination. The antidotes effectively exchange Zn^{++} or Ca^{++} for the transuranium elements and excrete the chelated toxin in the urine. An additional strategy to decontaminate individuals exposed to toxic doses of cesium or thallium (other radioactive nuclides associated with dirty bombs) uses Prussian blue. Prussian blue traps these radioactive nuclides within its crystal structure. Being highly insoluble, the complex is excreted via the biliary mechanisms into the feces.

Cyanide Poisoning

Antidote: hydroxocobalamin, sodium thiosulfate, amyl or sodium nitrate

Cyanide causes lethal toxicity by binding to, and inactivating, cytochrome oxidase and uncoupling oxidative phosphorylation (even in the presence of O_2). Cyanide poisoning is often observed after smoke inhalation of burning plastics due to production of hydrogen cyanide. Cyanide poioning may also result from rapid infusion of high doses of the vasodilator nitrate, nitroprusside. Infrequently, cyanide toxicology is oberved after ingestion of cyanide-containing supplements (illegally purchased laetrile products [mistakenly thought to prevent cancer]) or foods like cassava (yuca), apricots, or papayas (pits). Approved antidotes include hydroxocobalamin, which combines with cyanide to form nontoxic cyanocobalamin (vitamin B_{12}), or sodium thiosulfate, which converts cyanide to less toxic thiocyanate or amyl or sodium nitrate, which converts hemoglobin to methemoglobin that binds with cyanide to form cyanate hemoglobin.

●●● COMPLEMENTARY AND ALTERNATIVE MEDICINES

Patients often use natural products mistakenly believing that something "natural" will not be harmful. However, natural products may also produce toxic responses, especially when combined with prescription medications that have narrow therapeutic windows. For instance, a natural compound that interferes with the metabolism of a prescription drug might increase its concentration in the blood and drive it to toxic levels. St. John's wort is frequently used for depression and anxiety. This herbal alternative induces many cytochrome P450 enzymes and thus affects metabolism of other drugs. In particular, toxicologic effects of St. John's wort can increase metabolism of sex steroids and render birth control less effective.

●●● TOP FIVE LIST

1. In situations of accidental poisoning or overdose, first stabilize the patient before seeking general or specific antidote therapy.
2. The best antidote for a toxin is an antagonist of the toxic agent. Unfortunately, antagonists are rarely available.
3. Carbon monoxide and methanol poisoning are treated with agents that are themselves considered toxic (high concentrations of O_2 and ethanol, respectively).
4. Antidotes for heavy metals are generally chelators that form stable complexes with the metal and transport them from the body, trapping them in the urine.
5. Hepatotoxicity associated with acetaminophen poisoning is treated by restoring glutathione levels.

Self-assessment questions can be accessed at www. StudentConsult.com.

COMPLEMENTARY AND ALTERNATIVE MEDICINES

Patients often use natural products, mistakenly believing that something "natural" will not be harmful. However, natural products may also produce toxic responses, especially when combined with prescription medications that have narrow therapeutic windows. For instance, a natural compound that interferes with the metabolism of a prescription drug might increase its concentration in the blood and drive it to toxic levels. St. John's wort is frequently used for depression and anxiety. This herbal alternative induces many cytochrome P450 enzymes and this affects metabolism of other drugs, in particular toxicologic effects of St. John's wort can increase metabolism of sex steroids and render birth control less effective.

TOP FIVE LIST

Treatment of Infectious Diseases

4

CONTENTS

ANTIBACTERIALS
  Cell Wall Synthesis Inhibitors
  Protein Synthesis Inhibitors
  Folic Acid Synthesis Inhibitors
  Inhibitors of DNA/RNA Synthesis
ANTIMYCOBACTERIALS
  Treatment Options
ANTIFUNGALS
  Polyenes
  Azoles
  Other Antifungal Agents
ANTIPARASITICS
  Antimalarials
  Antihelmintics
  Head Lice Medications
ANTIVIRALS
  Inhibitors of Viral Uncoating
  Inhibitors of Viral Neuraminidase
  Inhibition of Intracellular Synthesis by Analogs
    of Viral Nucleic Acids
  Antivirals that Interfere with Viral Penetration into Host Cells
  Therapies for Human Papilloma Virus Management
MANAGEMENT OF HUMAN IMMUNODEFICIENCY VIRUS
  Nucleoside/Nucleotide Reverse Transcriptase Inhibitors
  Non-Nucleoside Reverse Transcriptase Inhibitors
  Protease Inhibitors
  Fusion Inhibitors
  Entry Inhibitors
  Integrase Inhibitors
COMPLEMENTARY AND ALTERNATIVE MEDICINE
  Treatment of Antibiotic-Associated Diarrhea
  Treatment of Yeast Infections
  Treatment of the Common Cold
TOP FIVE LIST

Treatment of infectious disease is all about death—selective cell death, that is. Agents that kill or inhibit growth of microorganisms are known as *antimicrobials*. The term *antibiotic* was initially reserved for describing substances produced by microorganisms that killed or inhibited the growth of other microorganisms. However, the terms *antimicrobial* and *antibiotic* are now used interchangeably. Antimicrobial agents used clinically are selectively toxic (i.e., the antibiotics preferentially destroy microorganisms rather than the patient).

Each antimicrobial may be described in terms of whether it has bacteriostatic activity or bactericidal activity. *Bacteriostatic* describes antimicrobials that inhibit growth of microorganisms, whereas *bactericidal* is a term that describes antimicrobials that kill microorganisms. In addition, each antimicrobial is associated with a particular spectrum of activity. The *spectrum of activity* describes the number of different types of organisms that are sensitive to the drug. Antibiotics have a broad spectrum if they target many different species of bacteria and a narrow spectrum if they are effective against only a few species of bacteria.

Resistance to antimicrobial agents is becoming increasingly problematic. Numerous antibiotics are no longer able to kill or suppress growth of microorganisms at plasma concentrations that are readily attainable because the microorganisms are no longer susceptible to the drugs. Microorganisms acquire resistance to antibiotics in numerous ways (Box 4-1).

Another important consideration is that not all bacteria in or on human bodies are disease causing. In fact, more than 90% of the cells in or on the human body are of prokaryotic origin. In other words, 90% of our bodies are normal flora. Infections from normal flora typically occur only when our defenses are impaired or these "normal" microorganisms translocate (move) to other parts of the body. Table 4-1 lists microorganisms that are normally found in various sites of the body, although these same bacteria can be pathogens if found in other areas of the body.

To select the most appropriate drug for treating an infection, several factors must be considered, including microorganism factors, host factors, and drug factors (Box 4-2). Microorganisms should be identified whenever possible by using microscopy coupled with Gram staining or direct culturing. Table 4-2 gives a generalization of "suspected" microbes based on site of infection. Empiric antimicrobial therapy against these organisms typically is initiated even before culture results are complete.

Culturing a microorganism from a site of infection is useful to determine the pharmacologic agents to which the microorganism is susceptible. Figure 4-1 depicts the methods by which microbial susceptibility is determined by using both quantitative (Fig. 4-1A) and qualitative (Fig. 4-1B) methods.

Box 4-1. OVERVIEW OF ANTIBACTERIAL RESISTANCE MECHANISMS

- Alterations in receptor target. Examples: mutations in penicillin-binding proteins (cell wall synthesis inhibitors); methylation of ribosomal subunits (protein synthesis inhibitors)
- Decreased entry or efflux of drug out of microorganism. Examples: altered porins (cell wall synthesis inhibitors); efflux pumps to remove drug (tetracyclines)
- Alterations in metabolic pathways. Example: microorganisms acquire alternative metabolic pathways to bypass a blocked pathway (sulfa drugs)
- Drug is inactive. Example: failure to convert a prodrug to active form (isoniazid); inactivation of drug (penicillins by β-lactamases)

Box 4-2. FACTORS TO CONSIDER WHEN SELECTING AN ANTI-INFECTIVE

Microorganism Factors

Identification of organism
Susceptibility (minimal inhibitory concentration, minimal bactericidal concentration)

Host Factors

Drug allergies
Pharmacokinetic variables
Effect of food on drug absorption
Diseases affecting drug absorption
Effect of other drugs that alter biotransformation

Renal/hepatic function
Pregnancy/lactation
Site of infection
Signs and symptoms
Fever, malaise, leukocytosis, purulent drainage, etc.

Drug Factors

Economics
Can patient afford the drug?
Tissue penetration
Drug toxicity
Preventing resistance
Are combinations of drugs indicated?

TABLE 4-1. Microbes Frequently Regarded as Normal at Various Body Locations

LOCATION	MICROBE
Skin	Diphtheroids (*Corynebacterium*) *Propionibacterium* Staphylococci Streptococci
Gastrointestinal tract	*Bacteroides* *Clostridium* Diphtheroids Enterobacteriaceae (*Escherichia coli, Klebsiella*) *Fusobacterium* Streptococci (anaerobic)
Upper respiratory tract	*Bacteroides* *Haemophilus* *Neisseria* Streptococci
Genital tract	*Corynebacterium* Enterobacteriaceae *Lactobacillus* Mycoplasma Staphylococci Streptococci

Quantitatively, the minimal inhibitory concentration is the lowest concentration of an antibiotic that inhibits microorganism growth in liquid culture. The minimal bactericidal concentration is the lowest concentration of an antibiotic that induces bacterial cell death. Qualitatively, disks that are impregnated with antibiotics can be laid onto agar plates that were previously seeded with bacteria. The relative "zone of inhibition" around the drug-impregnated disk gives a general indication of drug susceptibility. Although these susceptibility tests indicate which drugs can prevent growth of an organism in vitro, this information may not always translate to the in vivo situation if the drug cannot reach the site of infection at the necessary concentration.

This chapter describes hundreds of antibacterial, antifungal, antiparasitic, and antiviral agents. It is important to know the mechanisms of actions, contraindications, and side effects for each class of antimicrobials. Rote memorization of each organism targeted by each drug within each class is not as effective as simply appreciating the ways in which specific classes of antibiotics target different classes of microorganisms. Many drugs now used may not be used in the near future; it is important to be familiar with the mechanism of action so that when new antibiotics are introduced into clinical practice, placing them in the appropriate context will be a comfortable exercise.

MICROBIOLOGY

Gram Staining

Microscopy assists in classification of infectious organisms and may tell the shape (e.g., coccus, bacillus) of a bacterial species or differentiate bacteria from fungi or spirochetes. Gram staining with gentian violet is useful to determine whether bacteria are gram positive or gram negative. The cell walls of gram-positive bacteria retain a violet color when stained with gentian violet. Cells walls of gram-negative bacteria lose this violet color when destained with alcohol but turn red when counterstained with safranin.

●●● ANTIBACTERIALS

In the most simplistic sense, antibacterial agents work by four distinct major mechanisms of action (Fig. 4-2):

- Inhibition of cell wall synthesis
- Inhibition of protein synthesis
- Inhibition of folic acid biosynthetic pathways
- Inhibition of DNA/RNA synthesis

TABLE 4-2. Suspected Microorganisms, Based on Site of Infection

LOCATION	CONDITION	MICROORGANISM
Respiratory tract	Pharyngitis, bronchitis, sinusitis, otitis	Group A streptococci, gonococci
	Pneumonia	*Haemophilus influenzae, Moraxella catarrhalis, Streptococcus pneumoniae, Staphylococcus aureus*
	Community Acquired Pneumonia	
	Normal host	*S. pneumoniae*, viral; *Mycoplasma*
	Aspiration	Normal aerobic and anaerobic mouth flora
	Pediatric patient	*S. pneumoniae, H. influenzae*
	COPD	*S. pneumoniae, Klebsiella*
	Nosocomial Acquired Pneumonia	
	Aspiration	Mouth anaerobes, gram-negative aerobic rods, *S. aureus*
	Neutropenic	Fungi, *Pneumocystis, Legionella*
	AIDS patient	Nocardia, *H. influenzae*, pneumococcus
Urinary tract	Community acquired	*Escherichia coli*, other gram-negative rods, enterococci
	Hospital acquired	Resistant gram-negative rods, enterococci
Skin/soft tissue	Cellulitis	Group A streptococci
	Intravenous catheter site	*S. aureus, Staphylococcus epidermis*
	Surgical wound	*S. aureus*, gram-negative rods
	Diabetic ulcer	*S. aureus*, gram-negative aerobic rods, anaerobes
Intra-abdominal	Gastroenteritis	*Bacteroides fragilis, E. coli*, enterococci, *Salmonella, Shigella, Campylobacter, Clostridium difficile*, amoebiasis, *Giardia*, viral
Skeletal system	Osteomyelitis or septic arthritis	*S. aureus*, gram-negative aerobic rods
Central nervous system	Meningitis	
	<2 months	Group B streptococci, *E. coli, Listeria*
	2 months to 12 years	*H. influenzae, S. pneumoniae, Neisseria meningitidis*
	Adult	*S. pneumoniae, N. meningitidis*, gram-negative aerobic rods
	Hospital acquired	*S. pneumoniae, N. meningitidis*, gram-negative aerobic rods
	Postneurosurgery	Gram-negative aerobic rods, *S. aureus*

AIDS, acquired immunodeficiency syndrome; *COPD*, chronic obstructive pulmonary disease.

In some instances, it makes sense to combine drugs that work by different mechanisms of action to achieve synergistic killing effects (Table 4-3).

Cell Wall Synthesis Inhibitors

Multiple drug classes interfere with cell wall synthesis, including the penicillins, the cephalosporins, the carbapenems, and the monobactams.

Penicillins
Mechanism of action
Penicillins inhibit cell wall synthesis by interfering with formation of the peptidoglycan layer and are bacteriocidal. Specifically, penicillins bind to a transpeptidase enzyme whose function is to cross-link *N*-acetyl muramic acid and *N*-acetyl glucosamine (Fig. 4-3). This linkage provides bacteria with structural stability. This transpeptidase is one of several bacterial proteins that penicillin binds that are collectively referred to as *penicillin-binding proteins* (PBPs). Other PBPs

that penicillins activate are autolysins that hydrolyze and destroy components of the cell as well as carboxypeptidases and endopeptidases that break peptide bonds.

Resistance
For penicillins to gain access to microbial cells, these drugs must first permeate the cell wall. Bacteria may become resistant to penicillins by the following mechanisms:
- Modification of their PBPs
- Active pumping of the drugs back out of the cells
- Cleavage of the β-lactam ring structure of penicillins via β-lactamases (also called *penicillinases*) within the periplasmic space, rendering the drugs inactive
- Altered porins (gram-negative bacteria only) that prevent the drugs from reaching the PBP targets

Figure 4-3 illustrates the layers of a bacterium cell wall, including the peptidoglycan layer with which penicillins interfere and the periplasmic space where β-lactamases may reside.

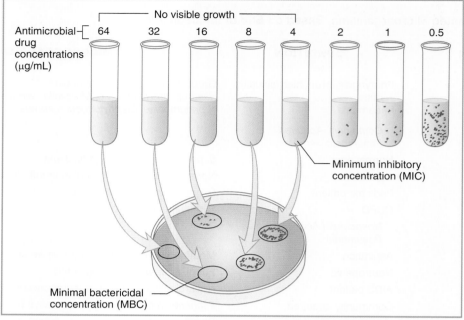

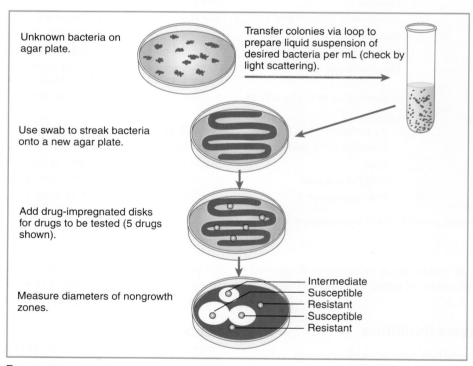

Figure 4-1. Susceptibility testing. **A,** Quantitative method. A single colony of bacteria is introduced into liquid cultures that vary in antibiotic concentration. The lowest concentration in which visible growth is absent (e.g., clear broth rather than cloudy) is the minimal inhibitory concentration. All subsequent liquid cultures are plated onto agar that contains no antibiotic. The lowest dose of the liquid antibiotic dilution that fails to exhibit growth on the petri dish is the minimal bactericidal concentration, indicating that the dose of antibiotic has killed the bacteria in culture. **B,** Qualitative method. Disks with impregnated drugs are placed onto a petri dish that has been seeded with bacteria. The zones of growth inhibition around the disks provide an indication of bacterial susceptibility to the drug.

Adverse effects

The major adverse effect associated with penicillins is hypersensitivity. Hypersensitivity reactions to penicillins range from mild to severe and may include hives, itching, or anaphylaxis. Most penicillins, with the exceptions of nafcillin and oxacillin, are excreted unchanged in the urine; therefore penicillin dosages must be lowered in patients with renal insufficiency. At high intravenous doses, penicillins may cause seizures or antiplatelet effects. Anemia, thrombocytopenia, and hypoprothrombinemia have also been reported.

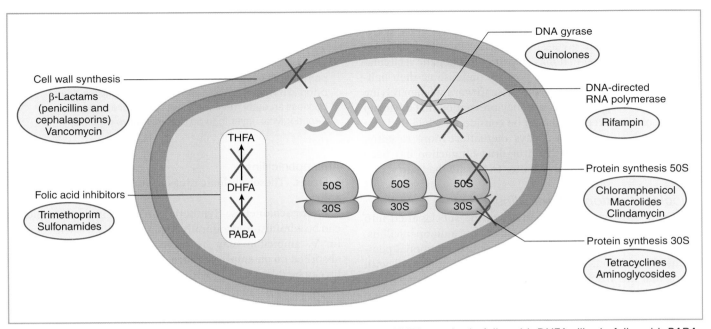

Figure 4-2. The four major mechanisms by which most antibiotics work. *THFA*, tetrahydrofolic acid; *DHFA*, dihydrofolic acid; *PABA*, para-aminobenzoic acid.

TABLE 4-3. Examples of Synergistic Drug Combinations

COMBINATION	DESCRIPTION
Penicillins + aminoglycosides	This combination is a cell wall synthesis inhibitor plus a protein synthesis inhibitor.
Sulfamethoxazole + trimethoprim	These agents act on sequential steps of the same microbial metabolic pathway.
Amoxicillin + clavulanic acid	Clavulanic acid inhibits a microbial enzyme that would otherwise inactivate amoxicillin.

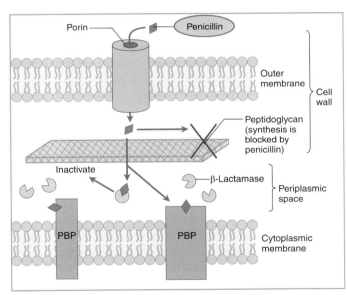

Figure 4-3. A gram-negative bacterial cell wall. Penicillins inhibit synthesis of bacterial cell walls by binding to penicillin-binding proteins (*PBPs*). PBPs are depicted as different enzymes because they have differing functions. Binding to PBPs (1) inhibits cell wall synthesis by blocking transpeptidation of peptidoglycan and (2) activates autolytic enzymes in the cell wall that cause lesions resulting in bacterial death. Actions of penicillins may be terminated by β-lactamase enzymes that reside in the periplasmic space. This is a mechanism by which bacteria become resistant to penicillins.

It is not uncommon for penicillins, especially broad-spectrum agents, to cause secondary infections by disrupting normal gut flora. This can lead to vaginal yeast infections as well as pseudomembranous colitis caused by overgrowth of *Clostridium difficile* in the gastrointestinal tract.

Drug interactions

When penicillins are combined with drugs that are bacteriostatic (e.g., tetracycline), pharmacologic antagonism results. For penicillins to be effective inhibitors of cell wall synthesis, microorganisms must be actively growing and dividing. Tetracyclines are bacteriostatic; therefore the growth of microorganisms is inhibited. As a result, the combination of a bacteriostatic drug such as a tetracycline with a bactericidal drug such as penicillin would not be expected to produce synergistic actions.

There has been a long-standing concern that combining penicillins (or any antibiotic) with oral contraceptives may lessen the efficacy of the oral contraceptive because estrogens are recycled via the enterohepatic recirculation pathway. Under normal circumstances, gut bacteria cleave estrogen-glucuronide conjugates, allowing the estrogenic component to be reabsorbed, thereby extending its duration of activity in the body. When antibiotics are given, normal gastrointestinal flora are disrupted, a situation that may impair enterohepatic recirculation of estrogenic compounds, possibly diminishing their half-life ($t_{1/2}$). As a result, it is probably wise to warn women relying on oral contraceptives for pregnancy prevention that a backup method of contraception should be considered while they are taking antibiotics and for 7 days thereafter. More recently, the clinical relevance of this drug-drug interaction has been questioned, yet it is probably better to be safe than sorry.

Subclassification of Penicillins

The numerous types of penicillins can be subclassified into four distinct categories: natural penicillins, aminopenicillins, penicillinase-resistant penicillins, and antipseudomonal penicillins. In addition, penicillins may be coadministered with drugs that are irreversible inhibitors of β-lactamase, which broadens the antimicrobial spectrum of coverage to include β-lactamase–producing organisms. As a general and probably oversimplified rule, natural penicillins and penicillinase-resistant penicillins tend to be used to treat gram-positive microorganisms, whereas aminopenicillins and antipseudomonal penicillins possess activity against gram-negative organisms as well. A list of microorganisms for which penicillins might be selected as drugs of choice is found in Table 4-4. This table is not an exhaustive list of all microorganisms for which penicillins are effective, and only drugs of choice are listed rather than complete sensitivity data for each penicillin.

Natural penicillins

Drugs. Penicillin G and penicillin V.

Pharmacokinetics. Because penicillin G is readily destroyed in acidic environments, such as that found in the digestive tract, the drug can only be administered intravenously or intramuscularly. Long-acting intramuscular depot injections of penicillin G are sometimes used to prevent rheumatic fever and to treat syphilis. Penicillin V is somewhat more stable than penicillin G in acidic environments and thus is administered orally; however, the drug still must be given on an empty stomach, 1 hour before meals or 2 to 3 hours after meals for maximal efficacy.

Clinical use. These antibiotics are primarily used for treating infections caused by susceptible gram-positive microorganisms. Some uses for penicillin G include serious streptococcal infections, neurosyphilis, and endocarditis. Penicillin V is the drug of choice for treating streptococcal pharyngitis. These drugs are inactivated by β-lactamases.

MICROBIOLOGY AND IMMUNOLOGY

Cell Walls

Unique to bacteria is a cell wall comprising a complex peptidoglycan that consists of cross-linked polysaccharides and polypeptides. The polysaccharide contains alternating amino sugars of *N*-acetylglucosamine and *N*-acetylmuramic acid which are connected by a peptide bridge. A penicillin-binding protein called transpeptidase, cross-links the peptidoglycan chains to form rigid cell walls. Such cross-links provide bacterial cell walls with structural rigidity. In addition to the peptidoglycan layer, gram-negative bacteria also possess an outer membrane that is permeated by porins, or channels, that provide access to the cytoplasmic membrane. Gram-positive organisms do not possess an outer membrane but have a much thicker peptidoglycan layer than do gram-negative organisms.

Aminopenicillins

Drugs. These synthetic drugs include ampicillin and amoxicillin.

Pharmacokinetics. Synthetic penicillins such as ampicillin can be administered enterally or parenterally. As with penicillin V, ampicillin may be prescribed orally, but it is best absorbed on an empty stomach. On the other hand, amoxicillin can be taken with or without food because it is stable even in the presence of gastric acids.

Clinical use. Although used primarily for treating gram-positive bacteria, these antibacterials have a broader spectrum against some gram-negative microorganisms than do the natural penicillins. However, aminopenicillins are ineffective for microorganisms that synthesize β-lactamases (i.e., penicillinases) and are often used in combination with β-lactamase inhibitors. Aminopenicillins are commonly used to treat infections of the ears, nose, throat, and lower respiratory tract and for prophylaxis against endocarditis.

Adverse effects. A nonallergic "ampicillin rash" is common, even in the absence of hypersensitivity to other penicillins. Ampicillin rashes occur most often in patients with mononucleosis or those using allopurinol concurrently.

Penicillinase-resistant penicillins

Drugs. Drugs include dicloxacillin, methicillin, oxacillin, and nafcillin.

Mechanism of action. Chemically, the penicillinase-resistant penicillins contain side groups that protect the drugs from being inactivated by bacterial β-lactamases.

Pharmacokinetics. Methicillin, oxacillin, and nafcillin are usually given parenterally; dicloxacillin is given orally.

Clinical use. Penicillinase-resistant penicillins are useful for treating infections caused by β-lactamase–producing staphylococci. Therapeutic applications for penicillinase-resistant penicillins include treatment or prevention of infections in the upper or lower respiratory tract, skin, bones, and joints. In addition, these antibiotics are used to treat meningitis, septicemia, and endocarditis.

It should be assumed that all staphylococci synthesize β-lactamases; hence, staphylococcal infections are best treated with pharmacologic agents that are resistant to the effects of these penicillin-inactivating enzymes. During the past decade, increasing staphylococcal resistance led to the term *MRSA* (methicillin-resistant *Staphylococcus aureus*). It should be noted that MRSA is resistant to all penicillins and cephalosporins but fortunately may be sensitive to other cell wall synthesis inhibitors such as vancomycin, antimetabolites

TABLE 4-4. Microorganisms for Which Penicillins Might Be Selected as Drugs of Choice

Organisms	NATURAL PENICILLINS		AMINOPENICILLINS ±β-LACTAMASE INHIBITORS				PENICILLINASE-RESISTANT PENICILLINS	ANTIPSEUDOMONAL PENICILLINS*
	Penicillin G	Penicillin V	Ampicillin	Ampicillin + Sulbactam	Amoxicillin	Amoxicillin + Clavulanate	Methicillin, Nafcillin, Oxacillin, and Others	Piperacillin/Tazobactam or Ticarcillin/Clavulanate
Gram positive								
Cocci								
Enterococcus faecalis, serious infection	X		X					
E. faecalis, urinary tract infection			X		X			
Staphylococcus aureus, S. epidermis				✓†		✓†	X†	
Streptococcus (groups A, B, C, G, and *S. bovis*)	X	X	X					
Streptococcus pneumoniae, penicillin-sensitive strains	X	X	X					
Streptococcus viridans group	X							
Bacilli								
Clostridium perfringens	X							
Gram negative								
Cocci								
Moraxella catarrhalis				X		X		
Neisseria meningitidis	X							
Bacilli								
Escherichia coli			X	✓		X		
Haemophilus influenzae				X	X	X		
Proteus mirabilis			X					
Pseudomonas aeruginosa								X

*Although the antipseudomonal penicillins could be used to treat infections caused by most of the microorganisms listed, they are reserved for treating only the infections for which other penicillins would be ineffective.
†Used as long as organism is methicillin sensitive.
This table is not all inclusive. It is a representation of common infectious microorganisms and the penicillins that might be selected as drugs of choice to treat a variety of different types of infections, either individually or as part of a combination treatment regimen.
X, Drug of choice; ✓, alternative therapy if first-line drugs cannot be used or are ineffective.

TABLE 4-5. Selected Adverse Effects Associated with Penicillinase-Resistant Penicillins

EFFECT	DRUG
Hepatitis	Oxacillin
Nephritis	Nafcillin

TABLE 4-6. Commercially Available Combination Products: Penicillins + β-Lactamase Inhibitors

PENICILLIN	β-LACTAMASE INHIBITOR
Amoxicillin	Clavulanic acid
Ticarcillin	Clavulanic acid
Ampicillin	Sulbactam
Piperacillin	Tazobactam

such as sulfamethoxazole/trimethoprim, and protein synthesis inhibitors such as linezolid.

Adverse effects. Thrombophlebitis, pain, and inflammation at the site of injection are common with parenteral administration. Additional adverse effects that are unique for penicillinase-resistant penicillins are shown in Table 4-5.

Antipseudomonal penicillins (extended-spectrum penicillins)

Drugs. Drugs include carbenicillin, ticarcillin, mezlocillin, and piperacillin.

Pharmacokinetics. These drugs are usually given parenterally. Carbenicillin is the only drug in this class that can be administered orally, but therapeutic levels of this drug are then found only in the urinary tract, limiting its enteral utility to treating urinary tract and prostatic infections.

Clinical use. Antipseudomonal penicillins are also called *extended-spectrum penicillins* because they provide better coverage of gram-negative microorganisms, including *Pseudomonas* and *Enterobacter* species, than other penicillins. These drugs are often reserved for treating serious gram-negative infections of the respiratory tract, soft tissues, bones, joints, and urinary tract as well as for treating sepsis. These drugs are frequently combined with aminoglycosides for synergistic effects in treatment of serious infections.

Adverse effects. Caution must be used when administering carbenicillin or ticarcillin to patients with cardiac disease because they contain large amounts of sodium, which may aggravate hypertension or congestive heart failure. Antipseudomonal penicillins have also been associated with antiplatelet activities.

Clinical use. Irreversible β-lactamase inhibitors have no antimicrobial activity by themselves. However, when these agents are combined with penicillins, expanded coverage against β-lactamase–producing microorganisms is provided. See Table 4-4 to compare situations in which amoxicillin versus amoxicillin + clavulanic acid might be selected as drugs of choice. Table 4-6 lists some common penicillin + β-lactamase inhibitor products.

Cephalosporins

Cephalosporins structurally resemble penicillins and, like penicillins, possess a β-lactam chemical backbone. Unlike the natural penicillins, cephalosporins are relatively stable to pH changes and may be taken with or without food. The clinical utility of cephalosporins is listed in Box 4-3. Cephalosporins are classified by generation. In general, gram-positive activity is lost with each succeeding generation, whereas gram-negative activity is gained. Table 4-7 lists microorganisms and selected situations in which cephalosporins may be selected as drugs of choice.

Mechanism of action. Same as that of penicillins.

Resistance. Porin alterations that prevent drug entry (especially among gram-negative species), mutations in PBPs, or lack of PBPs are mechanisms by which microorganisms become resistant to cephalosporins. As a group, cephalosporins are less likely to be degraded by β-lactamases than are penicillins.

CLINICAL MEDICINE

Keys to Prescribing Penicillin

- Amoxicillin/clavulanic acid is particularly effective for ear, nose, and throat infections.
- Nafcillin is the drug of choice for suspected staphylococcus aureus infections (unless cultures show methicillin-resistant *Staphylococcus aureus*, then vancomycin is used).
- Piperacillin/tazobactam is a broad spectrum antibiotic for empiric treatment. The drug combination is also used to treat pseudomonal infections.

Irreversible inhibitors of β-lactamases

Drugs. Drugs include clavulanic acid, sulbactam, tazobactam.

Box 4-3. CLINICAL UTILITY OF CEPHALOSPORINS

- Patients allergic to penicillin, when macrolides are not effective
- Drugs of choice for treating gram-negative infections, especially *Klebsiella*
- Drugs of choice for treating the three microorganisms that frequently cause pediatric meningitis (*Haemophilus influenzae, Streptococcus pneumoniae, Neisseria meningitidis*)
- Polymicrobial infections
- Empiric treatment of infections of unknown etiology
- Prophylaxis during surgery, especially if implants are involved

TABLE 4-7. Examples of Microorganisms for Which Cephalosporins Might Be Considered Drugs of Choice

Organisms	FIRST GENERATION				SECOND GENERATION					THIRD (AND FOURTH) GENERATION							
	Cefazolin (IV)	Cephalexin (Oral)	Cephradine (Oral)	Cefadroxil (Oral)	Cefuroxime (IV, Oral)	Cefaclor (Oral)	Cefprozil (Oral)	Cefoxitin	Cefotetan	Cefotaxime (IV)	Ceftriaxone (IV)	Cefixime (Oral)	Cefpodoxime (Oral)	Ceftibuten (Oral)	Cefdinir	Ceftazidime (IV)	Cefepime (IV)
Gram Positive																	
Cocci																	
Staphylococcus aureus/, epidermis methicillin sensitive	✓	✓	✓	✓													
Streptococcus (groups A, B, C, G and *S. bovis*)	✓	✓	✓	✓													
Streptococcus pneumoniae, penicillin sensitive	✓	✓	✓	✓													
Streptococcus pneumoniae, penicillin—intermediate level of resistance										X	X						
Streptococcus, viridans group	✓	✓	✓	✓						✓	✓						
Bacilli																	
Clostridium perfringens	✓																
Gram-Negative																	
Cocci																	
Moraxella catarrhalis					✓	✓	✓			✓	✓	✓	✓	✓	✓		
Neisseria gonorrhoeae										X	X		X				
Neisseria meningitides										✓	✓						
Bacilli																	
Bacteroides fragilis								✓									
Enterobacter spp.																	X*
Escherichia coli, meningitis										X	X						
Escherichia coli, systemic infection	✓	✓	✓							X	X						

Continued

TABLE 4-7. Examples of Microorganisms for Which Cephalosporins Might Be Considered Drugs of Choice—cont'd

Organisms	FIRST GENERATION				SECOND GENERATION					THIRD (AND FOURTH) GENERATION							
	Cefazolin (IV)	Cephalexin (Oral)	Cephradine (Oral)	Cefadroxil (Oral)	Cefuroxime (IV, Oral)	Cefaclor (Oral)	Cefprozil (Oral)	Cefoxitin	Cefotetan	Cefotaxime (IV)	Ceftriaxone (IV)	Cefixime (Oral)	Cefpodoxime (Oral)	Ceftibuten (Oral)	Cefdinir	Ceftazidime (IV)	Cefepime (IV)
Escherichia coli, urinary tract infection	✓	X	✓	✓													
Haemophilus influenzae, meningitis										X	X						
Haemophilus influenzae, other infections					✓												
Klebsiella pneumoniae					✓					X	X						
Other																	
Proteus (indole positive)					X	X	X	X	X								
Providencia stuartii					X	X											
Pseudomonas aeruginosa																X	X
Salmonella typhi					X	X											
Treponema pallidum,											X						
Borrelia burgdorferi					X					X	X						

*Use with an aminoglycoside
X, Drug of choice; ✓, alternative.

Adverse effects. Because of chemical structural similarities between cephalosporins and penicillins, there is a possibility that penicillin-allergic patients may also be hypersensitive to cephalosporins. However, recent data suggest that the incidence of this cross-reactivity is probably much lower than previously believed. As a rule, it is wise to refrain from prescribing cephalosporins to patients with a documented history of anaphylactic reactions to penicillins.

Gastrointestinal irritation is common with oral cephalosporins, but taking the medications with food may prevent this adverse effect. Parenterally administered cephalosporins cause local irritation at the site of injection. Because many cephalosporins are excreted by the kidneys, renal toxicity is possible; caution should be used in patients with preexisting renal disease (impaired creatinine clearance). As indicated later in this chapter, some second- and third-generation cephalosporins may cause disulfiram-like reactions and hypoprothrombinemia. Newer cephalosporins, especially those administered parenterally, may cause seizures, but this is usually only a concern for individuals with impaired kidney function because the drugs may accumulate. Because of disruption of normal flora, secondary infections, including pseudomembranous colitis and vaginal yeast infections, may also occur.

First-generation cephalosporins

Drugs. Drugs include cefadroxil, cefazolin, cephalexin, cephradine, and cephapirin (note that they all begin with "cef-" or "ceph-").

Clinical use. As a rule, first-generation cephalosporins possess excellent activity against gram-positive aerobic bacteria but are not effective against anaerobes. Groups A and B streptococcal organisms are typically sensitive to first-generation cephalosporins, but MRSA, enterococci, and penicillin-resistant *Streptococcus pneumoniae* are not.

Although these drugs have activity against some gram-negative organisms such as *Escherichia coli* and *Proteus mirabilis*, first-generation cephalosporins do not have reliable activity against *Moraxella catarrhalis* (a common culprit in upper respiratory infections). First-generation cephalosporins are most commonly used for treating uncomplicated skin and soft tissue infections.

Second-generation cephalosporins

Drugs. Drugs are cefoxitin, cefaclor, cefuroxime, cefotetan, cefprozil (again, notice that the drugs begin with "cef-").

Clinical use. As a group, second-generation cephalosporins possess wider activity against gram-negative bacteria and anaerobic microorganisms than do first-generation cephalosporins. Specifically, cefoxitin is effective against *Bacteroides fragilis* and other anaerobic organisms. In addition, cefuroxime is the only second-generation cephalosporin that enters the central nervous system and can be used to treat meningitis.

Adverse effects. The chemical side chain (N-methylthiotetrazole) on the chemical backbone of cefotetan inhibits aldehyde dehydrogenase; therefore disulfiram-like reactions may occur if alcohol is consumed within 72 hours of administration of this medication. Disulfiram is a drug that is used to discourage alcohol abuse by elevating plasma aldehyde levels, thereby resulting in unpleasant side effects. The N-methylthiotetrazole side chain may also cause hypoprothrombinemia and risk of bleeding. Cefaclor is associated with hypersensitivity, including a rash and serum sickness, but these reactions to cefaclor are not contraindications to the use of other cephalosporins or penicillins.

CLINICAL MEDICINE

Keys to Cephalosporin Prescribing

- Cefazolin (first generation) is commonly used for surgical prophylaxis.
- Cephalexin (first generation) is the most commonly prescribed cephalosporin for outpatient use.
- Ceftriaxone (third generation) is commonly used for treating sexually transmitted diseases; ceftriaxone is also a drug of choice for treating pediatric meningitis.
- Cefepime (third generation) is used to treat pseudomonal infections.

Third-generation cephalosporins

Drugs. Drugs include cefotaxime, cefpodoxime, ceftazidime, ceftibuten, ceftizoxime, ceftriaxone, cefdinir, cefditoren, cefepime, and cefixime. (Again, note that they all begin with "cef-." In addition, some texts classify cefepime by itself as a fourth-generation cephalosporin.)

Clinical use. As a group, third-generation cephalosporins have wide activity against gram-negative microorganisms. In addition, many of the drugs in this class (cefotaxime and ceftriaxone) also possess some coverage against anaerobic bacteria. Activity against gram-positive microorganisms is less reliable with third-generation cephalosporins than with previous generations. Some of these drugs are active against *Pseudomonas* (ceftazidime); others cross the blood-brain barrier and can be used to treat meningitis (ceftriaxone). Clinically, third-generation cephalosporins are used to treat infections caused by gram-negative bacteria, especially hospital-acquired infections or complicated community-acquired infections involving the respiratory tract, blood, skin and soft tissues, urinary tract, and intra-abdominal infections. Because of their activity against gram-negative bacteria, third-generation cephalosporins may be an alternative to aminoglycosides.

Adverse effects. Biliary sludging may also occur with third-generation cephalosporins as a result of inhibited bile outflow. In addition, cefditoren causes renal excretion of carnitine and should be avoided in carnitine-deficient individuals. Cefditoren should also be avoided in patients with a true hypersensitivity to milk (sodium caseinate).

Carbapenems

Drugs. Drugs include imipenem/cilastatin, doripenem, ertapenem, and meropenem.

Mechanism of action. As with penicillins and cephalosporins, carbapenems are bactericidal and inhibit cell wall synthesis. Unlike penicillins and cephalosporins, carbapenems have a different stereochemical structure in their β-lactam ring that renders them resistant to β-lactamases.

Clinical use. These drugs are parenterally administered, broad-spectrum antibiotics. Most are effective against gram-positive organisms such as staphylococci and streptococci, as well as gram-negative organisms including *Pseudomonas* (exception is ertapenem with little activity against this gram-negative organism) and anaerobes including *Bacteroides fragilis*. Imipenem is always given in combination with cilastatin. Cilastatin does not have antimicrobial activity; instead, it inhibits a renal dehydropeptidase enzyme that inactivates imipenem. Given their broad spectrum of activity, carbapenems may be used in treatment of mixed infections that otherwise would have required the use of at least two antibiotics.

Adverse effects. Seizures have been reported in a small percentage of patients, especially those who are predisposed such as patients with renal insufficiency, a recent history of head trauma, or epilepsy. Pseudomembranous colitis and bone marrow suppression have also occurred. Because of structural similarities, carbapenems should be used cautiously (if at all) in patients who are hypersensitive to penicillins.

Monobactams

Drug. The only choice is aztreonam.

Mechanism of action and clinical use. Currently, aztreonam is the only monobactam approved for use in the United States. Monobactams may be used in penicillin-allergic patients. Aztreonam is relatively resistant to β-lactamases. Aztreonam is a gram-negative–specific antimicrobial that interferes with cell wall synthesis. Clinically, aztreonam is used for treating respiratory, urinary, skin, gynecologic, and intra-abdominal infections. Aztreonam may antagonize the

TABLE 4-8. Adverse Effects Carbapenems Associated with β-Lactam Antibiotics (Penicillins, Cephalosporins, Monobactams, Penems)

EVENT	SYMPTOM OR CONDITION
Allergic reaction, anaphylaxis, urticaria, serum sickness, rash, fever	Ampicillin rash is common in absence of cross-reactivity to other penicillins; most common in those with mononucleosis or concurrent allopurinol use
	Cefaclor is associated with a higher than expected incidence of hypersensitivity reactions
	Cross-reactivity between penicillins and imipenem
	No cross-reactivity between aztreonam and penicillins
Diarrhea	Common with amoxicillin + clavulanic acid, ampicillin, ceftriaxone, cefoperazone
	Pseudomembranous colitis, caused by *Clostridium difficile* overgrowth, can occur with nearly any antibacterial agent
Anemia, thrombocytopenia, antiplatelet activity, hypoprothrombinemia	Hemolytic anemia is more common at higher doses
	Antiplatelet activity is most common with antipseudomonal penicillins and high serum levels of other β-lactams
Hepatitis	Most common with oxacillin
Seizure	Associated with high levels of β-lactams, particularly penicillins and imipenem
Sodium load	Carbenicillin, ticarcillin
Nephritis	Most common with methicillin, but reported with all β-lactams
Disulfiram reaction	Cephalosporins with methylthiotetrazole side chains (e.g., cefamandole, cefotetan, cefoperazone, cefmetazole)
Hypotension, nausea	Associated with fast infusion of imipenem

efficacy of other β-lactam antibiotics but is often used synergistically with aminoglycosides.

Table 4-8 lists the major adverse effects associated with antibiotics that possess β-lactam chemical structures.

Other antibiotics that disrupt cell walls

Drug. Telavancin, vancomycin

Mechanism of action. These drugs interfere with cell wall synthesis by blocking polymerization and cross-linking of peptidoglycan by binding to the D-Ala-D-Ala portion of cell walls. Additional mechanisms for telavancin involve disruption of membrane potential and changes in cell permeability because of the presence of a lipophilic side chain moiety.

Clinical use. Although the drugs are rapidly bactericidal, they are effective only against gram-positive microorganisms. These drugs are used parenterally to treat serious systemic staphylococcal infections (including MRSA), streptococcal, and enterococcal (if susceptible) infections. Vancomycin is also given orally for gastrointestinal-specific treatment of *C. difficile*–associated diarrhea and pseudomembranous colitis. Vancomycin is not absorbed systemically when administered orally; therefore, there are few adverse effects with enteral administration.

Adverse effects. A unique adverse effect termed *red neck syndrome,* characterized by itching, rash, fever, and chills, can occur if vancomycin is infused too rapidly. This is not an allergic reaction and is simply an infusion reaction that can be prevented by prior administration of antihistamines or slow administration of the drug. Other adverse effects include the possibility of nephrotoxicity, cardiac arrest, vascular collapse, and bone marrow suppression. Although current vancomycin formulations are not as nephrotoxic as they once were, it is wise to monitor kidney function, including blood urea nitrogen and serum creatinine, as well as serum vancomycin (peak and trough) levels. Extra precautions should be used to monitor renal function when vancomycin is administered concurrently with other drugs that are also potentially nephrotoxic. Telavancin is thought to be teratogenic according to preclinical data and should not be administered to a woman of child-bearing age unless a negative serum pregnancy test is obtained. Telavancin also prolongs the QT interval on electrocardiograms. Adverse effects associated with vancomycin are listed in Table 4-9. The potential emergence of vancomycin-resistant enterococci is always a concern.

Drug. Cycloserine.

Mechanism of action. Cycloserine inhibits cell wall synthesis in gram-positive and gram-negative microorganisms but it is usually reserved for treating *Mycobacterium tuberculosis* infections resistant to first-line antitubercular drugs.

Adverse effects. Cycloserine may cause central nervous system toxicities such as psychosis, headaches, visual disturbances, and seizures; these adverse effects appear to be dose related. As a result of its side-effect profile, cycloserine is contraindicated in patients with seizure disorders, renal disease, alcoholism, depression, and anxiety disorders.

Bacitracin. Because of serious nephrotoxicity, bacitracin is typically reserved for topical use in the treatment of ocular or skin infections. It is available for topical use as a single agent and is also one component of triple-antibiotic ointment, both of which are available without a prescription. In rare

TABLE 4-9. Adverse Effects Associated with Vancomycin

EVENT	SYMPTOM OR CONDITION
Ototoxicity	Of concern at high serum levels (>50 µg/mL)
Nephrotoxicity	May be increased with concurrent administration of aminoglycosides
Hypotension, flushing	Associated with rapid infusion
Phlebitis	Needs large volume dilution

TABLE 4-10. Adverse Pulmonary Effects Associated with Nitrofurantoin

ACUTE	SUBACUTE	CHRONIC
Dyspnea	Dyspnea	Pulmonary fibrosis
Chills	Tachypnea	Respiratory failure
Fever	Persistent cough	
Angina	Interstitial pneumonitis	
Cough	Chest pain	

circumstances, the antibiotic is used parenterally to treat systemic infections caused by drug-sensitive staphylococci that are resistant to other, safer antibiotics.

Drug. Polymyxin B.

Mechanism of action. This drug is bactericidal to nearly all gram-negative bacilli, with the exception of *Proteus*. It is a cationic detergent that disrupts lipoproteins in bacterial cell walls, thus increasing membrane permeability.

Clinical use. Polymyxin B is usually used topically for ocular and otic infections or bladder irrigations. As with bacitracin, polymyxin B is found in triple-antibiotic ointment. Although rarely used parenterally, it may be used intravenously, intramuscularly, or intrathecally to treat serious infections caused by *Pseudomonas, E. coli, Klebsiella,* or *Haemophilus influenzae* when other antibiotics cannot be used. However, parenteral use of polymyxin B has largely been replaced by aminoglycosides.

Adverse effects. When used parenterally, apnea has occurred, especially when combined with curare-type skeletal muscle relaxants.

Drug. Nitrofurantoin.

Mechanism of action. Once inside bacterial cells, nitrofurantoin exhibits a novel mechanism. It is reduced by flavoproteins to multiple reactive intermediates that damage ribosomal proteins, DNA, and other cellular molecules. At high doses, nitrofurantoin may be bactericidal against some strains of bacteria.

Resistance. Because of its unique mechanism of action, nitrofurantoin is not cross-resistant with any other antibiotics.

Clinical use. Nitrofurantoin is excreted unchanged into the urine. This drug reaches therapeutic concentrations only in the urine and is therefore used to treat urinary tract infections.

Adverse effects. Nitrofurantoin may discolor urine, causing it to darken. Gastrointestinal upset may also occur, which is minimized by taking the drug with food. This antibiotic is contraindicated in pregnant women near term and in glucose 6-phosphate dehydrogenase (G6PD)-deficient individuals because of the risk of hemolytic anemia. Hepatotoxicity and irreversible peripheral neuropathies have also been reported. Nitrofurantoin has also been associated with pulmonary problems, both short and long term (Table 4-10).

Protein Synthesis Inhibitors

In addition to drugs that target bacterial cell walls, other classes of antibiotics target pathways associated with bacterial, but not human, protein synthesis. Drugs that inhibit bacterial protein synthesis (aminoglycosides, macrolides, and tetracyclines) exert their effects at different locations along the pathway. These drugs directly interfere with the initiation phase of protein synthesis, the binding of tRNA, and the activities of peptidyl transferase. They also may cause inappropriate amino acid insertions into growing peptide chains (misreading errors), which ultimately interferes with essential protein functions (Fig. 4-4).

BIOCHEMISTRY

Prokaryotic Protein Synthesis

Prokaryotic protein synthesis begins with the initiation phase in which necessary components come together (30 S ribosomal subunit, 50 S ribosomal subunit, incoming tRNA, mRNA). An incoming tRNA binds to the A site of ribosomal subunits, in response to a codon that it recognizes. The new amino acid is then transferred to the P site, and peptidyl transferase catalyzes formation of a peptide bond between the new amino acid and the growing peptide chain. During the last step, movement of the incoming amino acid from the A site to the P site occurs, a process known as *translocation* (a process catalyzed by an enzyme translocase).

Aminoglycosides
Drugs

Drugs are amikacin, gentamicin, kanamycin, netilmicin, streptomycin, tobramycin, and neomycin.

Mechanism of action

Aminoglycoside binding to bacterial 30 S ribosomal subunits interferes with protein synthesis in at least three ways:
- Aminoglycosides interfere with formation of the initiation complex.
- Aminoglycosides misread mRNA and miscode amino acids in the growing peptide chain.
- Aminoglycosides cause ribosomes to separate from mRNA.

Blockade of movement of the ribosome may occur after formation of a single initiation complex, resulting in a mRNA chain

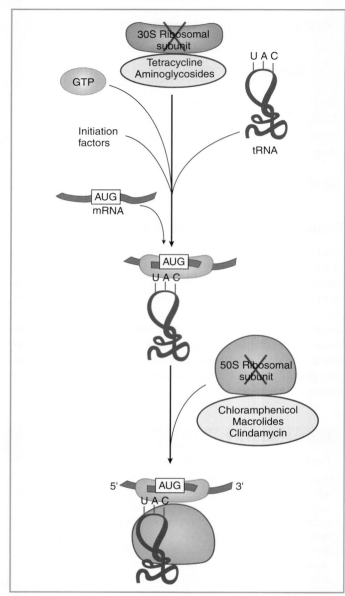

Figure 4-4. Prokaryotic protein synthesis. *GTP,* guanosine triphosphate.

with only a single ribosome, called a *monosome.* This causes inefficient protein synthesis, because many ribosomes (polysomes) typically work together during protein translation.

Pharmacokinetics

Aminoglycosides are too water soluble (because they are highly polar cations) to be absorbed if given orally; therefore they are usually used parenterally. Except in neonates, aminoglycosides exhibit marginal penetration of the central nervous system because of this high degree of hydrophilicity. Despite short half-lives in systemic circulation, accumulation occurs in the inner ear and renal cortex. Accumulation in these tissues accounts for the nephrotoxic and ototoxic side effects associated with aminoglycosides. Because of the translational mechanism of action, microorganisms continue to die even as plasma levels of the drug decline, a phenomenon referred to as the *postantibiotic effect.*

Clinical use

Aminoglycosides are usually reserved for treating severe gram-negative infections, and they are often added to cell wall synthesis inhibitors for synergistic effects (Table 4-11). Aminoglycosides are used parenterally to treat severe or hospital-acquired infections caused by *Enterobacter, Proteus, Pseudomonas, Klebsiella, E. coli,* and *Serratia* that affect the respiratory system, the gastrointestinal tract, urinary tract, bone, skin, blood, or soft tissues. Gentamicin is usually the parenteral aminoglycoside of choice, although it is available for topical and ophthalmic uses, too. Streptomycin may be used in combination with other antibacterials to treat mycobacterial infections. Tobramycin and amikacin may be given by inhalation to treat pseudomonal infections in patients with cystic fibrosis. Neomycin is used for topical skin infections and orally for its "topical" effects in the gastrointestinal tract to eradicate *E. coli, Klebsiella,* and *Enterobacter* before surgical bowel procedures.

Resistance

The aminoglycosides are reliably used only in treating gram-negative infections. Some bacterial species, especially anaerobes, have acquired resistance to aminoglycosides by way of alterations in receptor proteins on their ribosomes, which prevent aminoglycosides from binding. In addition, bacteria may enzymatically or posttranslationally alter aminoglycosides through phosphorylation, acetylation, or adenylation, which interferes with the drug's ability to bind efficiently to ribosomal subunits.

Adverse effects

High serum concentrations of aminoglycosides, especially at the nadir (trough) of the dosing cycle, have been associated with serious and irreversible vestibular and auditory ototoxicity as well as nephrotoxicity (usually reversible). In addition, neuromuscular blockade and acute muscle paralysis may occur, especially in

TABLE 4-11. Examples of Microorganisms for Which Aminoglycosides May Be Drugs of Choice	
GRAM-NEGATIVE BACILLI	**AMINOGLYCOSIDES**
Acinetobacter	X
Enterobacter	X
Escherichia coli, urinary tract infection	✓
Klebsiella pneumoniae, urinary tract infection	X
Pseudomonas aeruginosa	X
Pseudomonas, urinary tract infection	X
Serratia marcescens	X

This table is not all inclusive. It is a representation of common infectious microorganisms for which aminoglycosides may be the drugs of choice. Aminoglycosides are frequently combined with β-lactam antibiotics for treating serious infections caused by gram-negative bacilli.
X, Drug of choice; ✓, alternative choice if first-line agent cannot be used.

TABLE 4-12. Adverse Effects Associated with Aminoglycoside Antibiotics (Gentamicin, Tobramycin, Amikacin, Netilmicin)

EVENT	SYMPTOM OR CONDITION
Nephrotoxicity	10% to 15% incidence; generally reversible; usually occurs after 5 to 7 days of therapy
	Risk factors: advancing age, dehydration, duration of therapy, concurrent nephrotoxins, liver disease
Ototoxicity	1% to 5% incidence; often irreversible; both cochlear and/or vestibular toxicity may occur
Neuromuscular paralysis	Rare; most common with myasthenia gravis

patients with preexisting myasthenia gravis or when aminoglycosides are used in combination with succinylcholine or are used in dialysis fluid for peritoneal infections. Urinary output and serum peak and trough concentrations should be monitored. Audiometric testing may also be important with long-term therapy. Caution should be used when administering aminoglycosides with other drugs associated with nephrotoxicity (e.g., amphotericin, cephalosporins). Table 4-12 summarizes adverse effects associated with aminoglycoside antibiotics.

Tetracyclines
Drugs
Drugs are tetracycline, minocycline, doxycycline, demeclocycline, oxytetracycline, and tigecycline (all ending with "-cycline").

Mechanism of action
Tetracyclines inhibit protein synthesis through reversible binding to bacterial 30 S ribosomal subunits, which prevent binding of new incoming amino acids (aminoacyl-tRNA) and thus interfere with peptide growth (Fig. 4-5). Tigecycline

is sometimes designated as the first glycylcycline antibiotic; glycylcyclines are antibiotics derived from tetracycline that are designed to overcome two common mechanisms of tetracycline resistance—namely, resistance mediated by efflux pumps and ribosomal protection. Of all the tetracycline derivatives, tigecycline is most closely related structurally to minocycline. Despite the fact that tetracyclines are bacteriostatic against gram-negative and gram-positive bacteria, the modes of penetration are different: passive diffusion in gram-negative and active transport in gram-positive bacteria.

Pharmacokinetics
Gastric absorption of tetracyclines may be inhibited by chelation to divalent cations (iron; aluminum-, magnesium-, or calcium-containing antacids; milk) or to bile acid resins. As a result, it is best to administer tetracyclines on an empty stomach. Of the drugs in this class, doxycycline is metabolized hepatically and excreted in the feces, so it is the safest option in patients with renal dysfunction.

Clinical use
Tetracyclines were the first broad-spectrum antibiotics. These drugs are bacteriostatic against numerous microorganisms (Table 4-13). In addition to susceptible gram-positive and

TABLE 4-13. Examples of Microorganisms for Which Tetracyclines May Be Drugs of Choice

ORGANISM	DOXYCYCLINE
Gram Positive	
Cocci	
Staphylococcus aureus, S. epidermis	✓*
Bacilli	
Clostridium perfringens	✓
Gram Negative	
Cocci	
Moraxella catarrhalis	✓
Bacilli	
Legionella spp.	✓
Pasteurella multocida	✓
Miscellaneous	
Chlamydia pneumoniae	X
Chlamydia trachomatis	X
Mycoplasma pneumoniae	✓
Treponema pallidum	✓
Borrelia burgdorferi (Lyme disease)	X

*Could be selected as an alternative to first-line agents, pending susceptibility. This table is not all inclusive. It is a representation of common infectious microorganisms for which doxycycline may be the drug of choice.
X, Drug of choice; ✓, alternative choice if first-line agents cannot be used.

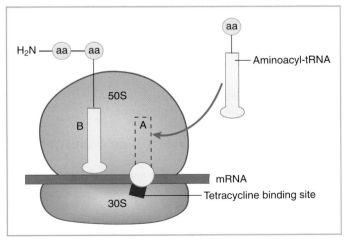

Figure 4-5. Site of action for tetracyclines.

gram-negative microorganisms such as *Borrelia burgdorferi* (Lyme disease), tetracyclines are also effective against rickettsia (typhus, Rocky Mountain spotted fever) and *Mycoplasma*. Tetracyclines are also active against *Propionibacterium acnes* and are commonly used to treat inflammatory acne vulgaris.

Resistance

Gram-positive microorganisms acquire resistance to tetracyclines by actively pumping the drugs out of the cells via an efflux pump. Gram-negative bacteria may acquire alterations in their outer membrane proteins that prevent tetracyclines from entering the microorganisms. Tigecycline is not affected by tetracycline resistance mechanisms, and cross-resistance between tigecycline and other antibiotics has not been observed.

Adverse effects

The most notable adverse effects associated with tetracyclines are discoloration of teeth when used in children younger than 8 years of age and disturbed fetal bone growth when used during gestation; therefore tetracyclines should not be used in young children or pregnant women. Photosensitivity, exfoliative dermatitis, secondary superinfections (yeast, pseudomembranous colitis), hypersensitivity, liver disease (jaundice, nausea, vomiting, darkened urine, abdominal pain), renal disease, bone marrow suppression, and pseudotumor cerebri are adverse effects that may be associated with tetracyclines (Table 4-14).

Chloramphenicol
Mechanism of action

As with the tetracyclines, chloramphenicol is bacteriostatic. At the molecular level, chloramphenicol binds to the 50 S ribosomal subunit and blocks linkage of incoming amino acids to the growing peptide chain by interfering with the enzyme peptidyl transferase (Fig. 4-6).

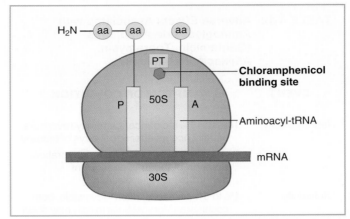

Figure 4-6. Site of action for chloramphenicol, the macrolides, and clindamycin. *PT*, peptidyl transferase.

Pharmacokinetics

Chloramphenicol is metabolized via glucuronidation. In infants as well as adults with hepatic disease, the drug accumulates because it is inefficiently glucuronidated, resulting in a "gray baby" (or "gray adult") syndrome in which infants fail to eat, fail to thrive, become pale and cyanotic, have abdominal distention, and may die of respiratory or vasomotor collapse. If any signs of this syndrome occur, the drug should be immediately discontinued.

Clinical use

Chloramphenicol is used to treat serious infections caused by *Salmonella*, *Haemophilus influenzae*, and anaerobic infections including those caused by *Bacteroides fragilis*. Chloramphenicol is also used whenever less dangerous antibiotics are ineffective for meningeal infections, rickettsiae, and gram-negative infections causing bacteremia. In addition to its systemic utility, chloramphenicol is used topically to treat otic and ophthalmic infections. This drug is rarely used in clinical medicine because safer effective antibiotics are usually available.

Adverse effects

Dose-related bone marrow suppression may occur as well as idiopathic aplastic anemia, which is unrelated to dose and may occur weeks or even months after the drug has been discontinued (Table 4-15). The drug is best avoided in patients with G6PD deficiency, which is the most commonly inherited

TABLE 4-14. Adverse Effects Associated with Tetracyclines

EVENT	SYMPTOM OR CONDITION
Allergic reaction	Rash Anaphylaxis Urticaria Fever
Teeth/bone deposition	Avoid in children and pregnant women
Gastrointestinal upset	Nausea Diarrhea
Hepatitis	Primarily seen with high intravenous doses in the elderly
Renal (azotemia)	Avoid in patients with renal dysfunction Lower incidence with doxycycline
Vestibular toxicity	Associated with minocycline
Photosensitivity	

TABLE 4-15. Adverse Effects Associated with Chloramphenicol

EVENT	SYMPTOM OR CONDITION
Anemia	Idiosyncratic irreversible aplastic anemia (rare) Reversible dose-related anemia
Gray syndrome	Because of inability of neonates to conjugate chloramphenicol

red blood cell enzyme deficiency and causes red blood cells to be particularly susceptible to oxidative stress and hemolysis.

Lincosamides
Drug

The common drug is clindamycin. Clindamycin interrupts protein synthesis by binding to 50 S ribosomal subunits and preventing translocation of incoming amino acids from the ribosomal A site to the P site (see Fig. 4-6).

Clinical use

Topically, clindamycin is used to treat acne vulgaris and rosacea and is also used vaginally for bacterial vaginosis. The antibiotic is administered systemically to eliminate numerous species of gram-positive bacteria, and it is the most active antibiotic for treating anaerobic infections, especially *Bacteroides fragilis* (Table 4-16). As a result of its broad spectrum, clindamycin is used to treat serious lung abscesses, skin and soft tissue infections, septicemia, intra-abdominal infections, and female pelvic infections. In children, clindamycin may be used for recurrent otitis media when other antibiotics have not been effective.

Adverse effects

Clindamycin potently eliminates numerous anaerobic and gram-positive microorganisms, facilitating opportunistic gastrointestinal infections caused by overgrowth of *Clostridium difficile*. This may lead to pseudomembranous colitis, which is characterized as potentially fatal diarrhea, coupled with abdominal cramping and excretion of blood or mucus (Table 4-17). Additionally, some formulations of clindamycin contain tartrazine (a yellow dye) and should be avoided in patients with asthma or aspirin allergies because of the possibility of allergic responses.

TABLE 4-16. Microorganisms for Which Clindamycin Might Be the Drug of Choice

ORGANISM	CLINDAMYCIN
Gram Positive	
Cocci	
Staphylococcus aureus, S. epidermidis, if methicillin sensitive	✓
Bacilli	
Clostridium perfringens	X
Gram Negative	
Bacilli	
Bacteroides fragilis	✓
Gardnerella vaginalis	✓

This table is not all inclusive. It is a representation of common infectious microorganisms for which clindamycin is the drug of choice.
X, Drug of choice; ✓, alternative choice if first-line agents cannot be used.

TABLE 4-17. Adverse Effects Associated with Clindamycin

EVENT	REASON
Diarrhea	High association with pseudomembranous colitis
Allergic	Tartrazine used as an inactive ingredient hypersensitivities

Macrolides
Drugs

Drugs include erythromycin base, erythromycin estolate, erythromycin stearate, erythromycin ethylsuccinate, clarithromycin, and azithromycin.

Mechanism of action

Macrolides inhibit protein synthesis by binding to the same site on prokaryotic ribosomal 50 S subunits as clindamycin and chloramphenicol bind. Macrolides prevent translocation of amino acids from the A site to the P site. Because they share the same binding site, clindamycin, chloramphenicol, and the macrolides may interfere with one another and cross-resistance may develop between these drugs. Activity may be either bacteriostatic or bactericidal depending on drug concentration.

Clinical use

Indications for macrolides are found in Box 4-4. Macrolides are broad-spectrum antibiotics, active against most gram-positive microorganisms, many gram-negative species, many anaerobes, a variety of mycoplasma species, including organisms such as *Borrelia, Chlamydia, Treponema, Helicobacter pylori*, and *Clostridium tetani* (Table 4-18). Macrolides may be used to treat soft tissue infections, genitourinary infections, Lyme disease, acne vulgaris, and ophthalmic infections. Compared with the erythromycins, clarithromycin has expanded activity, making it a suitable option for eliminating

Box 4-4. INDICATIONS FOR MACROLIDES

Amebiasis
Bacterial endocarditis
Chronic bronchitis
Conjunctivitis
Chronic obstructive pulmonary disease
Diphtheria
Genital ulcer disease
Legionnaires' disease
Listeria monocytogenes
Otitis media
Pelvic inflammatory disease
Pertussis
Pneumonia

Prevention of disseminated *Mycobacterium avium-intracellulare* complex in patients with advanced human immunodeficiency virus infection
Respiratory tract infections
Rheumatic fever
Sinusitis
Skin and skin structure infections
Syphilis
Urogenital infections

TABLE 4-18. Microorganisms for Which Macrolides Might Be Drugs of Choice

ORGANISMS	ERYTHROMYCIN	AZITHROMYCIN	CLARITHROMYCIN
Gram Positive			
Cocci			
Staphylococcus (groups A, B, C, G, and *S. bovis*)	✓	✓	✓
Streptococcus viridans group	✓	✓	✓
Gram Negative			
Cocci			
Moraxella catarrhalis	✓	✓	✓
Bacilli			
Haemophilus influenzae if β-lactamase–negative	✓	✓	✓
Legionella spp.	X	✓	✓
Miscellaneous			
Chlamydia pneumoniae	✓	✓	✓
Chlamydia trachomatis		X	
Mycoplasma pneumoniae	X	X	X
Borrelia burgdorferi		✓	✓

This table is not all inclusive. It is a representation of common infectious microorganisms for which a macrolide might be selected as a drug of choice.
X, Drug of choice; ✓, alternative choice if first-line agents cannot be used.

Helicobacter pylori. Similarly, both clarithromycin and azithromycin have expanded gram-negative actions for eliminating *Haemophilus influenzae.* These two newer macrolides also have better penetration into lung tissues and macrophages than does erythromycin. Azithromycin is a drug of choice for treating community-acquired pneumonia and is active against *Mycobacterium avium-intracellulare* in immunocompromised individuals. Clarithromycin also is an option for these indications. Additional reasons for selecting macrolides are listed in Box 4-5.

Resistance

Microorganisms become resistant to macrolides in the following circumstances:
- When their permeability for macrolides is altered
- When microorganisms methylate bacterial 50 S ribosomal subunits
- When bacteria develop mechanisms to enzymatically destroy the drugs

Adverse effects

Erythromycins are often associated with gastrointestinal distress, which can be minimized if the drugs are taken with food. The estolate salt of erythromycin may cause cholestatic hepatitis, characterized by elevated liver function enzymes, malaise, nausea, vomiting, abdominal cramps, jaundice, and fever. Liver function test results should be monitored if hepatotoxicity is suspected (Table 4-19). Erythromycins

Box 4-5. REASONS TO CHOOSE MACROLIDES

- Macrolides are the drugs of choice for penicillin/cephalosporin hypersensitivities
- Macrolides are the drugs of choice for infections caused by atypical microorganisms including *Legionella* and *Mycoplasma pneumoniae*
- Macrolides are the systemic drugs of choice for treatment of impetigo
- Macrolides may be drugs of choice for treating community-acquired pneumonia

may potentiate the actions of other drugs by inhibiting microsomal P450 3A4 metabolism, leading to toxicity of these other medications (Box 4-6). Erythromycin also prolongs the QT interval on electrocardiograms. This can lead to torsades de pointes, a fatal cardiac arrhythmia, especially when erythromycin is combined with other medications that also prolong the QT interval. As with erythromycin, clarithromycin also prolongs the QT interval and inhibits P450 3A4; however, clarithromycin is associated with less gastrointestinal distress than erythromycin. Unlike clarithromycin and erythromycin, azithromycin does not prolong the QT interval to a clinically relevant extent and does not inhibit hepatic microsomal P450 enzymes. In addition, azithromycin has only a minimal incidence of diarrhea associated with

TABLE 4-19. Adverse Effects Associated with Erythromycin

EVENT	SYMPTOM OR CONDITION
Nausea, vomiting, burning stomach	With oral administration
Cholestatic jaundice	Most common with estolate salt
Ototoxicity	Most common with high doses in patients with renal or hepatic failure

Box 4-6. DRUGS WHOSE METABOLISM IS POSSIBLY INHIBITED BY ERYTHROMYCIN

Benzodiazepines	Protease inhibitors
Calcium channel blockers	Quinidine
Carbamazepine	Sertraline
Cyclosporine	Statins
Digoxin	Theophylline
Disopyramide	Valproate
Ergotamine	Warfarin
Glyburide	

its use. Because of cross-sensitivity, azithromycin is contraindicated in patients who have a history of allergies to erythromycin.

Ketolides
Drug
Telithromycin.

Mechanism of action
As with the macrolides, telithromycin inhibits protein synthesis by inhibiting the 50 S ribosomal subunit. However, telithromycin binds to two separate domains within the 50 S ribosomal subunit. This means that two different mutations would be needed in two different domains for bacteria to develop resistance to this drug. In addition, telithromycin is a very poor substrate for bacterial efflux pumps. Together, these characteristics contribute to the effectiveness of telithromycin because it is more difficult for bacteria to acquire resistance to this drug.

Clinical use
Telithromycin offers an alternative to fluoroquinolones for treatment of multidrug-resistant streptococci. This ketolide can be used for treating bronchitis, mild to moderate community-acquired pneumonia, and sinusitis caused by multidrug-resistant *Staphylococcus pneumoniae*, *Haemophilus influenzae*, and *Moraxella catarrhalis*.

Adverse effects
Telithromycin is associated with the same concerns as erythromycin and clarithromycin with respect to QT interval prolongation and inhibition of CYP450 3A4. Drugs that are absolutely contraindicated with telithromycin, because of toxicities that result from P450 inhibition, are listed in Box 4-7. In addition, telithromycin is associated with visual disturbances such as blurred vision, difficulty focusing, and diplopia. Patients taking telithromycin should be cautioned about these visual disturbances and the dangers of driving while using this antibiotic. The drug is also contraindicated in individuals with myasthenia gravis because of reports of fatal and life-threatening respiratory failure. Because of hepatotoxicity and deaths associated with liver failure, the utility of this drug has become rather limited.

Protein Synthesis Inhibitors with Distinct Mechanisms of Action

Retapamulin
Mechanism of action
Available as a topical ointment, retapamulin is structurally considered to be a pleuromutilin antibiotic. Drugs in this class inhibit protein synthesis in bacteria by interfering with peptidyl transferase. Specifically, retapamulin inhibits bacterial protein synthesis by binding to a unique site on the ribosomal 50 S subunit, which prevents formation of active 50 S ribosomal subunits, inhibits peptidyl transferase, and blocks P-site interactions.

Clinical use
Retapamulin is used topically to treat skin infections caused by susceptible streptococci or staphylococci (e.g., impetigo).

Mupirocin
Mechanism of action
Available as a topical cream and ointment, mupirocin has a unique mechanism of action that results in no cross-resistance with any other antimicrobials. This antibacterial inhibits the tRNA that transports isoleucine.

Clinical use
Mupirocin is used topically to treat skin infections caused by streptococci or staphylococci (e.g., impetigo, nasal carriers of methicillin-resistant *S. aureus*).

Box 4-7. DRUGS CONTRAINDICATED WITH TELITHROMYCIN

Pimozide	Atorvastatin
Rifampin	Lovastatin
Type Ia and type III antiarrhythmics	Other drugs or risk factors that contribute to QT prolongation
Simvastatin	

Linezolid
Mechanism of action
Linezolid interferes with protein synthesis by binding to a unique RNA site on the 50 S subunit, preventing formation of the functional 70 S complex.

Clinical use
Linezolid is bacteriostatic against enterococci and staphylococci and is bactericidal for the majority of streptococcal strains. This antibiotic can be used for treating vancomycin-resistant *Enterococcus faecium*, MRSA, and community-acquired *Staphylococcus pneumoniae*.

Pharmacokinetics
The oral tablet formulation is 100% bioavailable; it can be used interchangeably with the parenteral form with no need for dosage adjustments.

Adverse effects
Linezolid inhibits monoamine oxidase; therefore all tyramine-containing foods (e.g., beer, wine, cheese, chocolate) and drugs such as selective serotonin reuptake inhibitors and pseudoephedrine must be avoided. The risk of myelosuppression occurs if linezolid is used for more than 2 weeks, so weekly blood counts are recommended.

Streptogramins
Drugs
The drug is a combination of quinupristin and dalfopristin.

Mechanism of action
The quinupristin/dalfopristin combination acts at bacterial ribosomes and interferes with protein synthesis. Quinupristin irreversibly blocks ribosomes and inhibits late phases of protein synthesis, whereas dalfopristin inhibits early phases of protein synthesis. The combination is used to treat life-threatening infections caused by vancomycin-resistant enterococci and complicated skin infections caused by MRSA.

Adverse effects
Injection site reactions (pain, inflammation, edema) are common, as are muscle/joint pain. Hyperbilirubinemia occurs frequently, and superinfections can occur from overgrowth of nonsusceptible microorganisms.

Folic Acid Synthesis Inhibitors

In addition to antibiotics that limit cell wall synthesis or protein synthesis, a third major class of antibiotics targets the synthesis of critical bacterial metabolites. Some antimicrobials capitalize on this fact by inhibiting bacterial folic acid synthesis. Bacteria synthesize their own folic acid. Unlike humans, who obtain this B vitamin from their diets, bacteria cannot use folic acid obtained from the environment. Figure 4-7 illustrates the folic acid biosynthetic pathway used by bacteria.

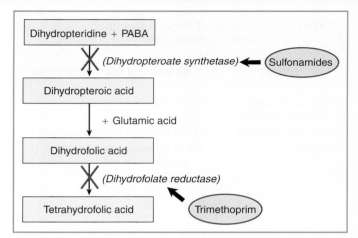

Figure 4-7. Biosynthesis of prokaryotic folic acid and sites of antimicrobial action for sulfonamides and trimethoprim. *PABA*, para-aminobenzoic acid.

Sulfonamides
Drugs
Sulfadiazine, silver sulfadiazine, sulfisoxazole, sulfamethoxazole, sulfacetamide, and sulfasalazine.

Mechanism of action
Sulfonamides compete with para-aminobenzoic acid at the first biosynthetic step of the folic acid pathway (see Fig. 4-7).

Pharmacokinetics
Sulfonamides are highly protein bound, so drug interactions may occur if sulfonamides displace other drugs from plasma protein-binding sites. This can lead to adverse effects when used with drugs such as warfarin, nonsteroidal antiinflammatory drugs, and sulfonylureas. Sulfonamides are contraindicated in pregnant women near term and in infants younger than 2 months because these drugs displace bilirubin from protein-binding sites in neonates. Hyperbilirubinemia in neonates may cause kernicterus (central nervous system disorders caused by elevated bilirubin).

Clinical use
Initially, sulfonamides had a broad spectrum of activity against gram-positive cocci and gram-negative bacilli; however, antimicrobial resistance is increasingly becoming problematic. Sulfonamides are used to treat urinary tract infections, conjunctivitis, and toxoplasmosis. They also are used to prevent and treat burn-related infections and are used adjunctively with pyrimethamine for malaria. Indications for some sulfonamides are listed in Box 4-8.

Individual sulfonamides have unique actions. Sulfadiazine distributes widely to the central nervous system. Sulfisoxazole may be used to treat urinary tract infections and is also an option for prophylaxis of rheumatic fever if the child is allergic to penicillin. Sulfisoxazole is also administered in a formulation that is combined with erythromycin. Sulfamethoxazole is commonly used in conjunction with trimethoprim for synergistic effects in the treatment of urinary tract infections. Sulfacetamide is used topically in the eyes for treating

Box 4-8. COMMON INDICATIONS FOR SULFONAMIDES

Chancroid	Otitis media, acute
Inclusion conjunctivitis	Rheumatic fever
Malaria	Toxoplasmosis
Meningitis, *Haemophilus influenzae*	Trachoma
Meningitis, meningococcal	Urinary tract infections (pyelonephritis, cystitis)
Nocardiosis	

conjunctivitis or corneal ulcers. Sulfasalazine is used as a treatment for inflammatory bowel disease. Silver sulfadiazine is available as a topical cream for treating burn patients.

Resistance

Bacteria develop resistance to sulfonamides in the following ways:

- Reduced bacterial uptake of the drugs
- Development of alternative metabolic pathways to synthesize folic acid
- Production of excessive amounts of para-aminobenzoic acid (up to 70 times normal) to compete with the sulfonamides for folic acid synthesis
- Alterations or mutations in dihydropteroate synthase, the enzyme that catalyzes the rate-limiting step of folate synthesis

Pharmacokinetics

Sulfonamides are metabolized hepatically by acetylation, oxidation, and/or glucuronidation. Individuals who are genetically "slow acetylators" may be at an increased risk of hypersensitivity reactions. Oxidation of sulfonamides likely is responsible for many of the adverse effects associated with sulfonamides. After hepatic biotransformation, sulfonamide metabolites are excreted renally.

Adverse effects

Sulfonamides predispose patients to photosensitivity. Bone marrow suppression, including hemolytic anemia, leukopenia, and thrombocytopenia, may occur. There is an increased risk of adverse hematologic effects in patients who are genetically deficient in G6PD. Sulfonamides may precipitate in the kidneys, causing renal stones; good hydration prevents this. Other miscellaneous effects include hepatotoxicity, pseudomembranous colitis, and hypersensitivity reactions, including Stevens-Johnson syndrome (Table 4-20). Because of chemical similarities, patients who are allergic to sulfonamides may also be hypersensitive to sulfonylureas, thiazide diuretics, and sunscreens that contain para-aminobenzoic acid.

CLINICAL MEDICINE

Stevens-Johnson Syndrome

Stevens-Johnson syndrome is a type III immunocomplex-mediated hypersensitivity that usually begins within 2 weeks of taking a drug. Variable lesions, including macules, papules, vesicles, urticarial plaques, and confluent erythema, develop but usually do not itch. The palms of the hands, soles of the feet, corneas, and mucosa are most often affected. Mucosal involvement may include erythema, edema, sloughing of skin, blistering, ulceration, and necrosis. A sore throat, fever, chills, headache, and malaise usually occur coincidentally. Patients often suspect they have influenza, and chickenpox initially may be misdiagnosed in children. This is a potentially life-threatening reaction, and, pathologically, the exfoliative dermatitis that accompanies Stevens-Johnson syndrome is similar to a burn.

TABLE 4-20. Adverse Effects Associated with Sulfonamides

EVENT	SYMPTOM OR CONDITION
Gastrointestinal	Nausea, diarrhea
Hepatic	Cholestatic hepatitis, increased incidence in AIDS
Rash	Exfoliative dermatitis, Stevens-Johnson syndrome (more common in AIDS)
Bone marrow	Neutropenia, thrombocytopenia (more common in AIDS)
Kernicterus	Sulfonamide displaces bilirubin from protein, resulting in excessive free sulfonamide and kernicterus

AIDS, acquired immunodeficiency syndrome.

Trimethoprim

Mechanism of action

Trimethoprim inhibits dihydrofolate reductase, the enzyme that catalyzes the last step of bacterial folic acid synthesis (see Fig. 4-7).

Clinical use

Trimethoprim, although available as a single agent, is seldom used this way. Instead, trimethoprim is nearly always used in combination with sulfamethoxazole for synergistic effects. This antibacterial also possesses antimalarial properties. When used alone, trimethoprim is bacteriostatic, but it is bactericidal when combined with sulfonamides. Trimethoprim is used in combination with sulfonamides to treat urinary tract infections, prostatic infections, otitis media in children, elimination of *Shigella*, and treatment of *Pneumocystis carinii* pneumonia. When combined with polymyxin B, trimethoprim is also used for acute conjunctivitis. Although rarely used alone because of bacterial resistance, trimethoprim may be used to treat uncomplicated urinary tract infections caused by *Escherichia coli*, *Proteus mirabilis*, *Klebsiella pneumoniae*, *Enterobacter* species, and coagulase-negative *Staphylococcus*. Despite interfering with bacterial folate synthesis, patients taking trimethoprim (and sulfonamides) may use folic acid supplements without the supplements interfering with the activity of the antimicrobials.

Resistance

Bacteria may become resistant to trimethoprim by the following:

- Reduced bacterial uptake
- Alterations or mutations in dihydrofolate reductase
- Overproduction of dihydrofolate reductase

Adverse effects

Trimethoprim is associated with adverse effects similar to those of the sulfonamides, including pruritic rashes, gastrointestinal distress, hematologic abnormalities, and fever. Patients with HIV who take trimethoprim have an unusually high incidence of rash and fever.

Inhibitors of DNA/RNA Synthesis

Inhibition of DNA/RNA synthesis is the fourth and final major mechanism by which antibacterial agents work.

Fluoroquinolones
Drugs

Drugs are besifloxacin, ciprofloxacin, gatifloxacin, gemifloxacin, levofloxacin, moxifloxacin, norfloxacin, and ofloxacin (all ending in "-floxacin").

Mechanism of action

Fluoroquinolones are bactericidal and interfere with bacterial DNA synthesis by inhibiting one of two enzymes. Some fluoroquinolones inhibit DNA gyrase, the enzyme responsible for relaxing supercoiled DNA. This enzyme is essential for replication, transcription, and DNA repair. Other fluoroquinolones inhibit topoisomerase IV, an enzyme involved with separating DNA into daughter cells during replication. One fluoroquinolone, gemifloxacin, is especially effective at inhibiting both enzymes; therefore for resistance to develop to this antibiotic, bacteria must acquire mutations in two different enzymes.

Pharmacokinetics

Food or cations such as calcium, iron, aluminum, magnesium, and zinc may impair absorption of fluoroquinolones. In addition, sucralfate interferes with fluoroquinolone absorption.

Although drug penetration into the central nervous system is minimal, fluoroquinolones distribute to nearly all other body compartments, including the lungs, gallbladder, sputum, bronchi, bones, muscle, genitourinary tissues, lymph, skin, and prostate.

Clinical use

Early fluoroquinolones such as ciprofloxacin predominantly possessed coverage for gram-negative microorganisms such as Enterobacteriaceae, *Pseudomonas aeruginosa*, *H. influenzae*,

and *Moraxella catarrhalis* and were used primarily for treating urinary tract infections. However, newer fluoroquinolones (levofloxacin, moxifloxacin, gemifloxacin) have a wider spectrum of activity, with actions against gram-positive microorganisms such as *Streptococcus* and atypical bacteria such as *Mycoplasma pneumoniae*, *Chlamydia pneumoniae*, and *Legionella pneumoniae*. As a result of their expanded coverage, newer fluoroquinolones may also be used treat respiratory infections. In addition, fluoroquinolones are used to treat infections of the skin, bone and joints, and prostate as well as intra-abdominal infections, infections caused by *Salmonella* or *Shigella*, and inhalational anthrax. Several fluoroquinolones are also available as ophthalmic drops for treating conjunctivitis and otic drops for external otitis; however, it is probably best to reserve use of these agents to prevent or delay emergence of fluoroquinolone-resistant strains.

Resistance

Microorganisms develop resistance to fluoroquinolones by altered membrane permeability or through mutations in the DNA-binding region.

Adverse effects

Photosensitivity, rash, and, rarely, Stevens-Johnson syndrome may occur with fluoroquinolones. (Rash is most common with gemifloxacin.) In addition, some patients experience dysgeusia, an unpleasant taste in the mouth (Table 4-21).

Fluoroquinolones, especially moxifloxacin, prolong the QT interval and should be used cautiously in patients with risk factors for prolonged QT syndrome (Box 4-9) and patients who are taking medications that also prolong the QT interval (Box 4-10). Elderly patients seem to be particularly susceptible to the central nervous system side effects (psychosis, tremor, stimulation, nightmares, confusion, seizures, elevated intracranial pressure) of fluoroquinolones. Central nervous system adverse effects may occur because fluoroquinolones prevent γ-aminobutyric acid from binding to its receptors. There are also increasing numbers of reports of peripheral nervous system effects (tingling, numbness, twitching pain, spasms) associated with fluoroquinolones.

Fluoroquinolones frequently cause tendinitis, muscle or joint pain, and tendon rupture, which may be apparent immediately

TABLE 4-21. Adverse Effects Associated with Fluoroquinolones	
EVENT	**SYMPTOM OR CONDITION**
Gastrointestinal upset	Nausea, vomiting, diarrhea
Central nervous system disorder	Altered mental state, confusion, seizures
Cartilage toxicity	Teratogenic; avoid in children and pregnant/lactating women

after therapy begins or may not appear for up to 90 days afterward. Tendon and joint problems typically resolve after the drugs are discontinued, but pain and discomfort may last for up to 3 months. Because of possible cartilage damage, fluoroquinolones are contraindicated during pregnancy and lactation and in children younger than 17 years of age.

Lipopeptides
Daptomycin

Mechanism of action. The mechanism of daptomycin differs from that of all other antibacterials. Daptomycin binds to bacterial membranes, causing rapid depolarization of the cell. Loss of membrane potential brings DNA, RNA, and protein synthesis to a halt, resulting in cell death. Because of its unique mechanism, cross-resistance with other antibiotics has not been observed.

Pharmacokinetics. Daptomycin is primarily excreted unchanged in the urine.

Clinical use. Daptomycin is approved for parenteral treatment of staphylococcal (including MRSA), streptococcal, and enterococcal (vancomycin-susceptible strains) infections.

Adverse effects
Some patients have muscle pain and weakness associated with elevations of creatine phosphokinase. Thus creatine phosphokinase levels should be monitored at least weekly. As a result of muscular adverse effects, it is best to temporarily discontinue statin therapy in patients who are taking daptomycin.

Infrequently, the drug has been associated with peripheral neuropathies (e.g., paresthesias, Bell palsy).

Three Drugs with Distinct Mechanisms
Metronidazole, nitazoxanide, tinidazole

Mechanism of action. Metronidazole is selectively absorbed by anaerobic bacteria and sensitive protozoa. Once taken up by anaerobes, it is nonenzymatically reduced by reacting with reduced ferredoxin, which is generated by pyruvate/ferredoxin oxido-reductase. This reduction causes the production of metabolites that are toxic to anaerobic cells, resulting in inhibition of DNA synthesis, degradation of existing DNA, DNA strand breaks, and inhibition of nucleic acid synthesis, all of which lead to bacterial cell death. Similarly, nitazoxanide interferes with pyruvate/ferredoxin oxidoreductase enzyme-dependent electron transfer, a reaction essential for anaerobic metabolism. Tinidazole is believed to cause cytotoxicity by damaging DNA and inhibiting further DNA synthesis. Because of their actions, these drugs may be mutagenic and possibly carcinogenic. Both tinidazole and metronidazole are contraindicated during the first trimester of pregnancy.

Pharmacokinetics. Metronidazole penetrates the central nervous system and can be used to treat meningitis and brain abscesses caused by anaerobes. Absorption through skin or mucus membranes is low when used topically.

Clinical use. Metronidazole is used topically to treat acne or rosacea; bacterial vaginosis caused by *Trichomonas, Gardnerella vaginalis*, or other anaerobic infections; and orally or intravenously to treat *Helicobacter pylori* (peptic ulcer disease), amebiasis, *Giardia, Clostridium difficile* (pseudomembranous colitis), or *Bacteroides* species. Notice that metronidazole is approved for treating bacterial infections as well as parasites (e.g., *Giardia*, amebiasis). Nitazoxanide and tinidazole have fewer indications than metronidazole. Nitazoxanide is approved to treat *Cryptosporidium* and *Giardia* infections. Tinidazole is used to treat *Giardia* infection and amebiasis.

Adverse effects. Patients commonly experience peripheral neuropathies and a metallic taste in the mouth. Severe disulfiram-like reactions may occur, and alcohol must be strictly avoided during therapy and for 1 to 3 days afterward. Metronidazole may cause urine to darken in color.

Rifaximin

Mechanism of action. Rifaximin is a rifampin derivative that inhibits bacterial RNA synthesis by binding to bacterial DNA-dependent RNA polymerase.

Pharmacokinetics. Compared with rifampin (see section on Antimycobacterials), rifaximin is not absorbed from the gastrointestinal tract; therefore most drug is excreted unchanged in feces. Furthermore, rifaximin does not interfere with hepatic cytochrome P450 enzymes as rifampin does.

Clinical use. Rifaximin is used to treat traveler's diarrhea caused by noninvasive *Escherichia coli*.

Adverse effects. Because rifaximin is not absorbed, the drug is very well tolerated.

●●● ANTIMYCOBACTERIALS

Mycobacterial are rodlike gram-positive aerobic bacteria that can form filamentous branching structures. Infections caused by mycobacteria (e.g., tuberculosis, leprosy) are notoriously difficult to treat for a variety of reasons, including the following:

- Mycobacteria grow slowly. Even during periods of active growth, they may take 18 hours or longer to divide.
- Mycobacteria can lie dormant.
- Mycobacterial cell walls are thick and impermeable; therefore it is difficult for antibiotics to attain access intracellularly.
- Mycobacteria can reside inside host cells, making it even more difficult to reach therapeutic drug levels inside the mycobacterial cells.
- Mycobacteria become resistant to antibiotic therapies rather quickly.

For these reasons, it is necessary to treat mycobacterial infections for long periods, with several different antibiotics simultaneously, to prevent emergence of resistant strains. It is important to eradicate the organisms to obtain a cure. The drugs that treat mycobacterial infections work by several different mechanisms and include isoniazid, rifampin, pyrazinamide, ethambutol, and clofazimine.

Treatment Options for Mycobacterial Infections

Isoniazid
Mechanism of action
Isoniazid inhibits synthesis of mycolic acids, essential components of mycobacterial cell walls.

Pharmacokinetics
Isoniazid diffuses throughout total body water, even the central nervous system. Metabolism of isoniazid occurs by acetylation. In patients who are genetically "fast acetylators," isoniazid may not reach therapeutic levels and will have a short plasma $t_{1/2}$ compared with that of "slow acetylators." Slow acetylators are at a greater risk for drug-related toxicities because of the drug's long $t_{1/2}$.

Clinical use
At therapeutic levels, isoniazid is bactericidal against actively growing intracellular and extracellular *Mycobacterium tuberculosis*; therefore the drug is primarily used in treatment or prophylaxis of tuberculosis.

Adverse effects
Neuropathies may occur with isoniazid as a result of pyridoxine (vitamin B_6) deficiency, but supplementation with vitamin B_6 often prevents or minimizes this. Severe, even fatal, hepatitis may occur, and patients should avoid taking acetaminophen or drinking alcohol when taking isoniazid.

Rifampin
Mechanism of action
Rifampin inhibits bacterial RNA polymerase, which prevents transcription by suppressing initiation of RNA chain formation.

Pharmacokinetics
Rifampin is a potent inducer of drug metabolism and alters the plasma levels of many drugs (e.g., digoxin, quinidine, warfarin, oral contraceptives, methadone, theophylline, antifungals, β-blockers, calcium channel blockers). Therefore drug-drug interactions are a major concern.

Clinical use
At therapeutic levels, rifampin is bactericidal against intracellular and extracellular *Mycobacterium tuberculosis* organisms and is used in combination with other antimycobacterials to treat tuberculosis. Rifampin is effective against many gram-positive and gram-negative microorganisms. This antimicrobial is the drug of choice for prophylaxis of meningococcal meningitis. Rifampin is used prophylactically in close contacts of patients affected by epiglottitis or meningitis caused by *Haemophilus influenzae*. The drug is also used prophylactically against leprosy and in combination with other drugs to treat *Legionella*.

Adverse effects
Hepatotoxicity may occur with rifampin. For this reason, acetaminophen should be avoided. Rifampin also discolors body fluids, turning urine, sweat, saliva, and tears red-orange. Contact lenses may be permanently stained. Oral contraceptive efficacy may be severely lessened by induction of hepatic P450 microsomal enzymes, and patients should consider alternative contraceptive measures.

Pyrazinamide
Mechanism of action
The mechanism of action of pyrazinamide is unclear. It may be that pyrazinamide lowers the pH in the tubercle cavity and inhibits growth of mycobacterium.

Clinical use
This drug is often added to isoniazid and rifampin when treating tuberculosis.

Adverse effects
Pyrazinamide is associated with gastrointestinal distress, elevated uric acid, and hepatotoxicity. Patients should be monitored for hyperuricemia and signs of hepatotoxicity.

Ethambutol
Mechanism of action
Ethambutol inhibits RNA synthesis and decreases replication of tubercle bacilli.

Clinical use
This drug may be added as a fourth drug to the antitubercular cocktail while awaiting drug-susceptibility data in patients with tuberculosis. Ethambutol is also used to treat

Mycobacterium avium-intracellulare infections in patients with AIDS.

Adverse effects
Ethambutol may cause optic neuritis, which decreases visual acuity. In addition, ethambutol may lead to an inability to see the color green. For these reasons, eye examinations are recommended every 2 to 3 months. Gout, joint pain, liver impairment, and cataracts may also occur.

Clofazimine
Mechanism of action
Clofazimine binds to mycobacterial DNA and inhibits RNA polymerase actions. The bactericidal activities of this drug are very slow, and patients are treated for a minimum of 2 years and possibly for life.

Clinical use
Clofazimine is used to treat leprosy, but it should always be used in combination with other antimycobacterial drugs to prevent emergence of resistant strains.

Adverse effects
Clofazimine colors body secretions reddish brown-black, which may last for years after the drug is discontinued. The drug has been associated with gastrointestinal intolerance and dry skin.

●●● ANTIFUNGALS
Although their mechanisms of action differ slightly, antifungals often interfere with lipid biosynthesis and therefore the integrity of the fungal membrane (Fig. 4-8). A variety of antifungals are used to treat fungal infections, depending on whether the infection is cutaneous or systemic. Major antifungals include the polyenes (amphotericin B, nystatin) and the "azoles" (voriconazole, ketoconazole, and fluconazole).

Polyenes
Amphotericin B
Mechanism of action
Amphotericin B is an example of a "polyene" type of antifungal. Polyenes bind to fungal ergosterol (the primary sterol in fungal cell membranes). This alters cell membrane permeability, and intracellular components leak from the cell. Depending on the concentration attained in the body, amphotericin B can be either fungistatic or fungicidal.

Pharmacokinetics
Amphotericin B does not penetrate the central nervous system well. This drug has a very long $t_{1/2}$.

Clinical use
Amphotericin B may be used to treat serious, life-threatening systemic fungal infections. It is administered intravenously or intrathecally for systemic fungal infections including systemic *Candida, Cryptococcus*, blastomycosis, and histoplasmosis.

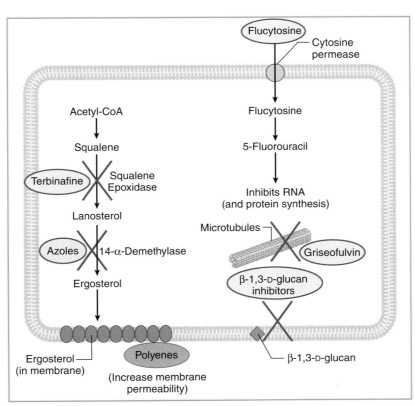

Figure 4-8. Mechanisms of action for common antifungal drugs. *CoA*, coenzyme A.

Box 4-11. TOXICITIES ASSOCIATED WITH AMPHOTERICIN B

Liver disease	Seizures
Renal failure	Intra-alveolar hemorrhage
Hypokalemia	Blood dyscrasias
Hypomagnesemia	Fever, chills, headache, rash
Hypersensitivity including	in 50% (prevented by
anaphylaxis	premedicating with
Phlebitis	acetaminophen,
Cardiac arrest	diphenhydramine, and
Cardiac arrhythmias	corticosteroids)

Adverse effects

Numerous toxicities are attributed to amphotericin B (Box 4-11). Serum creatinine, blood urea nitrogen, complete blood counts, serum potassium, serum sodium, serum magnesium, and liver function test results must be monitored. When amphotericin B is used with aminoglycosides or neuromuscular blockers, prolonged skeletal muscle paralysis may result.

Nystatin
Mechanism of action

Nystatin is a polyene antifungal that is effective only against *Candida*.

Clinical use

It is poorly absorbed and thus reserved for topical treatment of oral thrush, vaginal infections, intestinal infections, and cutaneous infections.

Adverse effects

Gastrointestinal upset is common when nystatin is taken orally.

Natamycin
Mechanism of action

Natamycin is a polyene antifungal that is used for ocular infections.

Azoles

"Azole" antifungals (imidazoles and triazoles) have slightly different chemical structures, but they all inhibit biosynthesis of ergosterol, the main sterol in fungal cell membranes (see Fig. 4-8). Disruption in ergosterol synthesis, by inhibiting the enzyme 14-α-demethylase, ultimately increases cellular permeability and causes cell leakage. Some of these drugs (e.g., ketoconazole) also interfere with human cortisol and testosterone biosynthesis, which explains side effects such as gynecomastia in men and menstrual irregularities in women. Azoles are potent inhibitors of P450 hepatic metabolism and have the potential to cause many severe and even life-threatening drug interactions. Additionally, all azoles have been associated with liver toxicity when used systemically.

Voriconazole
Pharmacokinetics

Voriconazole is metabolized hepatically and inhibits P450 enzymes.

Clinical use

Voriconazole is an option for treating serious fungal infections including those caused by *Aspergillus* and *Scedosporium*.

Adverse effects

Visual disturbances and hallucinations may occur; therefore patients are warned not to drive at night. Some patients experience a rash. Liver function test results may be elevated and should be periodically monitored. Prolongation of the QT interval on electrocardiograms may occur. Despite these side effects, overall, voriconazole is better tolerated than amphotericin B.

Ketoconazole
Pharmacokinetics

Ketoconazole requires an acidic environment for dissolution and systemic absorption. It does not enter the central nervous system. Ketoconazole is a potent inhibitor of hepatic P450 enzymes; thus dosage adjustments may be necessary to prevent adverse drug interactions. Table 4-22 contains a partial listing of potentially serious drug interactions.

Clinical use

Ketoconazole is used to treat severe recalcitrant infections such as mucocutaneous candidiasis, histoplasmosis, coccidioidomycosis, and chromomycosis. It is not active against *Aspergillus*. In addition to systemic formulations, ketoconazole is available as a topical cream and shampoo.

Adverse effects

Ketoconazole may cause hepatotoxicity. Because of the risk of liver toxicity, liver function test results should be monitored. Gynecomastia and impotence may occur in men (Table 4-23).

TABLE 4-22. Partial Listing of Serious Drug Interactions Associated with Ketoconazole

INTERACTING DRUG	ADVERSE REACTION
Statins	Rhabdomyolysis
Alcohol	Disulfiram-like reactions
Warfarin	Increased bleeding
Cyclosporine	Potential nephrotoxicity
Sulfonylureas	Hypoglycemia

TABLE 4-23. Adverse Effects Associated with Azole Antifungals (e.g., Ketoconazole, Fluconazole, Itraconazole)

EVENT	SYMPTOM OR CONDITION
Hepatitis	Ranges from mild liver dysfunction to fatal hepatitis
Gynecomastia	More common with high doses of ketoconazole (>400 mg/day) because of decreased testosterone synthesis; decreased libido and azoospermia

Fluconazole
Pharmacokinetics
A single dose of fluconazole has a long $t_{1/2}$; this property allows a one-time oral dose to be used for treating vaginal yeast infections. Eighty percent of the drug is cleared from the body renally. The drug also penetrates the central nervous system and is used prophylactically in immunocompromised patients. Numerous drug interactions are likely because fluconazole inhibits P450 hepatic enzymes.

Clinical use
Fluconazole has a greater activity and spectrum than other azoles (Box 4-12). Because of its penetration of the central nervous system, fluconazole may be used to treat cryptococcal meningitis.

Adverse effects
Toxicities associated with fluconazole include hepatic disease and exfoliative skin disorders.

Itraconazole
Pharmacokinetics
As with ketoconazole, itraconazole is best absorbed in an acidic environment. By inhibiting P450 hepatic enzymes, numerous severe drug interactions may occur.

Clinical use
Itraconazole was initially used orally for treating fungal infections of the nails; however, parenteral forms are also available for treating life-threatening infections caused by blastomycosis, histoplasmosis, and aspergillosis. This drug may be an alternative to amphotericin B. Itraconazole has greater activity against *Aspergillus* than either ketoconazole or fluconazole.

Adverse effects
Itraconazole may exacerbate preexisting congestive heart failure and may cause liver failure.

Posaconazole
Pharmacokinetics
As with voriconazole, posaconazole is a triazole. The bioavailability and maximum plasma concentration of posaconazole are three times higher when administered with food; therefore it is recommended that the drug be taken with a meal or liquid nutritional supplement. Similar to other azoles, posaconazole inhibits P450 enzymes and dose adjustments should be made for affected drugs.

Clinical use
Posaconazole is used to treat *Candida* infections that are resistant to other antifungals and is the first drug approved for prophylaxis of invasive *Aspergillus* in severely immunocompromised adults and adolescents. It is more potent at inhibiting 14-α demethylase than itraconazole and has been shown to decrease the incidence of breakthrough *Aspergillus* infections compared with other azoles.

Adverse effects
Gastrointestinal effects are commonly observed, and the risk of hepatotoxicity warrants routine monitoring of liver function test results. Patients taking other prescription and nonprescription medications should be assessed for potentially severe drug interactions because the drug inhibits hepatic P450 enzymes.

Other Azole Antifungals
Other azole antifungals include butoconazole, clotrimazole, econazole, miconazole, oxiconazole, sertaconazole, sulconazole, terconazole, and tioconazole. Some of these drugs require a prescription, whereas others are available for purchase by consumers without a prescription. These drugs may be used topically to treat tinea pedis, tinea cruris, tinea versicolor, tinea corporis, and candidal infections of the vagina, vulva, and throat.

Other Antifungal Agents

Caspofungin, Micafungin, and Anidulafungin (β-[1,3]-ᴅ-Glucan Inhibitors)
Mechanism of action
Caspofungin was the first in a new class of antifungals, the glucan synthesis inhibitors, which inhibit the synthesis of β-(1,3)-ᴅ-glucan, a necessary component of fungal cell walls.

Pharmacokinetics
All three drugs in this class are administered by intravenous infusions.

Box 4-12. SPECTRUM OF ACTIVITY FOR FLUCONAZOLE

Aspergillus
Blastomyces dermatitidis
Candida albicans
Candida kefyr
Candida tropicalis
Coccidioides immitis
Cryptococcus neoformans
Histoplasma capsulatum
Torulopsis glabrata

Clinical use

Caspofungin is effective for treating invasive aspergillosis in patients who cannot tolerate, or whose infections are refractory to, other therapies. In clinical studies, caspofungin appears to have a lower incidence of adverse effects compared with amphotericin B. Both micafungin and anidulafungin may be used to treat patients with esophageal candidiasis and other types of candidal infections, and micafungin is used prophylactically in patients at risk of *Candida* infection while undergoing hematopoietic stem cell transplantation. Micafungin and anidulafungin are less likely to interact with cyclosporine compared with caspofungin, which may be an important distinction in transplant patients.

Adverse effects

Serious hypersensitivity reactions (rash, itching, facial swelling, vasodilation) and elevated bilirubin levels have been reported with micafungin.

Flucytosine
Mechanism of action

After penetration of fungal cells, flucytosine is converted to fluorouracil, which competes with uracil and interferes with fungal RNA and protein synthesis.

Clinical use

Flucytosine is used adjunctively to treat serious systemic fungal infections caused by susceptible strains of *Candida* or *Cryptococcus*. It is not used alone because of rapid emergence of resistant fungal organisms.

Adverse effects

Flucytosine has been associated with bone marrow depression as well as elevations in hepatic enzymes and bilirubin because of acute liver injury. Unlike most antifungals, the drug is primarily eliminated unchanged in the urine. As a result, the dose of flucytosine must be decreased in patients with renal dysfunction; these patients must be monitored closely.

Griseofulvin
Mechanism of action

Griseofulvin deposits in the stratum corneum layer of skin, hair, and nails. It inhibits fungal mitosis by blocking assembly of microtubules. The drug is gradually exfoliated and replaced by uninfected tissues.

Clinical use

Griseofulvin is used to treat infections of the hair, nails, and skin.

Adverse effects

The most common side effects are hypersensitive skin reactions and hives. Although rare, more serious reactions may occur including angioneurotic edema, gastrointestinal bleeding, leukopenia, menstrual irregularities, and hepatotoxicity. The drug is contraindicated in patients with liver disease and should not be used in pregnant women because of carcinogenic and teratogenic effects in animal studies. Griseofulvin may decrease the efficacy of warfarin and oral contraceptives.

Terbinafine
Mechanism of action

This drug inhibits the enzyme (squalene epoxidase) that is required for sterol synthesis.

Pharmacokinetics

Terbinafine undergoes extensive first-pass metabolism in the liver. Because of its inhibition of hepatic P450 enzymes, numerous drug interactions are possible.

Clinical use

Terbinafine has a spectrum of action similar to that of griseofulvin and is used to treat nail fungus.

Adverse effects

Terbinafine may cause patients to temporarily lose their sense of taste.

Ciclopirox
Mechanism of action

Ciclopirox chelates polyvalent cations (aluminum, iron), resulting in inhibition of metal-dependent enzymes that are responsible for degrading peroxides inside fungal cells.

Clinical use

Ciclopirox is an option for treating topical fungal infections. The drug is formulated as a topical cream, gel, and solution. The topical solution is applied daily (like nail polish) to fingernails and toenails that are affected by fungus. Each day, a new layer of drug is applied over existing layers; once per week, previous layers of drug are removed. Although it takes a year for ciclopirox to eliminate the nail fungus, it is an option for patients who are unable or unwilling to tolerate the potential hepatotoxicity of azoles.

●●● ANTIPARASITICS
Antimalarials

Malaria is a mosquito-transmitted illness caused by parasitic protozoans that is mainly found in tropical and subtropical areas. Transmitted via a variety of *Plasmodium* species, the illness is characterized by bouts of shivering, fever, sweating, and red blood cell lysis. After a diagnosis of malaria has been confirmed, the infecting species of *Plasmodium* must be identified so that an appropriate therapy can be selected. Therapy is based on (1) the clinical status of the patient and (2) the drug susceptibility of the parasite as determined by the geographic area where the infection was acquired. Treatments include chloroquine, mefloquine, primaquine, atovaquone-proguanil, and quinine as well as some antibacterials that have already been discussed (Table 4-24). The latest treatment guidelines compiled by the Centers for Disease Control and Prevention can be found at http://www.cdc.gov. Therapeutic recommendations change regularly because *Plasmodium* resistance patterns to antimalarial drugs constantly change.

TABLE 4-24. Treatment Options for Malaria

PLASMODIUM SPECIES	DRUG OPTIONS
P. falciparum, P. malariae	Chloroquine or Quinine sulfate plus doxycycline, tetracycline, or clindamycin or Atovaquone-proguanil or Mefloquine
P. vivax, P. ovale	Chloroquine plus primaquine or Quinine sulfate plus either doxycycline or tetracycline plus primaquine or Mefloquine plus primaquine

Chloroquine and Hydroxychloroquine
Mechanism of action
Chloroquine and hydroxychloroquine are taken up more readily into affected cells than into noninfected cells. Their exact mechanism is unknown. Inside cells, the antimalarials may raise the internal pH inside parasite vesicles and may also interfere with parasite nucleoprotein synthesis.

Clinical use
These drugs are used for prophylaxis and acute attacks of malaria. They are effective for treating the erythrocytic (blood) stage of malaria; however, they have no effect on exoerythrocytic (tissue) forms of malaria.

Adverse effects
Resistance to these drugs is increasing in many parts of the world. These drugs may cause hemolysis in patients with G6PD deficiency. In addition, these drugs have been associated with seizures, electrocardiographic changes, agranulocytosis, and irreversible retinal damage. Ophthalmic examinations are recommended.

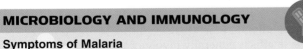

MICROBIOLOGY AND IMMUNOLOGY

Symptoms of Malaria

Malaria is transmitted by mosquitoes in tropical areas. Early symptoms are nonspecific and include malaise, headache, fatigue, abdominal discomfort, muscle aches, fever, nausea, vomiting, orthostatic hypotension, and anemia. These symptoms are followed by the classic symptoms of malaria, which include high fever, chills, and rigors occurring at regular intervals. Four different species of *Plasmodium* may cause malaria. *P. falciparum* can rapidly progress to severe illness or death, whereas the other species (*P. vivax*, *P. ovale*, and *P. malariae*) rarely cause severe illness. *P. vivax* and *P. ovale* infections may require treatment for the hypnozoite forms that lie dormant in the liver and cause relapsing infections.

Mefloquine
Mechanism of action
The mechanism of mefloquine is unknown.

Clinical use
Mefloquine is used for treatment and prevention of malaria.

Adverse effects
Mefloquine is associated with gastrointestinal upset, circulatory disturbances, rash, and musculoskeletal weakness and cramps. In addition, disorientation or confusion as well as psychiatric symptoms of depression, hallucinations, or suicidal thoughts may occur.

Primaquine
Mechanism of action
Primaquine disrupts parasitic mitochondria and binds to DNA.

Clinical use
Primaquine is used to treat tissue (exoerythrocytic) and blood (erythrocytic) forms of *Plasmodium vivax* malaria.

Adverse effects
Primaquine causes drug-induced hemolysis and gastrointestinal upset.

Atovaquone-Proguanil
Mechanism of action
Atovaquone-proguanil interferes with two different pathways in pyrimidine biosynthesis that are required for parasitic nucleic acid replication.

Clinical use
This combination of drugs is used to treat and prevent malaria.

Adverse effects
Of all the antimalarials, atovaquone-proguanil is probably the safest, although it is also the most expensive.

Quinine
Mechanism of action
The precise mechanism of quinine is unknown but may involve elevating the pH of intracellular organelles inside parasites.

Adverse effects
A conglomeration of symptoms called cinchonism (headache, tinnitus, nausea, blurred vision, diplopia, disturbed color vision) may occur as well as hepatitis and other gastrointestinal disturbances and cardiac arrhythmias. This drug is contraindicated in patients with G6PD deficiency because of the risk of hemolysis.

Artemether and Lumefantrine
Mechanism of action
In the United States, these drugs are not marketed individually, but only together as a combination product for treatment of acute, uncomplicated malaria infections caused by

Plasmodium falciparum. Both drugs are active against erythrocytic stages of the infection. Artemether and its major metabolite are rapid schizonticides (selectively destroying the schizont of a sporozoan parasite), with activity attributed to the endoperoxide component common to each substance. Artemether inhibits an essential calcium adenosine triphosphatase. The exact mechanism of lumefantrine is unknown, but it may inhibit β-hematin formation by complexing with hemin. Both artemether and lumefantrine inhibit nucleic acid and protein synthesis.

Pharmacokinetics

Food, especially a high-fat meal, increases absorption of both drugs considerably. Taking the drugs with meals is therefore important to achieving adequate antimalarial efficacy. When the drugs are used soon after mefloquine, plasma levels of lumefantrine are decreased; this is thought to be secondary to reduced absorption resulting from a mefloquine-induced decrease in bile production. In this situation, consumption of food with artemether/lumefantrine becomes even more important.

Adverse effects

The most important concern with artemether/lumefantrine is prolongation of the QT interval on electrocardiograms. Both drugs are metabolized primarily by CYP3A4; therefore the malarial treatment must be used with caution in individuals taking CYP3A4 inducers or inhibitors simultaneously.

Antihelmintics

Numerous types of helminths (flatworms, round worms, flukes, and tapeworms) are particularly problematic in areas of the world where sanitation is poor. In addition, some worm infections may be obtained by eating poorly cooked pork. Drugs of choice are listed in Table 4-25. Note that some of these medications are available only outside the United States or through the Centers for Disease Control and Prevention. The following discussion features a few of the medications used to treat worm infections.

TABLE 4-25. Parasitic Infections and Drugs of Choice

INFECTION (COMMON NAME)	DRUGS OF CHOICE
Intestinal nematodes	Mebendazole, pyrantel pamoate, albendazole, or diethylcarbamazine
Tissue nematodes	Thiabendazole, albendazole, flubendazole, mebendazole, ivermectin, suramin, or diethylcarbamazine
Cestodes	Praziquantel, niclosamide, or albendazole
Trematodes	Praziquantel, oxamniquine, or bithionol

Mebendazole
Mechanism of action

Mebendazole and thiabendazole block assembly of tubulin polymers. By disrupting microtubule assembly, the formation of mitotic spindles is disrupted. In addition, glucose uptake into the parasite is disrupted with mebendazole, causing worms to starve to death.

Clinical use

These drugs may be used to treat the enteric stages of pinworm, roundworm, hookworm, and whipworm infections but not larvae after they have migrated to muscle tissues.

Adverse effects

These drugs may cause gastrointestinal upset. In addition, these agents are embryotoxic and should be avoided during pregnancy.

Ivermectin
Mechanism of action

Ivermectin causes a tonic paralysis of worms, probably by activating a glutamate-activated chloride channel. This leads to hyperpolarization of invertebrate nerve and muscle cells, which causes paralysis. Fortunately, ivermectin does not cross the mammalian blood-brain barrier.

Clinical use

Ivermectin is effective for treating nematodes.

Adverse effects

Because of its rapid killing effects, an inflammatory response termed the *Mazzotti reaction* (itching, rash, fever, swollen lymph nodes, and arthralgias) may occur as the worms are eliminated.

Praziquantel
Mechanism of action

Praziquantel increases cell membrane permeability, causing a loss of intracellular calcium, massive contractions, and paralysis.

Clinical use

Praziquantel is effective against a broad spectrum of helminths, including cestodes and many flukes.

Adverse effects

Adverse effects generally involve gastrointestinal discomfort and are short lived.

Head Lice Medications

Other than the common cold, head lice affect more school-aged children than any other communicable illness.

Lindane
Adverse effects

Although the gold standard for many years in treatment of head lice was lindane, a drug that is ovicidal by absorbing directly into the parasites and their ova, this drug has been banned from use in many countries and even in some states because of possible neurotoxicity (seizures and death). As a result, lindane is rarely used and, if it is prescribed, should definitely not be used in those with a history of seizure disorders. In addition, it should never be applied more than one time.

Permethrin
Mechanism of action
Permethrin keeps sodium channels opened for prolonged periods, thus delaying repolarization, resulting in paralysis of scabies.

Clinical use
Permethrin is a safer alternative to lindane. It is available over the counter as a lotion and cream rinse and is available with a prescription in a more concentrated cream formulation. Unfortunately, permethrin may not kill lice eggs, called nits. Nits are best removed with special combs. Permethrin may be applied again 2 weeks after initial use, but excessive application contributes to lice resistance (which may be as high as 50% to 98%).

Adverse effects
Permethrin is contraindicated in patients allergic to ragweed and chrysanthemums. Irritation at the site of application may occur.

Benzyl Alcohol
Mechanism of action
Benzyl alcohol is thought to inhibit lice from closing their respiratory spiracles, allowing the lotion to obstruct the spiracles and causing the lice to asphyxiate.

Clinical use
Because of the mechanism of action of benzyl alcohol, lice are less likely to develop resistance to the drug compared with permethrin. Patients with long hair may need up to six bottles of lotion to completely cover their hair during a single application. Because benzyl alcohol does not eliminate lice eggs, a second treatment, 1 week after the first, is necessary.

Adverse effects
Although unlikely with topical application, intravenous products containing benzyl alcohol have been associated with neonatal gasping syndrome, with manifestations including gasping respiration, metabolic acidosis, and hypotension. As a result of the risk of neonatal gasping syndrome, this drug should not be administered in infants younger than 6 months.

Other Options
Other alternatives for treating head lice include malathion, ivermectin, and even sulfamethoxazole/trimethoprim, all of which are covered elsewhere in this book.

●●● ANTIVIRALS

It is important to keep in mind that antivirals are not a cure. Antivirals simply shorten the duration, decrease the severity, and reduce the sequelae associated with viral infections. Antivirals are most efficacious when they are initiated at the first sign of infection.

Several classes of antivirals that work through distinct mechanisms have been approved (Fig. 4-9). Antivirals inhibit viral replication by the following mechanisms:
- Inhibiting viral uncoating
- Inhibiting viral neuraminidase
- Serving as "foreign" or nonfunctional analogs of DNA/RNA nucleotides
- Interfering with viral penetration of the host cell, or inhibiting fusion of viral and host membranes
- Inhibiting reverse transcriptases
- Inhibiting proteases responsible for cleaving viral precursor proteins

Inhibiting the Integrase Necessary for Integrating Viral DNA into Host Nucleic Acids

Some antiviral drugs ensure specificity of the response by becoming "activated" only inside virally infected cells. For example, some drugs that are analogs of nucleosides are administered in an unphosphorylated form. When these drugs are taken up by infected cells, the viral enzyme, thymidine kinase, phosphorylates the drug. (Note that because the host enzyme does not add the first phosphate, the drug does not become activated in uninfected cells.) The host cell

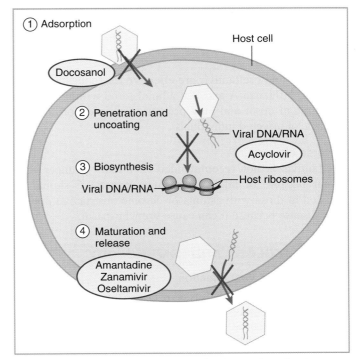

Figure 4-9. Drug targets for viral infection and replication.

subsequently adds two additional phosphates to the virally produced monophosphorylated drug. The triphosphorylated drug may now be incorporated into DNA or RNA as a "nucleic acid." However, when the drugs have been incorporated into viral DNA or RNA, the end result is chain termination and disrupted viral replication (see Fig. 4-9).

Inhibitors of Viral Uncoating

Amantadine and Rimantadine
Mechanism of action
Amantadine and rimantadine appear to work, at least in part, by preventing newly synthesized viruses from being released from the host cell (see Fig. 4-9).

Clinical use
Amantadine and rimantadine are effective for reducing the duration of influenza A if given within 24 hours of symptom onset and may prevent the infection in close contacts of affected individuals.

Adverse effects
Amantadine is associated with central nervous system side effects (nervousness, lightheadedness, insomnia, and seizures), especially in the elderly. In addition, amantadine is associated with anticholinergic side effects and may promote dopamine release. Because of these additional mechanisms, amantadine is sometimes used for managing symptoms associated with Parkinson disease. Use caution and consider dose reductions in patients with renal impairment.

Inhibitors of Viral Neuraminidase

Zanamivir and Oseltamivir
Mechanism of action
Zanamivir and oseltamivir inhibit viral neuraminidase, an enzyme essential for release of newly formed virus particles from infected cells and further spread of the infectious virus.

Clinical use
Zanamivir and oseltamivir are effective for reducing the duration of influenza A and B if administered within 48 hours of symptom onset and may prevent viral infection in close contacts of affected individuals.

Adverse effects
Oseltamivir is not recommended in infants younger than 1 year because of fatalities in mice. Zanamivir should be avoided in those with asthma or chronic obstructive pulmonary disease because it can cause bronchospasm.

MICROBIOLOGY AND IMMUNOLOGY

Mechanics of Viral Infection
Viruses are obligate intracellular parasites that usurp the metabolic processes of the hosts they invade for their own replication purposes. In brief, viruses must attach to and penetrate susceptible host cells—that is, cells that have appropriate receptors for viral binding and the necessary intracellular machinery for viral replication. Next, the virus uncoats, a process by which the viral DNA/RNA separates from the viral capsid. The virus then exploits the host's RNA/DNA/protein synthesis machinery. Viral subunits are then assembled, allowing the progeny viruses to be released, as the host cell disintegrates.

Inhibition of Intracellular Synthesis by Analogs of Viral Nucleic Acids

Ribavirin, Acyclovir, Valacyclovir, Ganciclovir, Valganciclovir, Famciclovir, Penciclovir, Foscarnet, Adefovir Dipivoxil, Entecavir, and Telbivudine
Many antivirals end in "-ovir."

Mechanism of action
Ribavirin and the other drugs interfere with intracellular viral replication processes. Most of these drugs are guanosine analogs (acyclovir, valacyclovir, ganciclovir, valganciclovir, famciclovir, penciclovir, and entecavir). Adefovir dipivoxil and telbivudine are analogs of adenosine monophosphate and thymidine, respectively. Adefovir dipivoxil is phosphorylated to its active metabolite, adefovir diphosphate, and telbivudine is phosphorylated to its triphosphate form, both of which inhibit hepatitis B virus (HBV) DNA polymerase (reverse transcriptase). The exact mechanism of ribavirin is not known, but it may act as an analog of guanosine or xanthosine. These drugs are first phosphorylated by a viral thymidine kinase and subsequently phosphorylated by the host cell before drug incorporation into viral nucleic acids. When the phosphorylated drugs are encountered by viral polymerases, the drugs are recognized as "foreign" and viral polymerase action is halted.

Unlike other antivirals in this class, foscarnet, although still an inhibitor of viral DNA polymerases, does not need to be activated (or phosphorylated) for its activity. Foscarnet binds directly to viral DNA polymerases and inhibits their activity.

Pharmacokinetics
Valacyclovir, valganciclovir, and famciclovir are simply prodrugs of acyclovir, ganciclovir, and penciclovir, respectively, with superior bioavailability over the parent compounds. These antivirals are excreted renally, so dosage adjustments are necessary at low glomerular filtration rates.

Clinical use
Ribavirin is approved as an aerosol for treating respiratory syncytial virus, a leading cause of pneumonia in infants; however, the aerosolized drug has cumbersome requirements (e.g., endotracheal intubation) because sometimes patients, especially infants, suddenly get worse with inhalation. In addition, strict isolation is necessary to prevent drug exposure to pregnant visitors and caregivers. This drug is also used in

combination with peg-interferon α-2b for treatment of hepatitis C in patients with decompensated liver disease.

Penciclovir is available only as a topical cream for treating oral cold sores caused by the herpesvirus. Acyclovir is used to treat herpes simplex virus (mucosal, cutaneous, encephalitis, recurrent genital infections, shingles, and varicella); the drug may also be used to reduce the risk of cytomegalovirus in high-risk patients. When used to treat chickenpox, acyclovir reduces the number of lesions, shortens the healing time, and decreases the duration of fever. The drug does not appear to have any pain-relieving properties when used for management of shingles. Famciclovir and valacyclovir are also used in treatment and management of herpes infections. Ganciclovir and valganciclovir are used to treat life-threatening or sight-threatening cytomegalovirus infections, and foscarnet is also used to treat herpes infections as well as cytomegalovirus in immunocompromised patients.

Adefovir dipivoxil, entecavir, and telbivudine are used for the treatment of HBV, acting to slow progression of the disease, ameliorate liver injury, and even decrease viral load. Lamivudine and tenofovir, discussed later in this chapter, are also pharmacologic components of HBV therapy.

Adverse effects

The primary toxicity associated with ribavirin is hemolytic anemia, which may worsen cardiac disease, even leading to death. The drug is mutagenic, carcinogenic, and teratogenic and should not be administered via the inhalation route by pregnant health care workers. Acyclovir is associated with rashes and photosensitivity. Granulocytopenia, anemia, and thrombocytopenia are limiting side effects of ganciclovir and valganciclovir, and these drugs are also thought to be carcinogenic and teratogenic (Table 4-26). Foscarnet may cause nephrotoxicity and electrolyte imbalances, so close monitoring is essential. Agents used for HBV treatment, entecavir, adefovir, and telbivudine, are associated with lactic acidosis, severe hepatomegaly with steatosis, and acute exacerbations of hepatitis upon discontinuation. In addition, adefovir is associated with nephrotoxicity. Patients taking telbivudine are more likely to experience myopathies and should be monitored appropriately.

Antivirals that Interfere with Viral Penetration into Host Cells

Docosanol
Mechanism of action
Docosanol interferes with viral penetration of host cells and subsequent migration of the virus to the nucleus (see Fig. 4-9).

Clinical use
This agent is available over the counter, without a prescription, as a cream that is applied topically to external cold sores.

Therapies for Human Papilloma Virus

Human papilloma viruses (HPV), a family of highly infectious, sexually transmitted, double-stranded DNA viruses, manifest clinically as anogenital warts and are the most common sexually transmitted viruses in the United States. Papillomavirus types are distinguished from one another by the degree of nucleic acid sequence homology. More than 100 HPV types are recognized, and individual types are often associated with specific clinical manifestations. Approximately 90% of anogenital warts are attributed to HPV types 6 and 11, whereas types 16, 18, 31, 33, and 45 have been linked to cervical cancers. Treatment of existing genital warts depends on the number and severity of lesions and may include surgical or pharmacologic approaches. Topical pharmacologic treatment options are available to patients for self-administration. It is important to note that these therapies do not eradicate HPV or affect the history of infection but merely aid in the destruction of warts. In fact, latent or subclinical HPV infection can persist and recurrence of visible warts is common.

CLINICAL MEDICINE

Human Papilloma Virus Vaccine

HPV, a family of highly infectious, sexually transmitted, double-stranded DNA viruses, manifests clinically as anogenital warts and includes the most common sexually transmitted viruses in the United States. Papillomavirus types are distinguished from one another by their degree of nucleic acid sequence homology. More than 100 HPV types are recognized, and individual types are often associated with specific clinical manifestations. Approximately 90% of anogenital warts are attributed to HPV types 6 and 11, whereas types 16, 18, 31, 33, and 45 have been linked to cervical cancers. Much controversy has surrounded the marketing of an HPV vaccine (Gardasil) that immunizes against four HPV strains: 6, 11, 16, and 18. Currently, the vaccine is approved for boys and girls beginning at 9 years of age. The length of protection offered by the HPV vaccination is not known; in clinical studies, it has prevented genital warts for 3 years, but this length is too short to determine efficacy in protecting from cervical cancer.

MEDICATION	SYMPTOM OR CONDITION
Acyclovir	Phlebitis: 15% to 20% incidence; because of poor solubility
	Renal failure: dehydration predisposes to toxicity
	CNS: 1% incidence (confusion, headache, lethargy, seizures, disorientation)
Ganciclovir	Neutropenia, thrombocytopenia: increased incidence in AIDS
	Hepatitis: usually mild to moderate increase in liver function test results

TABLE 4-26. Adverse Effects Associated with Common Antivirals

AIDS, Acquired immunodeficiency syndrome

Imiquimod, Podofilox, and Sinecatechins
Mechanism of action

Imiquimod is an immune response modifier and acts by inducing local cytokines such as interferon-α, tumor necrosis factor-α, and interleukins 1, 6, and 8, actions assumed to aid in the clearance of warts. The exact mechanism of podofilox is unknown, but it begins to cause necrosis of wart tissue within 24 hours after application, with sloughing of the wart occurring within 72 hours. This may be attributed to its induction of cytokines, interference with microtubule formation, and general immunosuppressive properties. Sinecatechins is a new alternative derived from green tea leaves. The mechanism of sinecatechins in treatment of HPV is unknown, but green tea has been shown to possess antioxidant, anticarcinogenic, and antimicrobial properties.

Pharmacokinetics

All three drugs are applied topically to warts. Imiquimod has the greatest potential for systemic absorption.

Adverse effects

Local irritation such as redness, burning, itching, and discomfort are common. These agents have the potential to weaken contraceptive devices such as condoms and diaphragms, thus lowering efficacy. The three formulations are intended for external use only and sexual contact should be avoided when these drugs are used. Special care must be taken to be certain that podofilox is applied only to wart tissue; it will cause necrosis of healthy skin if it comes into contact with it.

●●● MANAGEMENT OF HIV

Currently, six classes of antiretrovirals are used to manage HIV:

- Nucleoside-dependent reverse transcriptase inhibitors
- Non-nucleoside reverse transcriptase inhibitors
- Protease inhibitors
- Fusion inhibitors
- CCR5 antagonists
- Integrase inhibitors

Combinations of drugs are always used to delay the emergence of drug-resistant viral strains. Regimens can be highly complicated, with some patients ingesting 15 pills daily. Some medications must be taken with food, whereas other medications cannot be taken with food and should even be taken with an antacid. Numerous drug interactions and contraindications are associated with these drugs, and clinicians prescribing these medications must be thoroughly versed in these interactions, with appropriate safeguards in place. This brief review is not intended to provide a detailed discussion of each antiretroviral drug but instead provides an overview of each of the six major drug classes.

CLINICAL MEDICINE

Human Immunodeficiency Virus

HIV is the retrovirus that causes acquired immunodeficiency syndrome. Lymphocytes are infected first. Initially, patients may experience mononucleosis- or influenza-like symptoms while the virus spreads to lymphoid and other body tissues. It may take years before the patient becomes clinically ill. During this time, CD4+ T-cell numbers decline and patients become highly susceptible to opportunistic infections. Patients are monitored for CD4+ T-cell counts as well as the level of HIV RNA in plasma. Viral replication rates predict what will happen to CD4+ cell counts in the future.

Nucleoside/Nucleotide Reverse Transcriptase Inhibitors

Zidovudine, Zalcitabine, Stavudine, Lamivudine, Emtricitabine, Didanosine, Abacavir, and Tenofovir

Tenofovir is the only nucleotide reverse transcriptase inhibitor.

Mechanism of action

These drugs are structurally related to the sugars and nucleotides that comprise nucleic acids. As with many other antivirals, these drugs are phosphorylated and inserted as nonfunctional nucleotides. They inhibit viral DNA polymerase (reverse transcriptase) so that viral DNA synthesis is inhibited and viral replication is decreased.

Clinical use

Frequently, two nucleoside reverse transcriptase inhibitors are combined with a protease inhibitor to prevent development of resistant strains. The only indication for monotherapy is when one of these drugs is used to prevent perinatal transmission of the virus from mother to infant during labor and delivery. These drugs may also be used prophylactically to prevent infection in health care workers who have sustained accidental needle sticks.

Adverse effects

Adverse effects associated with this class of medications are listed in Box 4-13. In addition, emtricitabine may cause skin discoloration (hyperpigmentation of palms of hands or soles of feet).

Box 4-13. ADVERSE EFFECTS ASSOCIATED WITH NUCLEOSIDE REVERSE TRANSCRIPTASE INHIBITORS

Pancreatitis
Peripheral neuropathy
Granulocytopenia
Myopathy

Lactic acidosis with hepatic steatosis (rare, but potentially fatal)

Non-Nucleoside Reverse Transcriptase Inhibitors

Nevirapine, Delavirdine, Efavirenz, and Etravirine

Mechanism of action

These drugs are direct noncompetitive inhibitors of HIV-1 reverse transcriptase. Non-nucleoside reverse transcriptase inhibitors block RNA-dependent and DNA-dependent polymerase activities by inducing a conformational change that disrupts the enzyme's catalytic site. Unlike the nucleoside reverse transcriptase inhibitors, these drugs do not require intracellular phosphorylation for their actions. These drugs potentiate the actions of other antiretroviral drugs.

Clinical use

Non-nucleoside reverse transcriptase inhibitors are used in combination with other antiretroviral agents to treat HIV infections.

Pharmacokinetics

These drugs are metabolized by the P450 enzymes and are susceptible to numerous drug interactions by drugs that induce or inhibit the hepatic P450 microsomal enzymes.

Adverse effects

This drug class has been associated with potentially fatal hepatotoxicity, although etravirine appears to be the safest in this regard. Efavirenz has been associated with adverse psychiatric effects. Severe, life-threatening skin rashes, including Stevens-Johnson syndrome and toxic epidermal necrosis, may also occur.

Protease Inhibitors

Amprenavir, Atazanavir, Darunavir, Fosamprenavir, Indinavir, Lopinavir/Ritonavir, Nelfinavir, Ritonavir, Saquinavir, and Tipranavir

These drugs end in "-avir."

Mechanism of action

These drugs inhibit the protease responsible for cleaving viral precursor proteins, which are essential for HIV maturation, replication, and infection of new cells. Inhibition of the protease enzyme produces immature viral particles. When used in combination with other antiretroviral drugs, protease inhibitors lead to clinical improvements and prolonged patient survival. Rapid HIV resistance emerges if protease inhibitors are used as monotherapy.

Clinical use

Protease inhibitors are used in combination with other antiretrovirals for treating HIV infections. Unlike other drugs in this class that are large peptides, tipranavir does not have a

peptide structure and may be beneficial for patients with resistance to other protease inhibitors.

Pharmacokinetics

All drugs in this class are metabolized by hepatic microsomal enzymes and are susceptible to many severe, even life-threatening drug interactions.

Adverse effects

All protease inhibitors can cause gastrointestinal intolerance, increased bleeding, hyperglycemia, insulin resistance, hyperlipidemia, and hepatitis. As a result of the "metabolic syndrome" associated with these drugs, some practitioners suggest delaying administration of these drugs rather than using them as part of initial treatment regimens. In addition, tipranavir contains sulfonamide in its chemical structure; patients allergic to sulfonamide antibiotics may also be hypersensitive to this antiviral. Darunavir has been associated with serious rashes. Atazanavir may prolong the PR interval on electrocardiograms.

Fusion Inhibitors

Enfuvirtide

Mechanism of action

Enfuvirtide interferes with entry of HIV-1 into CD4+ cells by inhibiting fusion of viral and cellular membranes.

Pharmacokinetics

Enfuvirtide is a 36-amino-acid synthetic peptide administered twice daily by subcutaneous injections into the arm, thigh, or abdomen.

Adverse effects

Adverse effects include hypersensitivity reactions and injection site discomfort. Overall, enfuvirtide may have an improved safety profile compared with other antiretrovirals because it does not exert its effects inside host cells. Because the drug is metabolized to individual amino acids, there are no interactions with other medications or with the P450 hepatic enzymes. Adverse effects are primarily gastrointestinal (diarrhea, nausea).

Entry Inhibitors

Maraviroc

Mechanism of action

Maraviroc blocks HIV entry into human cells by acting as an antagonist at the chemokine receptor 5 (CCR5). CCR5 is a chemokine receptor present on the surface of some immune cells. It is a co-receptor used by HIV-1 to enter uninfected cells. The drug has no effect for HIV-1 strains that use the other co-receptor, CXCR-4, to gain cell entry. Before initiating maraviroc in a patient, tropism testing of the HIV strain is necessary (e.g., to identify which receptor

CCR5 or CXCR-4) to determine whether the drug will be of benefit.

Pharmacokinetics
Maraviroc is a P450 substrate and the dose may need to be adjusted if taken with drugs that induce or inhibit hepatic P450 enzymes.

Adverse effects
Maraviroc has been associated with liver toxicity, which is often preceded by evidence of a systemic allergic reaction (e.g., pruritic rash).

Integrase Inhibitors

Raltegravir
Mechanism of action
Raltegravir inhibits the viral integrase enzyme. This enzyme is produced by retroviruses (including HIV), enabling viral genetic material to be integrated into DNA of infected cells.

Pharmacokinetics
Raltegravir is eliminated mainly by metabolism by a uridine diphosphate glucuronosyltransferase-1A1–mediated glucuronidation pathway. Its metabolism may be slowed by concurrent use of drugs that inhibit this pathway (e.g., rifampin).

Adverse effects
Raltegravir is less likely to cause serious adverse effects or interact with other medications compared to other antiretroviral agents.

●●● COMPLEMENTARY AND ALTERNATIVE MEDICINE

Treatment of Antibiotic-Associated Diarrhea

Nearly all antibacterials disrupt normal gastrointestinal flora. This can lead to overgrowth of undesirable species including *Clostridium difficile*. The incidence of severe, life-threatening diarrhea caused by overgrowth of *C. difficile* is increasing, and some estimates from the Centers for Disease Control and Prevention indicate that the incidence doubled between 2000 and 2002 in the United States.

Probiotic supplements that replace the "good" gastrointestinal flora have been shown to prevent antibiotic-associated diarrhea and "cure" severe *C. difficile* diarrhea even in patients who are refractory to therapy with metronidazole and vancomycin. Most often, the bacterial species contained in probiotic supplements belong to members of the *Lactobacillus* or *Bifidobacterium* genera.

It is becoming increasingly apparent that for maximal benefit probiotic supplements must remain refrigerated, must contain tens or hundreds of billions of good bacteria, and are more likely to exert beneficial effects when multiple species are contained in a single product. These healthy bacterial supplements eliminate harmful *Clostridia* species via several mechanisms,

including competitive exclusion for space and nutrients, production of short-chain fatty acids, production of peroxides and bacteriocins, and stimulation of immunoglobulin A secretion.

Numerous probiotic products are available. Recommend products that have been shown effective in clinical trials, and shy away from products that have no data to back up their claims.

Another type of probiotic that has been shown extremely beneficial for treating *C. difficile* diarrhea is the yeast strain *Saccharomyces boulardii*. Although not normally part of our endogenous flora, this strain of yeast secretes an enzyme that selectively inactivates *C. difficile* toxins.

Treatment of Yeast Infections

For difficult to eradicate yeast infections, especially thrush in infants, a 0.5% gentian violet solution painted onto affected oral tissues with a cotton-tipped swab twice daily for 5 days can be effective at eliminating the infection. If the infant is breast fed, the mother's nipples may also require treatment. Alternatively, if the baby is bottle fed, nipples and bottles should be boiled daily to prevent reinfection at subsequent feedings.

Probiotics containing *Lactobacillus acidophilus* may also be effective at preventing chronic, recurrent vaginal yeast infections, including those that occur secondarily to antibiotic use. These probiotic supplements can be taken orally or inserted vaginally.

Treatment of the Common Cold

There is some evidence that *Echinacea* may shorten the duration of upper respiratory tract infection symptoms; however, there is no evidence that it *prevents* colds. Furthermore, some studies suggest that repeated use of *Echinacea* may actually suppress the immune system. Adverse reactions are rare, although people with allergies may be more susceptible to allergic effects (bronchospasm; itchy, watery eyes; hives). Recent evidence suggests that *Echinacea* may decrease fertility and should not be used by couples who are trying to conceive.

●●● TOP FIVE LIST

Although at first glance, memorization of the antibiotics seems a daunting task, the most important thing to learn is to match the drug with the bug. Remember that antibacterials can be divided into four major categories: those that interfere with cell wall synthesis, those that interfere with folic acid synthesis, those that interfere with protein synthesis, and those that interfere with transcription of DNA/RNA.

1. Understanding the mechanism of action allows for the rational combination of antibiotics to synergistically treat infections.
2. When selecting an antibacterial agent, always choose the most narrow-spectrum agent that is likely to eliminate the infecting microorganism. This practice helps decrease antibacterial resistance. Table 4-27 lists drugs of choice.
3. Emerging antimicrobial resistance is a major health concern in hospitals and the community (leading to secondary

TABLE 4-27. Common Pharmacologic Options for Various Microorganisms (Grouped by Morphology and Gram Staining)

MICROBE	OPTION
Gram-Positive Cocci	
Staphylococci (assume all make β-lactamases)	Penicillinase-resistant penicillins (e.g., nafcillin, methicillin, dicloxacillin) Amoxicillin/clavulanic acid Cephalosporins (first generation) Trimethoprim-sulfamethoxazole Doxycycline Vancomycin Clindamycin Linezolid Quinupristan-dalfopristan
Group A streptococci (*S. pyogenes*) (cause of pink eye and strep throat)	Penicillin Amoxicillin
Group B streptococci (possibly problematic for babies whose mothers are vaginal carriers)	Cephalosporins (first generation)
S. viridans (cause of bacterial endocarditis, persistent urinary tract infections)	Penicillin Gentamicin Cephalosporins (third generation) Macrolides Vancomycin
Gram-Negative Cocci	
Moraxella catarrhalis (one of three major causes of otitis media; secrete β-lactamases)	Amoxicillin/clavulanic acid or ampicillin/sulbactam Trimethoprim/sulfamethoxazole Macrolides Doxycycline Cephalosporins
Neisseria gonorrhoeae	Ceftriaxone or cefotaxime Ciprofloxacin or levofloxacin
Clostridium perfringens	Penicillin G Metronidazole Clindamycin Doxycycline Cefazolin Carbapenems
Gram-Negative Enteric Microorganisms	
Bacteroides fragilis	Metronidazole Clindamycin
Enterobacter	Carbapenem Cefepime ± aminoglycoside Ciprofloxacin or levofloxacin
Escherichia coli (meningitis or systemic infection)	Cephalosporin (third generation) Carbapenem Fluoroquinolone
Klebsiella pneumoniae (almost always acquired from hospital)	Third-generation cephalosporin Fluoroquinolone Carbapenem
Proteus mirabilis (frequent cause of urinary tract infections)	Ampicillin Trimethoprim/sulfamethoxazole
Salmonella typhi	Fluoroquinolones Ceftriaxone or cefotaxime Trimethoprim/sulfamethoxazole

and nosocomial infections). Physicians should be wary of prescribing third-generation cephalosporins and immediately using latest generation antibiotics as first-line therapies.

4. Secondary yeast infections (thrush and vaginal) often follow antibiotic therapy.

5. The major adverse effects or toxicities for antibacterials, antifungals, and antivirals are diarrhea, nephrotoxicity, hypersensitivity, and myelosuppression.

Self-assessment questions can be accessed at www. StudentConsult.com.

Cancer and Immunopharmacology

5

CONTENTS

ANTINEOPLASTIC CHEMOTHERAPY
CANCER DRUG RESISTANCE
CYTOTOXIC DRUGS
  Alkylating Agents
  Antimetabolites
  Cytotoxic Antibiotics
  Mitotic Inhibitors
BIOLOGICS AND SIGNAL TRANSDUCTION INHIBITORS
  Monoclonal Antibodies
ENDOCRINE THERAPY
INTRODUCTION TO IMMUNOPHARMACOLOGY
  Immunosuppressive Agents
COMPLEMENTARY ALTERNATIVE MEDICINE FOR CANCER PREVENTION
TOP FIVE LIST

●●● ANTINEOPLASTIC CHEMOTHERAPY

Immunopharmacology is all about combinatorial therapy—the use of multiple antitumor drugs that have different mechanisms of action. In addition, treatment regimens often combine drugs that target different phases of the cell cycle. Optimal treatment protocols combine drugs that have nonoverlapping toxicities. In this way, overall toxicity can be minimized, despite the use of a synergistic cohort of cytotoxic drugs. These cytotoxic cocktails provide maximal cell killing efficacy and may slow or prevent resistant cancer cells from developing.

Often, acronyms are used to describe these combinatorial treatment protocols. For example, MOPP, originally developed for Hodgkin lymphoma, uses *m*echlorethamine, *O*ncovin (trade name for vincristine), *p*rocarbazine, and *p*rednisone. More current combinatorial protocols are abbreviated FOLFOX, FOLFIRI, ABVD, and CHOP. However, memorizing these detailed protocols is not as important as understanding the overarching mechanisms of action of the drugs that preferentially target proliferating cancer cells. In fact, treatment protocols are continually modified or changed as more specific chemotherapeutics are developed and validated. Physicians often use the National Comprehensive

Cancer Network (www.NCCN.org) as a site to find clinical consensus guidelines and treatment protocols that are updated annually for treatment of all cancers.

Despite intense efforts over the last few decades, cancer continues to be a leading cause of death in the Western world. In the United States, lung neoplasms account for the largest percentage of cancer deaths among both males and females, although prostate and breast cancer are highest in incidence, respectively. Smoking, a modifiable risk factor, remains the single most common cause of cancer worldwide. At present, a curative or palliative approach to the treatment of cancer patients comprises five modalities: surgery, radiotherapy, chemotherapy, gene therapy, and immunotherapy. Often, two or more modalities may be combined in the hope of better clinical outcomes. When antineoplastic chemotherapy is given after surgery or irradiation (to diminish the risk of relapse from foci of microscopic lesions left behind by the initial therapy), the drug therapy is termed *adjuvant chemotherapy*.

The goal of antineoplastic therapy is to kill cancerous cells or inhibit their growth, with minimal effects on normal cells. Cancer cells differ from regular cells in one striking fashion—unlike untransformed cells, which undergo apoptosis (programmed cell death) after some finite number of cell divisions, cancer cells do not undergo apoptosis and are immortal. The rate of cellular division for cancer cells may also be unregulated. Antineoplastic drugs exploit this unchecked and possibly rapid rate of cell growth at the molecular level, allowing these drugs to work with some specificity. However, the same molecular mechanisms by which proliferative cancer cells are targeted also make normal cells with rapid turnover susceptible to cytotoxic actions of antineoplastic drugs. In fact, the hallmark toxicities of cytotoxic drugs—hair loss, neutropenia, and thrombocytopenia—are directly linked to the rapid growth rate of hair follicles and bone marrow. Additional common adverse side effects of cytotoxic drugs, including sterility and nausea, are listed in Table 5-1.

●●● CANCER DRUG RESISTANCE

Similar to bacteria and antibiotic resistance, some tumors are also relatively resistant to antineoplastic agents. Extracellular factors that account for such behavior include the location

TABLE 5-1. General Adverse Effects of Cytotoxic Drugs

TISSUE	SIDE EFFECTS
Bone marrow	Myelosuppression Leukopenia Infection Thrombocytopenia Anemia Hemorrhage Immunosuppression Secondary cancers
Gastrointestinal tract	Decreased mucosal cell division Anorexia Ulceration Diarrhea Nausea/vomiting
Skin	Alopecia Impaired wound healing
Reproductive organs	Sterility Teratogenesis Mutagenicity

TABLE 5-2. Distinctive Organ Toxicities of Cytotoxic Agents

ORGAN OR SYSTEM AFFECTED	DRUGS
Pulmonary	Bleomycin, procarbazine, busulfan
Cardiac	Doxorubicin, daunorubicin
Renal	Cisplatin, methotrexate
Hepatic	Mercaptopurine, cyclophosphamide, busulfan
Neurologic	Vincristine, cisplatin, paclitaxel
Immune	Cytarabine, dactinomycin, methotrexate, cyclophosphamide
Bladder	Cyclophosphamide
Leukocyte	Procarbazine
Pancreas	Asparaginase

of tumors within "safe havens" in the body, where large solid tumors are protected from the actions of drugs by a necrotic core and a dysfunctional capillary network, as well as physiologic barriers, such as the blood-brain barrier. In addition, tumor resistance to anticancer drugs is often the result of selection for resistant clones (i.e., antineoplastic drugs kill off the sensitive clones in the tumor, leaving behind resistant, virulent cells). Again, the major rationale for combinatorial drug therapies is to evade cancer cell resistance and minimize dose-limiting toxicity.

At the intracellular level, tumors can use numerous mechanisms to reduce their sensitivity to chemotherapeutic agents, such as

- Decreased drug influx from diminished binding affinity to receptors or decreased membrane permeability
- Increased drug efflux from increased expression of the multidrug resistance P-glycoprotein that actively pumps drug out of the cells
- Increased expression of enzymes that metabolize the drugs
- Abnormal intracellular binding to target proteins
- Enhanced nucleic acid repair mechanisms
- Diminished activation of pro-drugs

In general, chemotherapeutic drugs exert their effects via one of three mechanisms:

- Cytotoxic actions (the majority)
- Endocrine activities
- Immunotherapy

Each of these classes of chemotherapeutics, as well as their major organ-specific side effects (Table 5-2), are reviewed in the following sections.

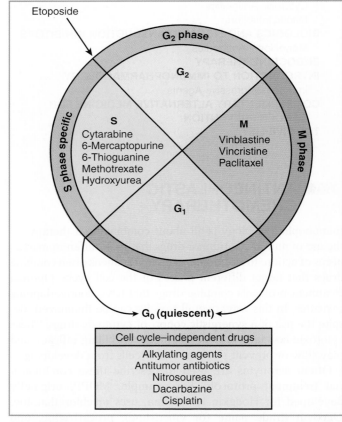

Figure 5-1. Sites of action of cell cycle phase–specific drugs.

●●● CYTOTOXIC DRUGS

Cytotoxic drugs work by affecting DNA synthesis and are classified according to their site of action within the cell cycle. As shown in Figure 5-1, some agents kill cells only during specific parts of the cell cycle as the cells replicate (these drugs are referred to as *phase specific*), whereas other drugs work throughout the cell cycle (*phase nonspecific*).

Cytotoxic agents usually follow first-order kinetics and, as a result, affect a fixed percentage of tumor cells per cycle. This is known as the *log-kill hypothesis*, and it provides another rationale for drug combinations—multiple drugs lead to a greater percentage of neoplastic cell death. A one-log drug kills 90% of the cells, a two-log drug kills 99%, and a three-log drug kills 99.9%.

By far, the majority of antineoplastic agents used in clinical practice today achieve their desired effects through cell cytotoxicity. This group of drugs can be further subdivided into four distinct categories (Fig. 5-2):

- Alkylating agents
- Antimetabolites
- Cytotoxic antibiotics
- Mitotic inhibitors

EMBRYOLOGY

The Cell Cycle

The G_1 phase is associated with synthesis of DNA, whereas the S phase is associated with increased activity of DNA-replicating enzymes, including thymidine kinase, DNA polymerase, dihydrofolate reductase, ribonucleotide reductase, RNA polymerase II, and the topoisomerases. Synthesis of machinery needed for mitosis (M phase) occurs during the G_2 phase. Mitosis divides the two sets of chromosomes. For rapidly dividing embryonic stem cells, the G_1 phase is minimized or significantly shortened. For dormant, nondividing cells, the G_1 phase is lengthened and is referred to as G_0. Cyclin-dependent kinases modify the phosphorylation state of cyclins to control the cell cycle.

BIOCHEMISTRY

Checkpoint Control and Telomerases

A hallmark of tumorigenic cells is increased proliferation as a result of loss of regulatory control and regulatory proteins. For example, many cancers are classified as p53 negative. p53 is a protein that extends the G_1 phase (growth arrest) to allow DNA repair or apoptosis to remove damaged cells. Thus, these p53-negative cancers have lost control of the mechanisms to rid the body of transformed cells. Cancer cells may also lose the ability to repair damaged DNA during the G_2/M transition (checkpoint). In several types of hereditary colon cancers, mutations in and/or loss of DNA repair genes that correct for mismatched base pairs are often observed.

Telomerases protect and maintain the structure of the telomere at the end of chromosomes, which is essential for chromosomal alignment during mitosis. All non-germ cells lose a portion of the telomere structure during cell division owing to diminished telomerase activity during growth and development. This leads to normal cellular senescence. Most cancer cells can reexpress telomerase, leading to cellular immortality. Often, the loss of checkpoint control mechanisms, including p53, leads to overexpression of telomerase.

EMBRYOLOGY

Angiogenesis

Solid tumors and their metastases must develop and maintain an adequate blood supply for rapid growth. Activation of tyrosine kinase receptors by vascular endothelial growth factor or fibroblast growth factor is a crucial step in angiogenesis (formation of new blood vessels). Understanding the molecular mechanisms of angiogenesis offers new therapeutic targets for chemotherapy.

Alkylating Agents

Altretamine, Bendamustine, Busulfan, Carboplatin, Carmustine, Chlorambucil, Cisplatin, Cyclophosphamide, Dacarbazine, Estramustine, Ifosfamide, Lomustine, Mechlorethamine, Melphalan, Mitomycin, Oxaliplatin, Procarbazine, Streptozocin, Temozolomide, Thiotepa, and Uracil Mustard

Mechanism of action

There are many alkylating agents. The main critical mechanism of action is that these drugs possess a reactive alkyl group that forms covalent bonds with nucleic acids, resulting in either DNA cross-linkage or strand breakage, both of which prevent further replication of nucleic acids. In fact, these cytotoxic drugs damage all cellular molecules (including proteins and RNA). However, DNA damage (exceeding repair mechanisms) is what kills the cells. For example, the nitrosoureas (carmustine and lomustine) and platinum compounds, such as cisplatin and carboplatin, directly interact with DNA to prevent proliferation. Cisplatin directly binds to guanine in DNA and RNA. Alkylating agents are phase nonspecific.

Clinical use

As examples of the wide use of alkylating agents for the treatment of multiple cancers, melphalan, cyclophosphamide, chlorambucil, and cisplatin will be discussed. Melphalan is typically used in the treatment of chronic leukemias, myelomas, and some solid tumors, whereas cyclophosphamide and chlorambucil are used to treat a variety of leukemias and lymphomas. Cyclophosphamide can be helpful in treating a variety of solid tumors and non-Hodgkin lymphoma and is also used to treat nonneoplastic diseases such as nephritic syndrome or severe rheumatoid arthritis. Cisplatin is used to treat lung, bladder, and testicular or ovarian carcinoma.

Bendamustine has been approved for chronic lymphocytic leukemia and was subsequently approved for the treatment of B-cell non-Hodgkin lymphoma. This unique agent combines two therapeutics into one molecule. It is a mechlorethamine derivative (alkylating agent) combined with a purine-like antimetabolite (see next section). The idea is to create a single bifunctional agent with two distinct mechanisms of action (and differing dose-limiting toxicities).

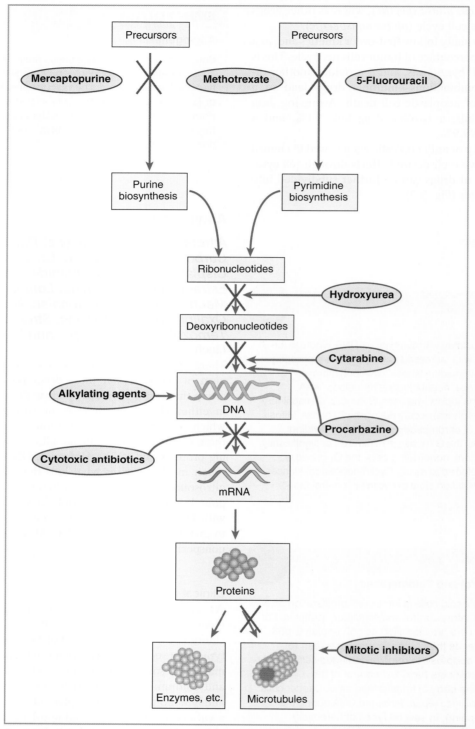

Figure 5-2. Site of action of four classes of cytotoxic drugs. These classes include: antimetabolites (mercaptopurine, methotrexate, 5-fluorouracil, hydroxyurea, cytarabine); DNA alkylating and modifying drugs (cisplatin, mechlorethamine, procarbazine); antibiotics (daunorubicin, doxorubicin, actinomycin, bleomycin); and natural products (vinblastine, vincristine, paclitaxel).

Adverse effects

The usual dose-limiting toxicity for alkylating agents is myelosuppression. These drugs may also be emetogenic. In addition to general side effects (see Table 5-1), the urinary metabolite of cyclophosphamide and ifosfamide, acrolein, is associated with serious hemorrhagic cystitis, which is prevented by adequate hydration or by administering MENSA (the Na^+ salt of methylethylsulfonate), which binds acrolein. Development of secondary acute nonlymphocytic leukemias and temporary sterility are also common problems associated with alkylating agents. Secondary malignancies and leukemia-related toxicities are not unexpected, because alkylating agents interact with DNA in highly proliferative noncancer cells also. Note that the dividing cells are most at risk because they have little time to repair DNA damage before mutations are passed to daughter cells. Nondividing cells have more time to repair alkylating damage. Cisplatin and carboplatin are associated with cumulative nephrotoxicity and ototoxicity.

Pharmacokinetics

Multiple alkylating agents are administered as pro-drugs. These pro-drugs include procarbazine and dacarbazine. Procarbazine is metabolized in the liver into an alkylating azoxy intermediate, whereas dacarbazine is metabolized to release an alkylating methyl diazonium ion. Procarbazine also inhibits monoamine oxidase; thus tyramine-containing foods must be avoided because patients could be put at risk of a hypertensive crisis. Additionally, disulfiram-like adverse reactions occur when procarbazine is used in combination with alcohol.

Antimetabolites

Azacitidine, Bendamustine, Capecitabine, Cladribine, Clofarabine, Cytarabine, Decitabine, Floxuridine, Fludarabine, Fluorouracil, Gemcitabine, Mercaptopurine, Methotrexate, Nelarabine, Pemetrexed, Pentostatin, Tegafur, Thioguanine, and Trimetrexate

Note: Most, but not all, of these drug names end in "-bine," "-dine," or "-tine."

These drugs are structural analogs of naturally occurring substances or metabolites within the body and thus compete with the endogenous metabolite, consequently interfering with specific cellular processes. For the most part, these drugs are mimetics of nucleotides, but because of their slightly altered structures they are actually inhibitors of purine or pyrimidine metabolism. These antimetabolites are cell cycle–specific drugs, and the major side effects are myelosuppression, diarrhea, and mucositis.

Fluorouracil, a pyrimidine (thymine) analog, acts via its conversion to a pseudopyrimidine nucleotide (fluorodeoxyuridine monophosphate) that inhibits thymidylate synthetase and impairs DNA synthesis. The difference between fluorouracil and thymidine is replacement of a fluorine atom with a methyl group. Fluorouracil is helpful for solid tumors and is used topically for some malignant skin conditions.

Cytarabine (ara-C) is a pyrimidine (cytosine) analog that undergoes intracellular conversion to a triphosphate form and competes with cytosine triphosphate for DNA polymerase. Cytotoxicity occurs when the mimetic is inappropriately incorporated into DNA. Again, the drug takes advantage of a subtle change in structure as the ribose sugar is replaced by D-arabinose in cytarabine. Gemcitabine also is a cytidine analog with slightly better pharmacokinetic and pharmacodynamic parameters. Cytarabine is used in treatment of various leukemias, whereas gemcitabine is used in solid tumors. In a similar vein, nelarabine is a pro-drug to an arabinose analog of guanosine (ara-G). As with ara-C, this molecule is incorporated into DNA and inhibits DNA synthesis. It is used for T-cell lymphoblastic leukemia and lymphoma.

Mercaptopurine and thioguanine are converted to pseudopurine nucleotides that feed back to inhibit the first step of de novo purine biosynthesis (glutamine 5-phosphoribosyl-pyrophosphate amino transferase). In addition, these drugs inhibit conversion of the purine precursor, inosinate, to adenylate or xanthylate, the precursor of guanylate. Dysfunctional RNA and DNA synthesis results. These drugs are also used to treat a variety of leukemias. As noted previously, bendamustine is a bifunctional agent containing a purine antimetabolite combined with a nitrogen mustard. Other purine analogs that work by incorporating into DNA and inhibiting DNA synthesis include cladribine, fludarabine, and clofarabine. Interestingly, despite similar mechanisms of action, these agents are approved for a variety of different cancers.

Two new antimetabolite drugs have been approved with a novel mechanism of action. Azacitidine and decitabine are two cytidine analogs that incorporate into DNA and inhibit DNA methyltransferase. This results in hypomethylated DNA (a key regulatory mechanism for global gene transcription). Both drugs have been approved for the treatment of myelodysplastic syndrome—a bone marrow disorder characterized by immature and abnormally functioning blood cells. Neutropenia, thrombocytopenia, and anemia are the most common side effects.

Methotrexate is structurally related to folic acid and competitively inhibits dihydrofolate reductase, preventing regeneration of tetrahydrofolate. Because tetrahydrofolate is an essential cofactor for synthesis of both purines and pyrimidines (thymidylate synthase), cellular DNA synthesis is diminished (Fig. 5-3). Methotrexate is used in the treatment of acute lymphoblastic leukemia and non-Hodgkin lymphoma. Interestingly, the drug is also used for symptomatic control of psoriasis and management of severe rheumatoid arthritis. Leucovorin, a derivative of folic acid, can be used as a rescue therapy to counteract adverse and sometimes life-threatening effects that high doses of methotrexate cause on the bone marrow. Methotrexate also has nephrotoxic effects at high doses, which can be minimized with good hydration and alkalinization of the urine to increase renal excretion of the drug. Pemetrexed is a newer generation dihydrofolate reductase inhibitor approved for mesothelioma and non–small-cell lung cancer.

Hydroxyurea, although not strictly a purine or pyrimidine analog, inhibits ribonucleotide reductase and prevents conversion of ribonucleotides to deoxyribonucleotides. Hydroxyurea is used to treat chronic myelogenous leukemia (CML).

Cytotoxic Antibiotics

Bleomycin, Dactinomycin, Daunorubicin, Doxorubicin, Epirubicin, Idarubicin, Mitomycin, Streptozocin, Valrubicin

Although each antibiotic in this category has a unique mechanism of action, they are cell cycle specific in their cytotoxicity, disrupting DNA function. In contrast to alkylating agents, these antibiotics *indirectly* damage DNA.

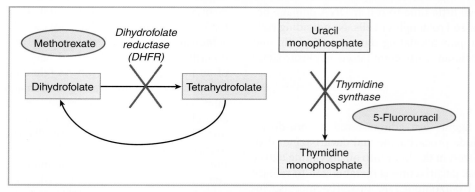

Figure 5-3. Multiple drugs inhibit thymidine synthesis. Tetrahydrofolate is a cosubstrate required for purine and pyrimidine biosynthesis (pyrimidine is shown here).

Dactinomycin interferes with RNA polymerase and thus prevents transcription. Dactinomycin is primarily used in the pediatric population and is approved for the treatment of Wilms' tumor, rhabdosarcoma, testicular carcinoma, and choriocarcinoma.

Bleomycin binds reduced iron and forms an intercalating complex with DNA (i.e., it inserts [intercalates] between adjacent bases in the double-stranded DNA). Upon oxidation of the iron complex, superoxide and hydroxyl radicals are formed that result in DNA strand breakage. Bleomycin is used for lymphomas, testicular carcinoma, and squamous cell carcinomas. In addition to general side effects (see Table 5-1), bleomycin is associated with the development of pulmonary fibrosis as well as hyperpigmentation of the hands. Bleomycin differs from most antineoplastic agents in that it rarely causes myelosuppression, but the drug does cause a high incidence of fever and chills.

Doxorubicin belongs to a class of antibiotics known as the *anthracyclines*, which inhibit transcription by impairing topoisomerase II, as well as by intercalating into DNA.

BIOCHEMISTRY

Topoisomerases

Topoisomerases help unwind intertwined DNA via transient cleavage of DNA strands. They are critical nuclear enzymes responsible for DNA replication, RNA transcription, and regulation of the tertiary structure of chromatin. Topoisomerases are elevated in multiple cancers and thus can be exploited as therapeutic targets. Antibiotic anthracyclines, such as doxorubicin, stabilize the topoisomerase cleavage sites in replicating DNA, leading to double-strand breaks and resultant apoptosis. Other nonantibiotic chemotherapeutics, including etoposide and teniposide, exert therapeutic efficacy by interacting with topoisomerases.

Doxorubicin and other anthracycline-like antibiotics (including daunorubicin, idarubicin, and epirubicin) intercalate nonspecifically between adjacent DNA pairs, thereby blocking DNA and RNA synthesis. Intercalation interferes with the normal DNA repair mechanisms of topoisomerase II. Doxorubicin is used widely in the treatment of acute leukemias, lymphomas, and various solid tumors. Doxorubicin (and other anthracyclines), at high doses, can produce irreversible, dose-dependent cardiotoxicity as a result of free radical damage. Idarubicin is a semisynthetic analog of daunorubicin and has been approved as an oral formulation outside the United States.

Mitotic Inhibitors

Docetaxel, Ixabepilone, Paclitaxel, Vincristine, Vinblastine, and Vinorelbine

Vincristine, vinblastine, and vinorelbine, often referred to as *Vinca alkaloids*, are metabolites derived from the periwinkle plant (*Vinca rosea*). These drugs inhibit polymerization of microtubules by binding to tubulin, leading to late G_2 growth arrest by disrupting mitotic filaments required for nuclear and cellular division. In contrast, paclitaxel, isolated from tree bark, enhances and stabilizes microtubule assembly. However, paclitaxel is equally cytotoxic, since it disrupts the dynamic equilibrium between tubulin monomers and dimers.

Vinca alkaloids are useful in management of acute leukemias, lymphomas, and some solid tumors. Vincristine is the "O" (for Oncovin, the trade name) in the MOPP and CHOP (cyclophosphamide + hydroxydaunorubicin + vincristine + prednisone) therapeutic regimens. Vinblastine is frequently used in combination with bleomycin and cisplatin for metastatic testicular carcinoma. Paclitaxel is used as primary or adjuvant therapy for ovarian and breast cancers. Ixabepilone, approved for the treatment of breast cancer, is a semisynthetic agent that binds directly to β-tubulin and suppresses microtubule dynamics.

In addition to myelosuppression and nausea and vomiting, vinca alkaloids can cause phlebitis and cellulitis. Additionally, peripheral neuropathy resulting in paresthesias, areflexia, or weakness occurs with vincristine. These neurologic and neuromuscular side effects, although reversible, often resolve very slowly. Interestingly, compared with most antineoplastic agents (including vinblastine), vincristine is associated with unusually low levels of bone marrow suppression. Paclitaxel can induce neutropenia and neuropathy. Hypersensitivity and cardiac reactions may also occur, caused by the excipient (polyoxyl castor oil), which solubilizes the intravenous formulation of the drug. Fortunately, this adverse effect can often be controlled with glucocorticoids or antihistamines.

BIOCHEMISTRY

Tubulin

Tubulin polymers and chromatin make up the mitotic spindle, which is part of the cytoskeleton and essential for internal movement of cellular components and organelles. The mitotic spindle is essential during cell division to ensure equal division of DNA into daughter cells. Tubulin polymers are composed of α- and β-monomers that elongate (the positive end) through dimerization and polymerization. The negative end of the tubulin polymer dissociates back into α- and β-tubulin monomers in a dynamic process. Drugs that are mitotic inhibitors impair this process by disrupting the equilibrium between polymerized and nonpolymerized microtubules. Ultimately, mitosis comes to a halt, and cell division is arrested at metaphase.

PATHOLOGY

Putting It Together—The ABVD Treatment Regimen for Stage III/IV Hodgkin Disease

A combinatorial therapy of a topoisomerase inhibitor (doxorubicin); a cytotoxic antibiotic (bleomycin); a tubulin-binding agent (vinblastine); and an alkylating agent (dacarbazine), together with radiotherapy, can lead to remission rates of greater than 80%. Potential adverse effects of bleomycin (pulmonary fibrosis) and doxorubicin (cardiomyopathy) may be lessened by use of drug combinations rather than high-dose monotherapy.

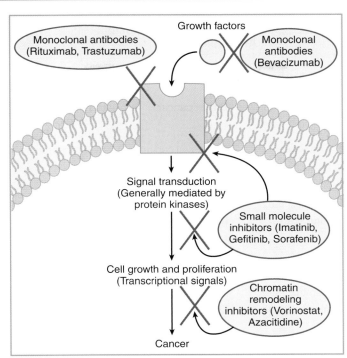

Figure 5-4. Biologics and signal transduction inhibitors. New generation anticancer drugs and immunomodulators are based on interruption of extra- and intracellular signaling. These newer agents bind to growth factors, growth factor receptors, signal transduction protein kinases, or factors responsible for regulating gene expression (chromatin and DNA modifiers).

⬤⬤⬤ BIOLOGICS AND SIGNAL TRANSDUCTION INHIBITORS

The latest generation of anticancer therapies focus not so much on killing dividing cells, but on depriving the cancer cells of key proliferation signals or environmental factors. In several of these new approaches, we are realizing a long-term goal of creating "magic bullets" that have the potential to specifically target the cancer cell while sparing the rest of the patient. Current therapies fall into two main camps. Biologics are agents produced by recombinant DNA technologies—primarily monoclonal antibodies or specific recombinant binding proteins—that deprive cells of specific growth signals or inhibit key receptors. Signal transduction modulators, on the other hand, are small molecule inhibitors (generally inhibitors of protein kinases) that shut off cell proliferation pathways (Fig. 5-4).

Monoclonal Antibodies

Alemtuzumab, Bevacizumab, Cetuximab, Gemtuzumab, Panitumumab, Rituximab, Tositumomab, and Trastuzumab

Note: Monoclonal antibody names always end in "-mab."

Use of monoclonal antibodies as therapeutics has revolutionized pharmacology, and these antibodies are now being extensively exploited as cancer therapies (Table 5-3). Gemtuzumab induces selective cytotoxicity of myelogenous leukemia cells by specifically interacting with the CD33 antigen, which is overexpressed on these cells. In a similar fashion, alemtuzumab interacts with the CD52 antigen to treat B-cell chronic lymphocytic leukemia.

Rituximab and tositumomab target non-Hodgkin B cells at their cell surface CD20 receptors. These two agents "flag" the B cells for destruction by the immune system. Rituximab enjoys widespread use in lymphomas, leukemias, and selected autoimmune diseases, as well as in transplant rejections. These extensive applications reflect the fact that this agent was the first of its kind and has a very favorable safety profile. Moreover, specifically targeting B cells obviously has uses in a variety of settings in which there is inappropriate proliferation of these cells or where the cells inappropriately target normal functions (e.g., rheumatoid arthritis). In an interesting modification, tositumomab is modified with radioactive iodine-131. Administration of this molecule "tags" the cells for imaging (I-131 releases gamma rays that can be detected) *and* destruction (I-131 also releases cytotoxic beta particles). This combinatorial approach is approved for use in non-Hodgkin lymphoma.

Trastuzumab targets overexpressed Her2/neu, an epidermal growth factor receptor for breast adenocarcinomas. The marked successes achieved with trastuzumab and breast cancer have been followed by the development of other epidermal growth factor receptor antibodies. Cetuximab and

TABLE 5-3. Clinical Uses of Monoclonal Antibodies (Mabs)

MAB	CLINICAL UTILITY	TARGET
Trastuzumab	Breast cancer	Her2/neu receptor (EGF receptor 2)
Cetuximab	Colorectal cancer and squamous cell carcinomas of the head and neck	EGF receptor 1
Panituximab	Colorectal cancer	EGF receptor 1
Rituximab	Non-Hodgkin lymphoma	CD20 (B-cell surface protein)
Tositumomab	Non-Hodgkin lymphoma	CD20
Gemtuzumab	Myeloid leukemia	CD33
Alemtuzumab	Chronic lymphocyte leukemia	CD52
Infliximab	Rheumatoid arthritis and Crohn disease	TNF
Abciximab	Antiplatelet therapy	IIb/IIIa receptors
Daclizumab	Transplant rejection	Interleukin-2 receptor
Muromonab	Transplant rejection	CD3
Bevacizumab	Non–small-cell lung cancer	VEGF

TNF, tumor necrosis factor; *VEGF*, vascular endothelial growth factor.

panitumumab bind to epidermal growth factor receptors and inhibit the growth and survival of tumors that express this particular receptor. Both agents have been approved for use in metastatic colorectal carcinoma, and cetuximab is also approved for squamous cell carcinoma of the head and neck.

Bevacizumab was the first angiogenesis inhibitor approved by the Food and Drug Administration. It acts by binding up circulating vascular endothelial growth factor—an important signal for new blood vessel formation and hence an important factor in the growth of solid tumors. Specifically, this is considered a neutralizing antibody in that it blocks natural growth factor signals. Used in combination with traditional alkylating agents and antimetabolites, bevacizumab has been approved for treatment of non–small-cell lung cancer as well as Her2-negative breast cancer.

Signal Transduction Inhibitors

Dasatinib, Erlotinib, Gefitinib, Imatinib, Lapatinib, Nilotinib, Sorafenib, Sunitinib, Vorinostat

Drug discovery has also begun to identify selective small molecule inhibitors of dysfunctional signaling targets in cancer cells.

As an example, imatinib (which is now more uniformly known internationally by its trade name, Gleevec) is the exemplar for the growing field of individualized medicine. Imatinib has revolutionized the treatment of CML. The majority of CML cases are characterized by an aberrant chromosome translocation (the Philadelphia chromosome) that produces a chimeric tyrosine kinase enzyme—bcr-abl. Imatinib is a selective kinase inhibitor that targets this specific dysfunctional enzyme by binding in the ATP site. Because of its selectivity, imatinib has a favorable side effect profile (minimal nausea, vomiting, edema). For those patients who develop resistance, two new drugs have been developed, dasatinib and nilotinib, which have a broader tyrosine kinase inhibition profile. Although these may provide cancer response, the broadened inhibition spectrum also produces more side effects (notably, myelosuppression).

As noted previously, monoclonal antibodies against the epidermal growth factor receptor (EGFR) have been developed as effective anticancer therapies. Similarly, small molecule inhibitors of EGFR have also been developed. Gefitinib was the first of these molecules and is an inhibitor of the tyrosine kinase activity of the EGFR receptor (also known as Her1 or ErbB1) and is approved for use in non–small-cell lung cancer. Given the lack of a long-term durable clinical response with gefitinib, it has been largely supplanted by erlotinib, which has a longer $t_{1/2}$ and is also approved for use in pancreatic cancer. The latest addition to this field is lapatinib, a molecule that inhibits both EGFR (ErbB1) and Her2 (ErbB2—the breast cancer trastuzumab target). As a result, lapatinib is currently approved for use in Her2-positive breast cancers that have not responded to trastuzumab therapy.

In recent years, several new drugs have been approved for treatment of renal cell carcinoma. The first two of these drugs were the multikinase inhibitors sorafenib and sunitinib. These two small molecules are closest in activity to erlotinib, the multikinase inhibitor approved for non–small-cell lung cancer described previously. They show a broad range of inhibitory activities including intracellular and extracellular kinases, as well as both tyrosine and serine/threonine kinases. Both compounds have potential adverse cardiac effects (cardiac ischemia and infarction for sorafenib; QT prolongation and torsades de pointes for sunitinib).

Finally, there are two new signal transduction modulators that do not fall into neat mechanistic categories. The first is vorinostat, a small-molecule histone deacetylase inhibitor. Histone acetylation in chromatin has recently been recognized as an important mechanism for regulating gene expression. Moreover, histone deacetylase activity is known to be upregulated in selected cancers. Vorinostat has been approved for use to treat cutaneous T-cell lymphoma—a general term for a selected group of T-cell non-Hodgkin lymphomas. Vorinostat is noteworthy in that it takes an extended period (2 to 6 months) to have a clinically beneficial effect. The second new class of compounds includes thalidomide (notorious for its association with birth defects in the 1950s and 1960s) and its analog lenalidomide. These compounds have been resurrected—and approved for use in multiple myeloma and myelodysplastic syndromes—based on their immunomodulatory, antiangiogenic, and antineoplastic activities. Given their known teratogenicity, these compounds are not to be used in pregnant women.

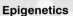

Epigenetics

The newest targets for anticancer therapies are focused on epigenetics. There is growing evidence that gene expression is regulated by events that happen to the DNA that are independent of mutations. That is, there are structural changes to the chromatin (posttranslational modification of histones [methylation and acetylation], and methylation of cytosine residues within CpG islands on DNA) that render genes more or less transcribable. New therapeutics (e.g., azacitidine, decitabine, and vorinostat) are targeted at these specific processes. These approaches remain largely nonspecific; in general, they do not target specific genes. Clearly, however, future generation agents will focus on the regulation of specific target genes.

●●● ENDOCRINE THERAPY

Some cancers are hormone dependent, and the growth of such tumors can be inhibited by surgically removing the source of the stimulating hormone. However, to avoid complications associated with surgical interventions, the use of hormonal antagonists (antihormones) is gaining preference (Table 5-4). Endocrine therapy can cause side effects, which generally are characterized by physiologic effects of the hormone being administered or antagonized. In general, side effects associated with endocrine therapy are considerably milder than those associated with cytotoxic agents.

As a case in point, patients with estrogen receptor–positive breast cancers have an approximately fivefold better outcome than patients with estrogen receptor–negative breast cancer.

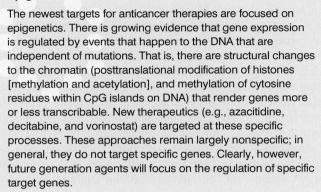

TABLE 5-4. Hormonal Agonists and Antagonists in Endocrine Therapy

HORMONE	CLINICAL USE
Estrogen antagonists (e.g., tamoxifen)	Competitive inhibition of estrogen receptors impairs stimulatory effect of estrogen on breast cancer cell division
Androgen antagonists (e.g., flutamide)	Useful in androgen-dependent prostate cancers
Estrogens (e.g., diethylstilbestrol)	Antiandrogenic effects can be used to suppress androgen-dependent prostate cancers
Progesterone derivatives	Useful in endometrial, prostate, and breast cancers
LHRH/GnRH	Used in androgen-dependent prostate cancers for their ability to inhibit LHRH/GnRH receptors via negative feedback (e.g., leuprolide)
Adrenocortical steroids (e.g., prednisone)	Inhibit growth of lymphoid tumors and hematologic neoplasms

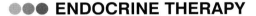

LHRH, luteinizing hormone–releasing hormone; *GnRH*, gonadotropin-releasing hormone agonist.

Tamoxifen, a selective estrogen receptor modulator, acts primarily as an estrogen receptor *antagonist* that competes for and blocks the promitogenic actions of endogenous estrogen in breast tissues. Tamoxifen may also exert *agonistic* estrogen-like actions in uterine tissue after long-term use (2 to 5 years) and is usually discontinued.

Circulating levels of estrogen can be maintained in postmenopausal women by a cytochrome P450 enzyme known as *aromatase*, which converts adrenal steroids (androstenedione and testosterone) to estrogens. Because breast cancer patients often have evidence of enhanced aromatase activity in tumors, drugs that inhibit aromatase are gaining popularity. Aromatase inhibitors (anastrazole, letrozole, exemestane) often are first-line therapies and have a lower risk of venous thromboemboli than does tamoxifen.

As another example of effective endocrine therapy, prostate tumors are particularly sensitive to antiandrogens or therapeutics that diminish endogenous concentrations of androgens. Flutamide is an androgen receptor antagonist that blocks androgen receptor function in the prostate, resulting in diminished DNA synthesis. Alternatively, subcutaneous administration of leuprolide, triptorelin, or goserelin, synthetic peptide analogs that act as luteinizing hormone–releasing hormone (LHRH; also known as gonadotropin-releasing hormone) receptor agonists, chronically downregulates LHRH receptors, resulting in low levels of testosterone and causing prostate-specific apoptosis. The adverse side effects associated with leuprolide and goserelin therapy include impotency, loss of bone mass, and immediate systemic allergic reactions. Whereas the LHRH agonists overstimulate and downregulate the LHRH receptors, abarelix and degarelix are synthetic decapeptides with strong LHRH antagonist activities. They therefore directly inhibit gonadotropin (and hence androgen) production. They have the advantage that they do not produce the initial testosterone surge characterized by the agonists (leuprolide, goserelin, and triptorelin).

Glucocorticoids are often integral components of combinatorial chemotherapeutic regimens (the final "P" in the CHOP and MOPP protocols is prednisone). For the most part, they are included as an immunosuppressant of white cells (Hodgkin disease). Moreover, they have ancillary benefits, including diminished inflammation, allergic reactions, neurologic side effects, and decreased emesis.

●●● INTRODUCTION TO IMMUNOPHARMACOLOGY

Relatively new in the arsenal against cancer, immunotherapy gained attention when it was observed that bacterial infections sometimes provoked regression of certain tumors. This is presumed to be due to indirect immunostimulation provided by the infection. Such observations have led to various immunologic approaches for cancer therapy, such as immunostimulatory cytokines, the use of tumor-specific monoclonal antibodies, and the potential of vaccines prepared from tumor cells.

Specifically, interferon-α has been used as an adjunctive therapy for chronic myelogenous leukemia and T-cell lymphomas.

Immunostimulation may be mediated by an increase in major histocompatibility complex expression, as well as by an increase in immune effector T and natural killer cells. In addition to immunostimulation, interferon-α may stimulate ribonucleases via 2′5′-oligoadenylate synthase activity. Major side effects of interferon therapy are malaise, fatigue, and fever. Interleukin (IL)-2 (aldesleukin) is also being used for melanoma and renal cell carcinoma.

Interestingly, recombinant human granulocyte colony–stimulating factor (filgrastim), and granulocyte-macrophage colony–stimulating factor (sargramostim) are now being used to reduce the severity and duration of neutropenia after successful cytotoxic therapy. In addition, IL-11 (oprelvekin), thrombopoietin, and erythropoietin are being evaluated to maximize platelet and red blood cell counts after chemotherapy (Table 5-5).

Immunosuppressive Agents

Cyclosporine, Pimecrolimus, Tacrolimus, Sirolimus, and Temsirolimus

Suppression of the immune system via pharmacologic agents is not only helpful for cancer therapy but also is used to treat autoimmune diseases, preventing host immune rejection to donor organ or transplant and suppressing donor immune responses against host antigens (graft-versus-host disease). For the most part, these agents (monoclonal antibodies, immunoglobulins, antibiotics, recombinant proteins, or receptors) restrict the proliferation or differentiation of B lymphoid cells, mediators of antibody formation and humoral immunity, as well as T lymphoid cells, responsible for cellular immunity. Various agents modulate components of the immune system as their primary targets, and an even larger number of drugs list "altered immune function" in their side effect profiles. Commonly used immunosuppressive agents include cyclosporine derivatives, mycophenolate mofetil, glucocorticoids, and modulators of tumor necrosis factor (TNF) activity.

Cyclosporine is a cyclic peptide derived from fungi that selectively inhibits T-cell receptor–mediated signal transduction (and therefore T-cell function). Cyclosporine enters T cells and specifically binds to cyclophilin, which leads to inhibition of a calcium-regulated cytoplasmic phosphatase known as calcineurin (Fig. 5-5). The resultant inhibition of the phosphatase leaves transcription regulators such as nuclear factor for activated T cells in a phosphorylated/inactive state (i.e., retained in cytosol), which can no longer facilitate the nuclear transcription of genes regulating the production of T-cell activators such as IL-2, IL-3, and interferon-γ. Because it suppresses overall T-cell function, the net effect of cyclosporine is impaired cell-mediated and antibody-specific immune responses. Tacrolimus functions similarly to cyclosporine to inhibit calcineurin, but its intracellular binding protein is known as FK-BP. The tacrolimus/FK-BP complex directly inhibits calcineurin. (This notation is derived from an earlier tacrolimus derivative, FK-506, which bound and activated a heat-shock protein, given the name FK-binding protein.) Sirolimus also binds to FK-BP but through undefined mechanisms does not inhibit calcineurin, instead inhibiting the promitogenic kinase m-TOR, which itself is regulated by IL-2. In a similar fashion, everolimus shares the primary mechanism of action as tacrolimus and sirolimus and has been approved for both preventing transplant rejection and treating cancer. Sirolimus is the principal active metabolite of the new pro-drug, temsirolimus, that has been approved as a cancer therapy. Temsirolimus and everolimus have been approved for the treatment of renal cell carcinoma.

Cyclosporine analogs are the drugs of choice to prevent graft or transplant rejection and graft-versus-host disease. Tacrolimus and pimecrolimus (a very similar compound) are also used topically to treat eczema. As an aside, sirolimus and paclitaxel have recently been approved as adjuvants to coronary stents for local drug delivery to limit vascular smooth muscle proliferation at the sites of coronary stent–induced restenosis (reblockage).

In contrast to most other immune suppressants, cyclosporine and tacrolimus do not cause myelosuppression. They do, however, exhibit marked nephrotoxicity (proximal tubule). Sirolimus can induce hyperlipidemia. Caution must be used if cyclosporine is administered in conjunction with other immunosuppressants because of increased susceptibility to infections and possible development of lymphoma. Cyclosporine analogs sold by different manufacturers are not bioequivalent and cannot be used interchangeably. Long-term topical use of tacrolimus and pimecrolimus appears to be associated with an increased risk of cancer, paradoxically.

TABLE 5-5. Clinical Uses of Recombinant Cytokines

CYTOKINE	CLINICAL UTILITY
G-CSF (filgrastim)	Bone marrow suppression; increases granulocytes
GM-CSF (sargramostim)	Bone marrow suppression, increases granulocytes
Thrombopoietin	Thrombocytopenia
Erythropoietin (epo)	Anemias
Interferon-α	Leukemias, melanoma, hepatitis B and C
Interferon-β	Multiple sclerosis
Interferon-γ	Chronic granulomatous disease
Interleukin-2 (aldesleukin)	Renal cell carcinoma and melanoma
Interleukin-11	Thrombocytopenia

G-CSF, granulocyte colony–stimulating factor; *GM-CSF*, granulocyte-macrophage colony–stimulating factor.

CLINICAL MEDICINE

Drug-Eluting Coronary Stents

Drug-eluting stents permit direct, local delivery of small quantities of immunosuppressive agents. Low doses of sirolimus or paclitaxel, delivered via drug-eluting coronary stents, reduce restenosis rates after angioplasty by diminishing neointimal hyperplasia and preventing subsequent reocclusion of the artery.

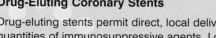

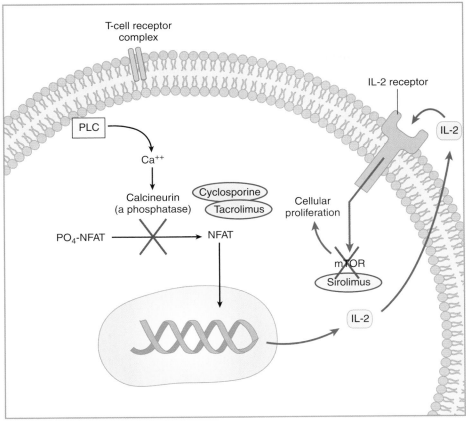

Figure 5-5. T-cell suppression by cyclosporine analogs. Analogs similar to sirolimus—temsirolimus (a sirolimus pro-drug) and everolimus—are used for renal cell carcinoma. In addition, everolimus is used for transplant rejection prophylaxis. *NFAT*, nuclear factor of activated T cells.

Mycophenolate Mofetil, and Azathioprine
Mechanism of action
These immunosuppressive drugs diminish B- and T-cell proliferation by inhibiting purine metabolism. Mycophenolate inhibits inosine monophosphate dehydrogenase, whereas azathioprine, through its metabolite mercaptopurine, impairs DNA replication by inserting itself into the replication fork as a pseudonucleotide.

Clinical use
Mycophenolate is one of the main drugs used to prevent transplant rejection, whereas azathioprine is used to treat various autoimmune illnesses.

Adverse effects
Myelosuppression is a major side effect with these drugs. Fortunately, the combination of mycophenolate with cyclosporine permits dosage of both drugs to be lower than if monotherapy were utilized, thus reducing the incidence of cyclosporine-induced nephrotoxicity.

Etanercept and Infliximab
Mechanism of action
Both these immunosuppressive agents decrease TNF activity and resultant activation of B and T cells. Etanercept is a circulating recombinant TNF receptor that serves as a reservoir to bind circulating TNF. Infliximab is a neutralizing monoclonal antibody that targets TNF.

Clinical use
Both agents are used to treat rheumatoid arthritis patients, and infliximab is also used to treat patients with Crohn disease.

Adverse effects
Both drugs can predispose patients to severe infections, cancers, or hypersensitivity reactions.

Glucocorticoids
A detailed discussion of glucocorticoids is found in Chapter 10. In terms of the immune system, glucocorticoids are used as adjunctive therapies in organ transplantation and autoimmune diseases. Glucocorticoids reduce activity of immune cells by inhibiting formation of proinflammatory phospholipase A_2 products, including prostaglandins, thromboxanes, and leukotrienes.

A summary of the use of monoclonal antibodies and recombinant cytokines in immune modulation was presented earlier in Tables 5-3 and 5-5.

●●● COMPLEMENTARY ALTERNATIVE MEDICINE FOR CANCER PREVENTION

The verdict is still out on the true effectiveness of complementary alternative medicines for cancer prevention. However, the following agents are routinely used by patients as putative preventative measures: garlic, green tea, folic acid, lycopene, saw palmetto, selenium, soy, St. John's wort, flaxseed, and wheat bran.

●●● TOP FIVE LIST

1. Most antineoplastic agents target dividing cells, whereas newer approaches target selectively overexpressed growth factors, growth factor receptors, or proliferation/survival signal transduction pathways.
2. Therapeutic regimens are often combinatorial, targeting multiple mechanisms of action to evade cancer cell resistance and dose-limiting toxicities.
3. Cancer cells have evolved multiple cellular mechanisms to evade the toxicities of antineoplastic agents.
4. Cytotoxic drugs damage DNA (disrupting DNA synthesis, replication, or repair) as well as alter microtubule function.
5. Immunotherapy is a double-edged sword: immunosuppression can be effective for myeloproliferative neoplastic disorders, whereas immunostimulation can be effective to reduce the severity of cytotoxic drug–induced neutropenia.

Self-assessment questions can be accessed at www. StudentConsult.com.

Autonomic Nervous System

6

CONTENTS

ORGANIZATION OF THE AUTONOMIC NERVOUS SYSTEM
Neurochemical Organization
Neuroreceptor Organization
Physiologic Responses
CHOLINERGIC SYSTEMS
Biochemistry of Cholinergic Systems
Cholinergic Receptor Subtypes
Nicotinic Drugs
Muscarinic Drugs
Acetylcholinesterase Inhibitors: Indirect-Acting
  Muscarinic and Nicotinic Receptor Agonists
ADRENERGIC SYSTEMS
Biochemistry of Adrenergic Systems
Adrenergic Receptor Subtypes
ADRENERGIC DRUGS
Alpha Drugs
Beta Drugs
CLINICALLY IMPORTANT INDIRECT EFFECTORS OF AUTONOMIC FUNCTION
TOP FIVE LIST

This chapter is all about diversity—diversity of receptors, that is. Similar receptor subtypes can produce differential effects if they are hard wired to different intracellular effectors and second messengers. In this way, the same neurotransmitter can have differing pharmacologic effects on target organs. This allows for specific drugs to target unique receptor subtypes. Nowhere is this more important than in the autonomic nervous system (ANS).

The ANS is the control mechanism for all automatic functions of the body. In essence, the ANS controls all the muscles of the body except skeletal muscles (the somatic nervous system). The difference between autonomic and somatic nervous systems is that the former controls functions that do not require conscious control (e.g., heart rate, blood pressure, gastrointestinal functions), whereas the latter is responsible for conscious control of movement (e.g., walking, driving, writing). Our minute-to-minute survival relies on coordinated control of autonomic functions; note that because the cranial nerves (representing a portion of the ANS) are intact, quadriplegic patients survive despite having no voluntary control from the neck down.

In general, there are two branches of the ANS that either speed or slow biologic processes. The *sympathetic* nervous system generally speeds things up ("fight or flight" functions), whereas the *parasympathetic* nervous system often slows things down ("rest and digest" functions). Key contrasting factors in the two branches of the ANS are summarized in Table 6-1.

It should be apparent from Table 6-1 that the branches of the ANS are fundamentally different in structure and function. In fact, the anatomy, neurochemistry, physiology, and pharmacology are distinct for each of the branches. Many of the neuropharmacologic and anatomic aspects of the ANS are summarized in Figures 6-1 and 6-2.

In general, both branches of the ANS are composed of a series of two nerve cells (a presynaptic neuron and a postsynaptic neuron) connected to each other at a ganglion synapse and connected to effector organs by another synapse. The key points to remember are (1) the specific neurotransmitter released at each anatomic location and (2) the corresponding receptor subtype to which neurotransmitters bind. With these pieces of information, the pharmacologic responses of organs can generally be predicted in light of the facts summarized in Table 6-1.

●●● ORGANIZATION OF THE AUTONOMIC NERVOUS SYSTEM

Neurochemical Organization

Figure 6-2 summarizes the structural organization of the ANS. Anatomic compartments of the ANS can be defined by the neurotransmitter used at each location. Surprisingly, there are only two major neurotransmitters at end organs in the ANS (acetylcholine [ACh] and norepinephrine). There is a single major neurotransmitter at every autonomic ganglion in the body (regardless of whether it is parasympathetic or sympathetic)—the neurotransmitter is ACh. This includes the specialized ganglion that is the adrenal medulla. In addition, the neurotransmitter at parasympathetic effector organs is also ACh. Although it is not the subject of this chapter, the somatic motor nervous system is also briefly discussed because the neurotransmitter at the neuromuscular junction is also ACh. How can so many different physiologic functions be driven by the same simple neurochemical—ACh? This critical question can be answered by the various ACh receptor subtypes that receive this chemical signal.

TABLE 6-1. Autonomic Nervous System

SYMPATHETIC	PARASYMPATHETIC
Fight or flight	Rest and digest
Stress responder	Resting homeostasis
"Whip" ("driving" the system)	"Reins" (tonic control)
Systemic "fire alarm"	Discrete localization of control

ANATOMY

Central Nervous System

Recall that the nervous system is composed of unique cell types. Whereas the typical liver cell might be 20 μm on a side, a single autonomic cell might be 10 μm across at the cell body, but it sends a long fiber called an axon (less than 1 μm in diameter) literally tens of centimeters away. The sympathetic nervous system originates from the thoracolumbar regions of the spinal cord and travels a short distance to the paravertebral chain ganglia. After neurochemical communication from presynaptic fibers, a long axon from a postsynaptic cell travels to innervated organs where it synapses with muscle. Because there is signal amplification as the cells leave these ganglia (few preganglionic fibers in and many fibers out) and go out to numerous organs, the sympathetic nervous system has global effects on physiology (a global "fire alarm"). On the parasympathetic side, cells originate from craniosacral regions of the spinal cord and send long fibers to synapse in organ-specific ganglia where short postganglionic fibers innervate target organs. This specific innervation of a particular organ provides for point-to-point, discrete regulation of physiology by the parasympathetic nervous system. The adrenal medulla can be considered a specialized version of the sympathetic nervous system; signals from a long presynaptic axon trigger the release of a circulating hormone from the specialized ganglion-like cell in the gland.

The preceding paragraph deals with the preganglionic fibers and postganglionic parasympathetic fibers. On the other hand, the neurotransmitter at most sympathetic effector synapses is the chemical norepinephrine (or epinephrine in the case of the neurohormone released from the adrenal medulla). Note that specialized exceptions exist in the case of certain sweat glands (sympathetic ACh innervation) and renal vasculature (sympathetic dopamine).

Neuroreceptor Organization

There are essentially three classes of neurotransmitter receptors in the ANS, with a number of different receptor subtypes (Table 6-2):

- Nicotinic ACh
- Muscarinic ACh
- Adrenergic norepinephrine/epinephrine

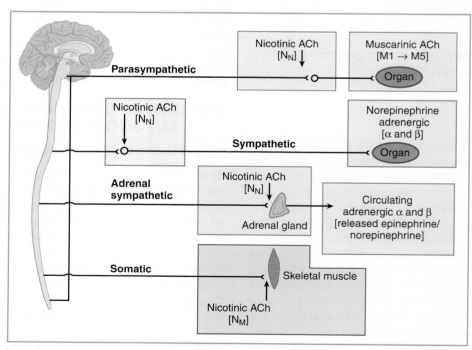

Figure 6-1. Autonomic and somatic physiology and pharmacology: neuroanatomic compartments. Note that the sympathetic and parasympathetic systems have two nerve components: presynaptic and postsynaptic. The adrenal gland functions as a neurohormone system that releases norepinephrine and epinephrine into the circulation where the neurotransmitters elicit the systemwide "fight or flight" response. The somatic nervous system uses a single long motor neuron that is functionally similar to a presynaptic autonomic neuron. *ACh,* acetylcholine; N_N, neuron-type nicotinic receptor; N_M, neuromuscular-type nicotinic receptor; *M,* muscarinic receptor (five subtypes); α/β, alpha-type and beta-type adrenergic receptors.

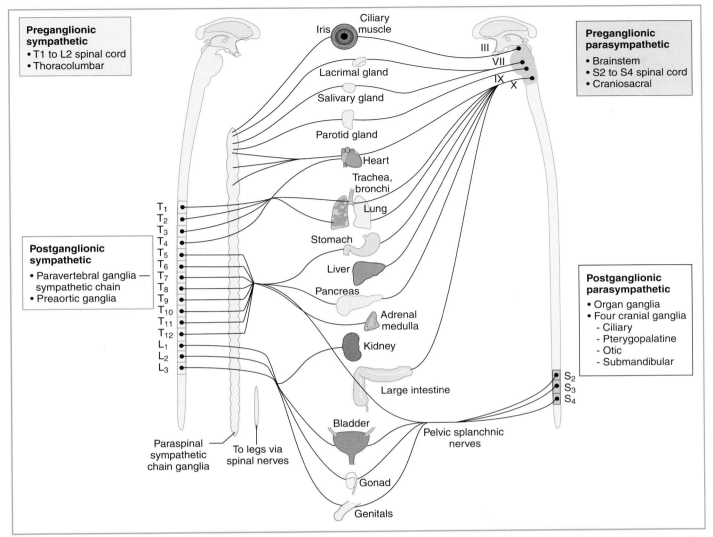

Figure 6-2. Anatomic organization of the autonomic nervous system. The sympathetic and parasympathetic systems are structurally distinct.

TABLE 6-2. Autonomic Receptor Subtypes

RECEPTOR CLASS	RECEPTOR SUBTYPES
Nicotinic	1. Ganglionic (N_N; neuronal) 2. Neuromuscular junction (N_M; muscle)
Muscarinic	1. M2 and M4 (M_{even}) 2. M1, M3, M5 (M_{odd})
Adrenergic	1. Alpha (α_1 and α_2) 2. Beta (β_1, β_2, and β_3)

For ACh, there are nicotinic receptors (defined by a prototypical agonist that activates these receptors—nicotine) and muscarinic receptors. Nicotinic receptors come in two types: (1) ganglionic nicotinic receptors found in ganglia/adrenal gland and (2) neuromuscular nicotinic receptors found at the end plate of the somatic (voluntary) motor nervous system. Parasympathetic end-organs contain different ACh receptors that are stimulated by the prototypical agonist muscarine; thus these receptors are called *muscarinic cholinergic receptors*.

Finally, the sympathetic nervous system contains two kinds of adrenergic receptor subtypes: (1) α-adrenoceptors and (2) β-adrenoceptors. Each of these classes has several receptor subtypes. Luckily for the clinician, although this seems to be a dizzying array of different receptor subtypes, a set of "rules" help master the underlying physiology and pharmacology.

Physiologic Responses

Table 6-3 is a simplified summary of organ responses to sympathetic and parasympathetic stimulation. Understanding this table helps predict pharmacologic responses to autonomic agonists and antagonists. For example, consider the heart—one of the simplest organs from an autonomic standpoint. The heart functions with an intrinsic pacemaker function. The ANS either speeds or slows this rhythm depending on need. Stimulation of the parasympathetic nervous

TABLE 6-3. Physiologic Response to Autonomic Nerve Activity

ORGAN OR SYSTEM	DOMINANT TONE	CHOLINERGIC RESPONSE (RECEPTOR)	ADRENERGIC RESPONSE (RECEPTOR)
Heart	Parasympathetic	Decreased rate (M_2) Decreased force (M_2)	Increased rate (β_1) Increased force (β_1)
Blood vessels	Sympathetic	Dilation Muscarinic receptors are present but not innervated Dilation mediated by nitric oxide	Biphasic Constriction (α_1): resting tone increases blood pressure Dilation (β_2): decreases TPR and blood pressure
Bronchial tree	Parasympathetic	Bronchoconstriction	Bronchodilation β_2-receptors are present but not innervated
Eye			
Iris, radial muscle	Sympathetic	—	Contraction (mydriasis; α_1)
Iris, sphincter	Parasympathetic	Contraction (miosis)	—
Ciliary muscle	Parasympathetic	Contraction (near vision)	Relaxation (β_2) (allows for far vision)
Gastrointestinal			
Motility	Parasympathetic	Increased motility	Decrease motility (α_1)
Sphincters	Parasympathetic	Relaxation	Constrict (α_1)
Secretions	Parasympathetic	Stimulation	Decrease (α_1)
Urinary bladder			
Detrusor	Parasympathetic	Contraction	Relaxation (via β_2)
Trigone and sphincter	Sympathetic	Relaxation	Contraction (via α_1)
Sweat and salivary glands	Parasympathetic	Increased secretion	Increased secretion (via α_1)

TPR, Total peripheral resistance.

system slows the heart and decreases contractility. Conversely, stimulation of the sympathetic nervous system increases heart rate and increases the force of contraction to effectively increase cardiac output. Injection of epinephrine, a sympathetic agonist, increases cardiac output, whereas administration of propranolol, a nonselective β-adrenergic blocker (sympathetic antagonist), decreases cardiac output. Table 6-3 therefore is an important resource for understanding underlying mechanisms that modulate autonomic function.

An important aspect of Table 6-3 is the designation of the autonomic branch that exerts the dominant tone at rest. This is generally the parasympathetic nervous system ("rest and digest"); however, there are several noteworthy exceptions. Foremost is the control of peripheral resistance and blood pressure. The dominant tone for blood pressure regulation is mediated via the sympathetic nervous system because there is no parasympathetic regulation of the peripheral vasculature. There are no parasympathetic nerves that communicate with receptors on the vasculature. On the other hand, there are sympathetic nerves that communicate with vasculature receptors (α_1) to constrict the vessels and increase peripheral resistance and blood pressure. This is how blood pressure is regulated in a resting state. In times of great stress, however ("fight or flight"), circulating epinephrine binds to a different set of receptors—the noninnervated β-receptors—leading to decreased resistance and greater delivery of blood and O_2 to the peripheral muscles. These important pharmacologic and physiologic concepts are explored in greater detail later in this chapter.

Thus, to review autonomic pharmacology, it is essential to review the underlying autonomic physiology to understand the following:

- What are the responses to sympathetic and parasympathetic stimulation?
- Which autonomic system exerts dominant neural control in various tissues?
- What types of receptors are present in each organ?

This last question provides the opportunity to design and develop selective pharmacotherapeutic agents.

●●● CHOLINERGIC SYSTEMS

Biochemistry of Cholinergic Systems

The synthesis and degradation of ACh are the same at all locations. Indeed, the synthesis/metabolism of ACh is elegant in its simplicity. Figure 6-3 describes the creation and destruction of ACh. This neurotransmitter is generated by a simple chemical condensation between choline (a chemical constituent of diet-derived lecithin [phosphatidyl choline]) and acetyl–coenzyme A (CoA) (a ubiquitous energy source derived from glycolysis via the pyruvate dehydrogenase complex reaction).

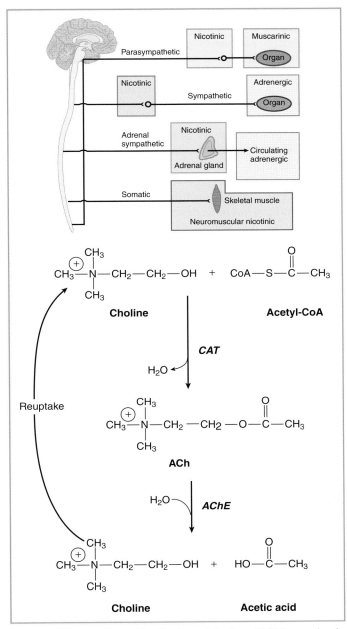

Figure 6-3. Parasympathetic (acetylcholine [*ACh*]) synthesis and degradation. ACh is synthesized from choline and acetyl–coenzyme A (*CoA*), a reaction that is catalyzed by choline acetyltransferase. Once released into the synapse, ACh is degraded by acetylcholinesterase into choline (which gets recycled for reuse) and acetate. This process takes place in all the colored boxes.

BIOCHEMISTRY

Two Forms of Acetylcholinesterase

An important pharmacologic aspect of the cholinergic system is that there are two forms of AChE. The first is a "true" cholinesterase that resides in the synapse and serves no role other than to break down the ACh neurotransmitter. On the other hand, there is also a nondiscriminating circulating esterase that has broad substrate specificity and essentially cleaves any ester bond. This latter enzyme appears to function

as a detoxifying enzyme and efficiently scavenges any circulating ACh. It is so efficient that it prevents detection of naturally circulating ACh and, more importantly, eliminates the possibility of using ACh directly as a pharmacologic agent. Any exogenous ACh injected is eliminated almost instantaneously.

BIOCHEMISTRY

Role of Amino Acids and Metabolic Intermediaries

Amino acids and metabolic intermediaries serve a variety of functions, in addition to being the building blocks of proteins and providing sources of energy, respectively. In the present context, acetyl-CoA is normally considered to be a product of glycolysis, and choline is a dietary molecule that becomes a part of structural lipids (phosphatidylcholine). However, in selected neurons, these substrates are diverted to neurotransmitter biosynthesis (ACh). Similarly, many amino acids (glutamate, aspartate, glycine, tryptophan, and tyrosine) are used as neurotransmitters directly or are converted to neurotransmitters. The key point to understand, however, is that this has to be a regulated process. Neurotransmitter products represent such a small percentage of the cellular need for these molecules that it would be detrimental to divert them in an unrestricted manner. Therefore neurotransmitter biosynthetic enzymes tend to be heavily regulated. Tyrosine hydroxylase, for instance, is the first and rate-limiting step in norepinephrine synthesis. This single enzyme is the subject of nearly every form of enzyme regulation that has been characterized (transcriptional, translational, and posttranslational regulation; feedback inhibition; allosteric modulation; protein stability; alternative RNA splicing). Therefore its tight regulation leads to a well-controlled diversion of tyrosine to neurotransmitter synthesis from its larger role in protein synthesis.

Choline and acetyl-CoA are condensed in neurons via the enzyme, choline acetyltransferase, and packaged as the neurotransmitter ACh. Neurons release the neurotransmitter on demand and a physiologic response is stimulated depending on the type of postjunctional receptor and its anatomic location. When the neuron completes its required stimulation—presumably after eliciting a physiologic response—further release of ACh is terminated. Neurotransmitter in the synapse is rapidly degraded by a highly efficient hydrolase, acetylcholinesterase (AChE). The products of hydrolysis are choline and acetate, which can both be reused. Both elegant and simple, this is the biologic equivalent of on-demand synthesis. It is worth noting that confusion commonly arises at this point from the unfortunate similarity in the names of the synthetic and degradative enzymes (choline acetyltransferase and AChE). Recall that the latter is an esterase that *degrades* ester bonds, whereas the former transfers a choline onto an acetate group (*creating* an ester bond).

Cholinergic Receptor Subtypes

Given the universal and widespread distribution of the ACh system, how does the body generate diversity in physiologic responses? The answer resides in the diversity of ACh receptor subtypes. Specifically, there are two major classes of ACh receptors (muscarinic and nicotinic) having different functions, different signal transduction mechanisms, and, significantly, differing pharmacologic characteristics (see Table 6-2). As noted in Figure 6-1, the neuronal synapse found at a ganglion contains one type of nicotinic receptor (N_N). The neuromuscular junction at the skeletal muscle within the somatic (voluntary) nervous system contains a different, but related, nicotinic receptor (N_M). Finally, parasympathetic end organs synthesize and express muscarinic ACh receptors with fundamentally distinct pharmacologic and cell biologic characteristics. Five different subtypes of muscarinic receptors (designated M1 through M5) are found in the end organs innervated by the parasympathetic system.

Nicotinic Receptors

The pharmacologic profiles of the receptors reside in different anatomic compartments within the ANS. When a neuronal action potential arrives at the nerve terminal, there is Ca^{++}-mediated release of ACh into the cleft. Target cells (postganglionic nerve cell or muscle) express nicotinic receptor subtypes. These receptors derive their name from the fact that they are stimulated by the tobacco plant alkaloid nicotine. Nicotinic ACh receptors (nAChR) form a pore and serve as ligand-gated ion channels (Fig. 6-4). When the nAChR is stimulated, the channel opens and allows Na^+ to rush into the cell. This triggers depolarization of the cell and elicits a neuronal action potential (in a postganglionic nerve) or muscle contraction (in skeletal muscle). Although the receptors on skeletal muscle and ganglionic nerves are both nicotinic, they are composed of different subunits. As distinct entities, they are therefore designated as neuronal (in this case ganglionic) nicotinic receptors (N_N AChR) or skeletal muscle nicotinic receptors (N_M AChR). Their physiologic functions are identical, but their pharmacologic responses can be discriminated through the use of selective ligands or through differential adaptations to stimulation.

Muscarinic Receptors

On reexamining Figure 6-1, it is apparent that there are yet other forms of ACh receptors—the muscarinic receptors—present on postganglionic target organs of the parasympathetic nervous system. These receptors are superficially different from nicotinic receptors because they are stimulated by the plant alkaloid muscarine instead of by nicotine. On a more fundamental level, however, these receptors act in a different manner from nicotinic receptors and elicit different kinds of physiologic effects. First, rather than being multimeric receptors that form ion channels, the muscarinic receptors are classical single subunit, 7-transmembrane-spanning domain, G-protein–coupled receptor proteins (7TM-GPCR) (see Fig. 6-4B). This information points out that these are proteins that elicit their actions through guanosine triphosphate–binding protein signal transduction

(cyclic adenosine monophosphate [cAMP] vs. phosphatidylinositides) (for review, see Chapter 2).

Studying the pharmacologic nature of muscarinic receptors is simultaneously a good news/bad news situation. The bad news is that there are five subtypes of muscarinic receptors, termed M1 through M5 AChR (numbered in order of their discovery). These receptors have different signal transduction mechanisms based on the G-protein to which they are coupled. However, the good news is that they fall into two broad categories: M1/M3/M5 stimulate inositol trisphosphate production, whereas M2/M4 inhibit cAMP production. Finally, although muscarinic receptors have differential anatomic distribution and physiologic functions, discriminating agonists and antagonists have yet to be developed (i.e., there are few drugs in clinical use that selectively interact with one muscarinic receptor over another).

To summarize, there are two broad classes of ACh receptors—nicotinic and muscarinic (Table 6-4). Nicotinic receptors are found in (1) the autonomic ganglion and (2) the neuromuscular junction. Nicotinic receptors are always excitatory (they are ligand-gated Na channels that cause depolarization). Although there are two distinct types of nAChR (N_N and N_M), they share the following pharmacologic feature: they are stimulated by the prototypical agonist nicotine.

At parasympathetic end-organs, ACh receptors are one of the five subtypes M1 through M5. These are all 7TM-GPCRs and couple either to phospholipase C (M1/M3/M5, leading to Ca^{++} mobilization and contraction; Fig. 6-5) or the inhibitory G-protein (M2/M4, leading to decreased cAMP and decreased activity; Fig. 6-6). As a result of their coupling mechanisms, muscarinic receptors can be either stimulatory or inhibitory. The muscarinic receptors are defined pharmacologically by the fact that they are stimulated by muscarine and blocked by the antagonist atropine.

Various pharmacologic compounds interact with and modulate the cholinergic aspects of the ANS. Prototypical agonists at nicotinic and muscarinic receptors are listed in Table 6-5.

Nicotinic Drugs

Drugs that modulate nicotinic receptors have limited applications because of the anatomic localization of these receptor subtypes (see Fig. 6-1). Specifically, pharmacologic stimulation of ganglionic neuronal AChR (N_N) has limited utility because it affects both branches of the ANS, eliciting opposing effects. Intentional stimulation would therefore be counterproductive. Moreover, any agent that lacks specificity for the N_N receptor and crosses, pharmacologically, to the N_M version of the receptor would have untoward side effects in terms of skeletal muscle stimulation.

In spite of these considerations, one nicotine agonist is among the most widely used drugs in the world (i.e., nicotine itself). Despite significant side effects and reinforcing/rewarding aspects of nicotine use, social pressures drive individuals to use this drug via tobacco to the point at which side effects become minimal because of tolerance. Pharmacologically, nicotine patches, inhalers, gums, and lozenges are used by patients in attempts to wean themselves from cigarette dependence.

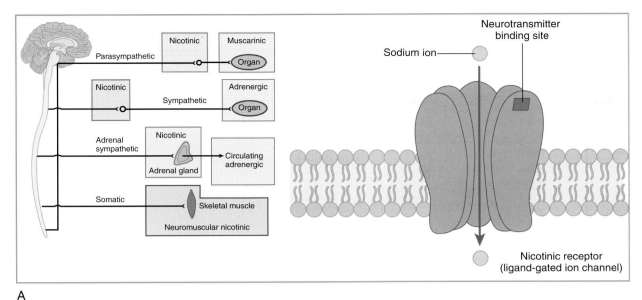

Figure 6-4. Schematic diagrams of the parasympathetic (acetylcholine) receptors. **A,** Nicotinic receptors (N_N or N_M) are ligand-gated ion channels. After stimulation, the resulting depolarization in neurons (N_N type) leads to a neuronal action potential, whereas depolarization in muscles (N_M type) leads to muscular contraction. **B,** Acetylcholine muscarinic receptors are 7-transmembrane domain G-protein–coupled receptors (*7TM-GPCR*) found at postganglionic terminals, representing the parasympathetic innervation of an end-organ. Note that the muscarinic receptor can be either stimulatory or inhibitory depending on the signal transduction mechanism to which it is coupled. As before (see Fig. 6-3) these two types of ACh receptors are in the colored compartments.

TABLE 6-4. Nicotinic Versus Muscarinic Receptors

RECEPTOR	STRUCTURE	FUNCTION	MECHANISM	AGONIST	ANTAGONIST
Nicotinic	Multisubunit channel (five subunits)	Excitatory	Ligand-gated Opens Na^+ channel	ACh; nicotine	Curare (neuromuscular only)
Muscarinic	7-Transmembrane receptor (one subunit)	Excitatory or inhibitory (depends on subtype and mechanism)	M1/M3/M5 GPCRs stimulate PLC M2/M4 inhibit cAMP synthesis and Ca^{++} while stimulating K^+ channels	ACh; muscarine	Atropine

ACh, acetylcholine; *GPCR*, G-protein–coupled receptor proteins; *PLC*, phospholipase C.

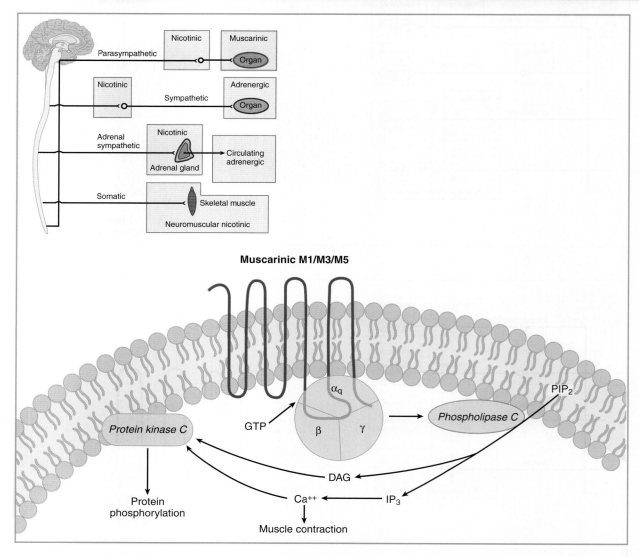

Figure 6-5. Muscarinic M1/M3/M5 acetylcholine receptors. The "odd" class of muscarinic receptors works through an α_q G-protein to activate a membrane-associated phospholipase C. *GTP*, guanosine triphosphate; *DAG*, diacylglycerol; *IP*, inositol triphosphate.

Nicotinic Agonists

Nicotine

Stimulation of nicotinic receptors can be accomplished in two ways: direct or indirect agonists. In the former case, nicotine can be administered as a direct pharmacologic agonist. In the latter case (indirect agonists), agents that inhibit degradation of ACh (AChE inhibitors) are powerful agents. Cholinesterase inhibitors are considered as a separate drug class because of their clinical uses, their potential uses as biochemical weapons, and because they have both muscarinic and nicotinic activities. In general, with the exception of recreational use of nicotine in tobacco (or its use in tobacco cessation), there are few applications for direct-acting nicotinic ganglionic (N_N) agonists. No matter how they are stimulated, nicotinic stimulation has a variety of side effects including nausea, vomiting, diarrhea, salivation, sweating, and dizziness.

Nicotinic Antagonists

Atracurium, Curare, Mecamylamine, Mivacurium, Pancuronium, Rocuronium, Succinylcholine, Trimethaphan, and Vecuronium

Nicotinic antagonists discriminate between the ganglionic (neuronal, N_N) and the neuromuscular nicotinic AChR (N_M) receptors. Several agents (e.g., mecamylamine, trimethaphan) act as ganglionic receptor antagonists (N_N) (see Fig. 6-1). Curare shows selectivity for the N_M neuromuscular junction receptor. (Historically, South American Indians used curare on the tips of their arrows while hunting to paralyze their prey.) There are very few uses for ganglionic antagonists; they are used only to elicit controlled hypotension during surgery or manage some cases of hypertensive crisis.

The N_M nAChR is an important target for inducing skeletal muscle paralysis for surgery and/or endrotracheal intubation. With skeletal muscle paralysis induced, less general anesthetic

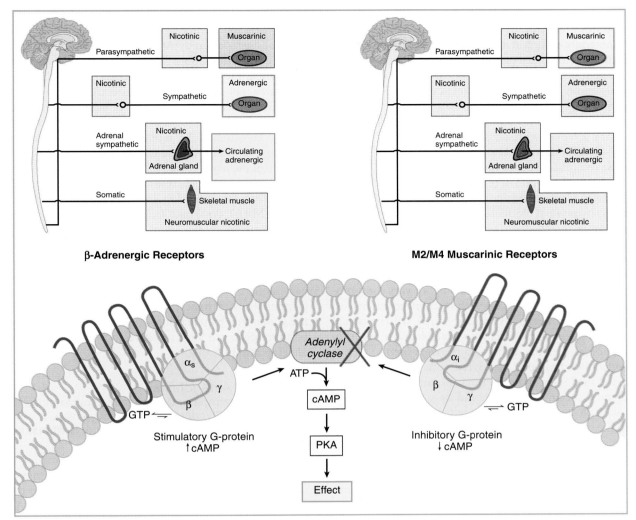

Figure 6-6. Reciprocal regulation of adenylyl cyclase by muscarinic and adrenergic receptors. **A,** The M2/M4 "even" class of muscarinic receptors works through an α_i-inhibitory G-protein to reduce synthesis of cyclic adenosine monophosphate (*cAMP*). This inhibition results in reduced intracellular signaling. **B,** The β-adrenergic receptors work through an α_s-stimulatory G-protein to activate adenylyl cyclase and increase the production of cAMP from adenosine triphosphate. These receptors frequently reside on the same organs to provide reciprocal regulation. *PKA,* protein kinase A; *GTP,* guanosine triphosphate.

TABLE 6-5. Pharmacology of Acetylcholine-like Agonists

AGONIST	DEGRADATION BY CHOLINESTERASE	MUSCARINIC RECEPTOR ACTIVITY	ATROPINE ANTAGONISM	NICOTINIC RECEPTOR ACTIVITY
Acetylcholine	+++	++	+++	++
Methacholine	+	++	+++	+
Carbachol	—	++	+	+++
Bethanechol	—	+++	+++	—
Muscarine	—	+++	+++	—
Pilocarpine	—	+++	+++	—

+++, Strong effect; ++, moderate effect; +, low effect; —, no effect.

may be required during surgery, which can reduce postoperative respiratory and cardiovascular depression. Two classes of N_M antagonists (succinylcholine and curare-like compounds) are used to induce paralysis (1) in situations in which controlled ventilation is needed and (2) to eliminate the muscular manifestations of tonic clonic seizures. Remember that these agents cause paralysis but have no analgesic properties.

Blockade of neuromuscular junction ACh receptors (N_M AChR) can be achieved with succinylcholine. This drug is essentially a tail-to-tail condensation of two ACh molecules. There is a two-phase response when succinylcholine binds to N_M AChR. Phase I involves stimulation of receptors, with associated muscle contraction. Continued stimulation, however, is followed fairly rapidly by phase II blockade. This produces a desensitization of receptors, making them refractory to subsequent stimulation. For this reason, succinylcholine is often referred to as a *depolarizing muscle relaxant*. When using succinylcholine, it is important to remember that the drug has a very short half-life ($t_{1/2}$)—less than 8 minutes—so it is used only for very short procedures. Skeletal muscle blockade with succinylcholine first affects muscles that move rapidly (e.g., eye, jaw), with limbs and the diaphragm affected last. Recovery from blockade occurs in the reverse order (i.e., the diaphragm recovers first).

Succinylcholine has been associated with transient hyperkalemia and malignant hyperthermia. Because of the risk of hyperkalemia, succinylcholine should be used cautiously in patients with electrolyte imbalances or those using certain antiarrhythmic drugs. Malignant hyperthermia can be managed by administration of dantrolene sodium, which uncouples excitation-contraction coupling in muscle cells by preventing release of Ca^{++} from the sarcoplasmic reticulum. Patients taking aminoglycosides may be at greater risk of prolonged paralysis. On the other hand, patients with myasthenia gravis may be resistant to the effects of succinylcholine.

Whereas succinylcholine binds to N_M AChR in a *noncompetitive* fashion (the drug cannot be displaced by increasing ACh concentrations), curare-like direct-acting N_M AChR antagonists (atracurium, mivacurium, pancuronium, vecuronium, and rocuronium) are *competitive* antagonists (effects of the drugs can be reversed by increasing ACh in the synapse). Compared with succinylcholine, the curare-derivatives have longer half-lives. Atracurium is somewhat unique in that it is spontaneously hydrolyzed. Likewise, mivacurium is inactivated by plasma cholinesterase. Therefore, the actions of these two drugs are terminated regardless of hepatic or renal function.

Muscarinic Drugs

Although nicotinic agents do not enjoy widespread clinical use, there are several important applications for muscarinic agents. However, there is a major limitation to the use of these drugs, because relatively few are selective for M2/M4 versus M1/M3/M5 receptor subclasses.

Muscarinic Agonists
Bethanechol, Carbachol, Muscarine, and Pilocarpine
Muscarine is the prototypical agonist for all muscarinic receptors (muscarine is an alkaloid derived from mushrooms and is associated with toxicity when poisonous mushrooms are

ingested). A few drugs that are derivatives of ACh have proven effective as therapeutic agents, in part because of their resistance to degradation by AChE (see Table 6-5).

Because of limitations in receptor specificity, applications for muscarinic agonists are limited. Notably, pilocarpine and carbachol are used ocularly to treat glaucoma because these drugs facilitate the outflow of aqueous humor, thereby reducing intraocular pressure. Pilocarpine is also used orally to treat xerostomia (dry mouth). Bethanechol is used to treat urinary retention (because it stimulates detrusor contraction [muscle of the bladder wall] and relaxes the trigone/sphincter) and nonobstructive gastrointestinal hypomotility.

However, muscarinic agonists have serious side effects, including SLUD syndrome (*s*alivation, *l*acrimation, *u*rination, *d*efecation). Moreover, they are contraindicated in patients with asthma because they cause bronchoconstriction and increase mucous secretions. Muscarinic-induced hypotension can lead to serious problems associated with reduced coronary blood flow. In addition, these drugs are contraindicated in patients with hyperthyroidism because the body reacts to hypotension by releasing norepinephrine. Patients with hyperthyroidism are very sensitive to norepinephrine and can develop atrial fibrillation.

Muscarinic Antagonists
Atropine, Benztropine, Darifenacin, Dicyclomine, Fesoterodine, Glycopyrrolate, Hyoscyamine, Ipratropium, Oxybutynin, Scopolamine, Solifenacin, Tiotropium, Tolterodine, and Trospium
Atropine, scopolamine, and the related muscarinic antagonists work by competitive antagonism. That is, they bind to muscarinic receptors, have no intrinsic activity after this binding, and block the ability of the endogenous ligand—ACh—to bind. However, few of these drugs demonstrate selectivity for any of the five muscarinic receptor subtypes. Interestingly, in spite of being similar in structure, atropine has fewer central nervous system (CNS) effects than scopolamine and is favored for peripheral applications. However, scopolamine continues to be used as a transdermal patch in the treatment of motion sickness and in postoperative nausea and vomiting.

A major use for muscarinic antagonists is in the treatment of AChE poisoning (see the next section), which produces a dramatic increase in ACh. In fact, atropine is the drug of choice for treating accidental poisoning (typically because of accidental insecticide poisoning or deliberate nerve gas poisoning). In addition, it has been issued in battlefield settings (both Gulf Wars) for use in the event of nerve agent attacks using anticholinesterase agents. Clinically, drugs that work by this mechanism may also be used in ophthalmology to produce mydriasis (dilation of the pupil) and cycloplegia (loss of accommodation or inability to focus).

In the respiratory system, ipratropium and tiotropium are used to block bronchoconstrictive muscarinic tone in the lungs and reduce bronchial secretions. These drugs are used in management of chronic obstructive pulmonary disease.

Numerous muscarinic receptor antagonists are also available to treat overactive bladder episodes. Antimuscarinic drugs reduce the number of incontinent episodes, increase the amount of urine the bladder can hold, reduce the frequency of urination, and decrease urgency. Drugs include oxybutynin, tolterodine, trospium, solifenacin, darifenacin, and fesoterodine. Each of these drugs is available in oral dose forms. Additionally, oxybutynin is available as a transdermal patch. The patch appears to have fewer adverse effects compared with the oral formulation, probably as a result of lower blood levels of the active metabolite that causes the anticholinergic adverse effects. Three of the drugs—solifenacin, trospium, and darifenacin—are said to be specific antagonists at M3 receptors. However, this reported selectivity does not manifest itself as improved efficacy or reduced side effects. (Because each of these agents slows voiding, they are not appropriate for individuals prone to urinary retention [e.g., men with benign prostatic hypertrophy].) In addition, the newest agent—fesoterodine—is closely related to tolterodine, and they are metabolized to the same active chemical compound.

Other muscarinic receptor antagonists include dicyclomine and hyoscyamine, which are used to treat the irritable bowel syndrome type of gastrointestinal hypermotility and spasticity. Benztropine, which crosses the blood-brain barrier, may be used to decrease tremors in Parkinson disease, whereas glycopyrrolate is used to dry glandular secretions (e.g., during surgical procedures, cerebral palsy).

Adverse effects of muscarinic receptor antagonists include dry mouth, mydriasis (causes blurred vision), tachycardia, hot and flushed skin, agitation, urinary retention, constipation, and delirium. A mnemonic to remember these side effects is "red as a beet, dry as a bone, blind as a bat, and mad as a hatter."

Acetylcholinesterase Inhibitors: Indirect-Acting Muscarinic and Nicotinic Receptor Agonists

Ambenonium, Donepezil, Echothiophate, Edrophonium, Galantamine, Neostigmine, Physostigmine, Pyridostigmine, Rivastigmine, Sarin, Soman, Tabun, and Tacrine

Another potent class of muscarinic mimetics includes the cholinesterase inhibitors that block the breakdown of ACh. For the effects of ACh to be rapidly and exquisitely regulated, the actions of the neurotransmitter need to be terminated by AChE. The inhibition of AChE results in the indirect increase in ACh, so these drugs are termed *indirect-acting cholinomimetics*.

There are two classes of anticholinesteras inhibitors. The first class is composed of *reversible* compounds that have significant clinical utility (edrophonium, ambenonium, neostigmine, physostigmine, and pyridostigmine). The second class is largely *irreversible* agents that often have more "toxic" roles as insecticides and chemical weapon agents (nerve gases). Members of this latter class share the characteristic of being reactive organophosphates and include echothiophate (used ocularly for treatment of glaucoma) and nerve gas agents such as sarin, soman, and tabun.

Endogenous AChE is susceptible to these pharmacologic inhibitors. ACh binds to the active site of AChE, where the acetyl group of ACh is transferred to a serine hydroxyl residue within the enzyme's active site. Then, H_2O rapidly cleaves the acetate and regenerates the active enzyme. For the anticholinesterase pharmacologic agents, a reactive group is transferred to the serine that is slower to come off. With the *irreversible* organophosphates, the phosphorylated serine is very slowly reversed and, if given time, "ages" into a permanent modification that cannot be reversed and hence inactivates the enzyme. With AChE inactivated, large excesses of cholinergic activity occur that can kill the affected individual.

Treatment of AChE inhibition toxicity or poisoning relies on the use of muscarinic antagonists. However, in the case of nerve gas poisoning, rapid intervention with an additional substrate called *pralidoxime* provides a strong nucleophilic center that strips the phosphate moiety from the enzyme. However, pralidoxime needs to be administered within several hours of the exposure (before it "ages"); otherwise, the AChE cannot be regenerated.

Clinically, the most common use for anticholinesterase agents is in diagnosis and treatment of myasthenia gravis, a neuromuscular disease in which the body makes antibodies against the N_M AChR. Of the various neuromuscular disorders presenting as muscle weakness, myasthenia gravis is the one that responds to anticholinesterase therapy. Therefore, diagnosis is made with the "Tensilon test," a short-acting challenge with ultra-short-acting edrophonium (Tensilon) ($t_{1/2}$ in minutes). After definitive diagnosis, treatment is initiated with the use of longer acting agents such as pyridostigmine, neostigmine, or ambenonium. Use of these drugs causes local synaptic concentrations of ACh to increase within the neuromuscular junction of the skeletal muscle, which increases the activity at the remaining functional receptors.

Several of the newest AChE inhibitors do not *covalently* bind to the AChE; rather, they bind as *noncovalent*, competitive inhibitors, and these drugs are used to treat Alzheimer disease (tacrine, donepezil, rivastigmine, and galantamine). Observations in brains affected by Alzheimer disease reveal that cholinergic neurons are among the earliest to be lost. Thus, the rationale for this treatment is that administration of anticholinesterase inhibitors increases central cholinergic tone to partially reverse the effects of lost cholinergic neurons. Unfortunately, these drugs have only modest effects in improving overall cognition in patients with Alzheimer disease, and all are associated with adverse gastrointestinal symptoms (e.g., diarrhea) because of excess ACh activity.

●●● ADRENERGIC SYSTEMS

Biochemistry of Adrenergic Systems

The term *adrenergic* refers to the fact that these neurotransmitters are found in the adrenal medulla, where epinephrine content predominates over that of norepinephrine. As shown in Figure 6-7, these neurotransmitters are synthesized from the amino acid precursor tyrosine. This single precursor (tyrosine) gives rise to three different catecholamine neurotransmitters: dopamine (primarily in the kidney and CNS), norepinephrine (autonomic sympathetic nerves and CNS), and epinephrine

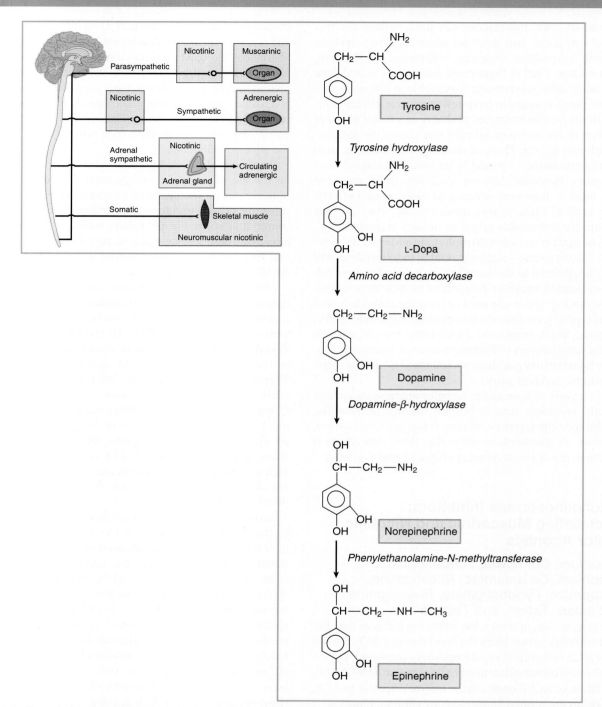

Figure 6-7. Catecholamine biosynthesis. Adrenergic biosynthesis begins with an essential amino acid—tyrosine—and its hydroxylation by the rate-limiting enzyme tyrosine hydroxylase. This reaction produces a benzene ring with neighboring hydroxyl groups. This chemical is called *catechol* and is the reason this class of molecules (all of subsequent molecules in the pathway) is collectively referred to as the *catecholamines*.

(primarily adrenal gland with a small CNS component). Therefore the biosynthetic enzymes described in Figure 6-7 are differentially expressed in different cells of the body.

Unlike cholinergic signals (and ACh), termination of adrenergic neuronal signals is not mediated by a simple hydrolysis reaction. Rather, at the neuron-organ synapse, 60% of norepinephrine is taken back into the nerve via a Na^+-dependent "pump" (Fig. 6-8A). (This reuptake transporter also happens to be the molecular target of cocaine.) Neurotransmitters can then be directly packaged for re-release. Of the remaining neurotransmitter in the synapse, 20% simply diffuses from the site of action, and 20% is degraded in situ. Degradation results in destruction of neurotransmitter function and excretion of metabolic products (Fig. 6-8B). As discussed in Chapter 13, drugs that inhibit catecholamine metabolism are used to treat several CNS disorders.

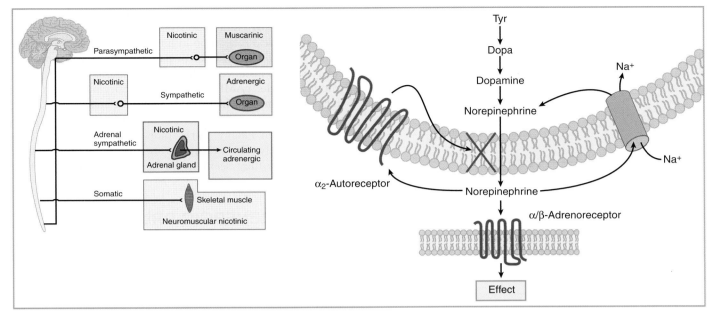

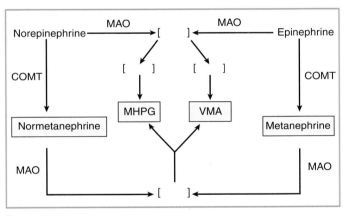

Figure 6-8. Termination of adrenergic responses. **A,** Most sympathetic signaling is terminated through reuptake (and repackaging and reuse) via a norepinephrine transporter. **B,** Enzymatic degradation of the catecholamines, a minor mechanism for signal termination, is also involved in terminating norepinephrine actions. The *empty brackets* represent less important chemical intermediaries. As noted in Chapter 13, several treatments in the central nervous system (especially for Parkinson disease) target these degradation enzymes. *COMT,* catechol-*O*-methyltransferase; *MAO,* monoamine oxidase; *MHPG,* 3-methoxy-4-hydroxyphenylglycol; *Tyr,* tyrosine; *VMA,* vanillomandelic acid.

Adrenergic Receptor Subtypes

As is the case for the cholinergic system, specific neurotransmitter receptor subtypes are found at various anatomic locations. In this case, there are again five different receptor subtypes: α_1, α_2, β_1, β_2, and β_3. Luckily, these receptors serve fairly discrete functions and can be functionally summarized by a relatively simplified table (Fig. 6-9). Moreover, they are all 7TM-GPCRs.

Alpha Receptors

The adrenergic receptors are classified into two main subgroups: alpha (α) and beta (β). In the case of the α-receptors, there are α_1 and α_2 (Figs. 6-8A, 6-9, and 6-10). These receptors

conveniently assume different functions and have different subcellular localizations. Adrenergic α_1-receptors are found on innervated organs and elicit a physiologic response to nerve signals (see Fig. 6-8A). In contrast, α_2-receptors are found primarily on *pre*synaptic neuronal cells. That is, α_2-receptors are located on nerve cells and function there as autoreceptors (see Fig. 6-8A). The functional role of these α_2-autoreceptors is to "sense" synaptic activity and "dampen" activity in situations in which there may be too much neurotransmitter in the synapse. Because they have different functions and anatomic locations, α_1- and α_2-receptors also display differing pharmacologic characteristics (see Fig. 6-10; see also Tables 6-6 and 6-7). Adrenergic α_1-receptors are coupled to the α_q-type subunit of G-protein and stimulate

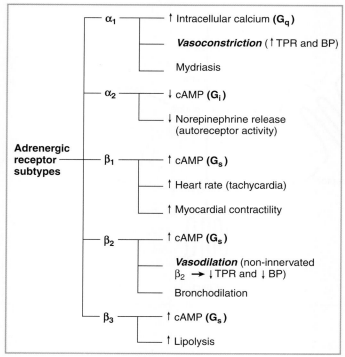

Figure 6-9. Physiology and pharmacology of adrenergic receptors. *cAMP*, cyclic adenosine monophosphate; *TPR*, temperature; *BP*, blood pressure.

phospholipase activity to release inositol triphosphate and diacylglycerol which ultimately trigger Ca^{++} release and cell stimulation (muscle contraction, much like the M1/M3/M5 muscarinic receptors).

Adrenergic α_2-receptors, as previously noted, function as autoreceptors. Working through a G_i/G_0 G-protein, these receptors inhibit adenylyl cyclase (much like the M2/M4 muscarinic receptors; see Fig. 6-10) and decrease cAMP levels. This produces a cascade of downstream events that ultimately results in decreased catecholamine neurotransmitter synthesis as well as decreased neurotransmitter release (see Fig. 6-8).

Beta Receptors

The β-receptors, like the α-receptors, are 7TM-GPCRs and are coupled to G-proteins. However, they are linked to G_s-proteins that stimulate adenylyl cyclase activity and ultimately increase cAMP levels. Depending on the cell type being innervated, stimulation of β-receptors produces vastly different results (see Table 6-6; see also Figs. 6-9 and 6-11).

Adrenergic β_1-receptors are found most notably on the heart, where they increase heart rate and cardiac contractility, leading to increased cardiac output. On the other hand, β_2-receptors are found on a variety of bronchial and vascular smooth muscles, where stimulation triggers muscle relaxation. In the peripheral vascular bed, β_2-receptor stimulation decreases total peripheral resistance and blood pressure.

In the case of β_2-receptors in the lungs, stimulation produces muscle relaxation and bronchodilation. For this reason, inhaled β_2-agonists are the drugs of choice for treating acute

asthma. The mechanistic reasons for the seemingly opposite effects of cAMP stimulation (increased contraction in the heart vs. muscle relaxation in lung and blood vessels) relate directly to the type of effector pathways engaged by specific cell types. For instance, in the case of pulmonary and vascular smooth muscle, cAMP leads to phosphorylation of myosin light chain kinase, which leads to smooth muscle relaxation; whereas in cardiac muscle, cAMP ultimately stimulates pacemaker function. Finally, β_3-receptors have been identified relatively recently. These receptors are found mainly on adipose tissue, where they seem to be involved in regulating fat metabolism.

●●● ADRENERGIC DRUGS

Unlike the cholinergic drugs currently available to modulate the parasympathetic (ACh) nervous system, many pharmacologic agents are available that allow discriminate modulation of individual adrenergic receptor subtypes. These characteristics of adrenergic receptors provide opportunities to treat selected disorders. The following section broadly considers the various classes of adrenergic drugs and their uses (Table 6-7). The pharmacologic details, however, are described in chapters on specific organ systems or therapeutic needs.

Alpha Drugs

There are highly selective agonists and antagonists for α-adrenoceptor subtypes (see Table 6-7 and Fig. 6-12). Indeed, given their selectivity, these drugs are used clinically in a variety of settings.

Alpha-Adrenergic Agonists
Clonidine, Dexmedetomidine, Methoxamine, Norepinephrine, and Phenylephrine

As shown in Figure 6-12, there are several α-selective drugs. Table 6-7 identifies the prototypical agonists for each receptor subtype. First, consider the main, naturally occurring, autonomic neurotransmitters (epinephrine and norepinephrine). Epinephrine is released from the adrenal medulla and interacts, via the circulation, with all adrenergic receptors. As a result of its actions, epinephrine raises blood pressure and increases cardiac output. It is therefore used to treat anaphylactic shock. In addition, epinephrine may be used clinically to treat status asthmaticus; symptomatic relief of serum sickness, urticaria, or angioedema; glaucoma; and prolongation of local/regional anesthetics by vasoconstrictive actions.

In contrast to epinephrine, norepinephrine is released from nerves, where it interacts with receptors in the synapse. Norepinephrine is the primary mediator of β_1 tone in the heart. Moreover, norepinephrine, released in the vasculature, interacts with α_1-receptors and is responsible for the maintenance of total peripheral resistance and blood pressure (Fig. 6-13).

Methoxamine is a synthetic catecholamine with selectivity for α-receptors (with a slight preference for α_1 over α_2). Methoxamine is used clinically to maintain blood pressure during

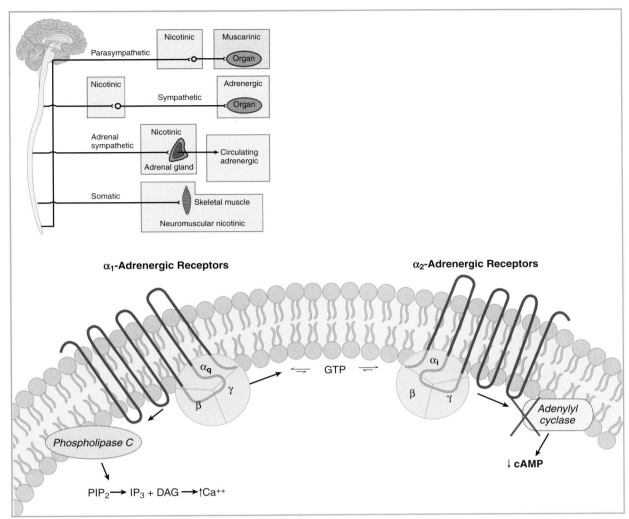

Figure 6-10. Reciprocal action by the α_1- and α_2-receptors. The α-receptors are 7-transmembrane-spanning domain, G-protein–coupled receptor proteins and are coupled to lipid metabolism or inhibition of cyclic adenosine monophosphate (*cAMP*) synthesis. *GTP*, guanosine triphosphate; *PIP_2*, phosphatidylinositol 4,5-bisphosphate; *IP_3*, inositol triphosphate; *DAG*, diacylglycerol.

TABLE 6-6. Mechanisms of Action of Adrenergic Receptors

RECEPTOR	G-PROTEIN (α SUBUNITS)	PRIMARY EFFECTS
α_1	G_q	↑ Phospholipase C ($\Rightarrow$ ↑ Ca^{++} and bioactive lipids)
α_2	G_i/G_0	↓ Adenylyl cyclase (↓ cAMP) ↑ K^+ channel activity ↓ Ca^{++} channel activity
$\beta_1/\beta_2/\beta_3$	G_s	↑ Adenylyl cyclase ($\Rightarrow$ ↑ cAMP)

cAMP, cyclic adenosine monophosphate.

anesthesia through its ability to stimulate α_1 and raise total peripheral resistance. (Do not forget, however, that the resulting increase in blood pressure leads to reflex activity of the baroreceptors, decreasing sympathetic outflow.)

Phenylephrine is the prototypical α_1 agonist. Because of its selectivity, phenylephrine has dramatic vasoconstrictor effects (see Fig. 6-9). It has historically been used as a nasal decongestant when topically applied to the nasal mucosa. It also has been used to overcome vascular failure in shock and supraventricular tachycardia.

On the other hand, clonidine is the prototypical α_2 agonist. This compound, which is predominantly thought of as an

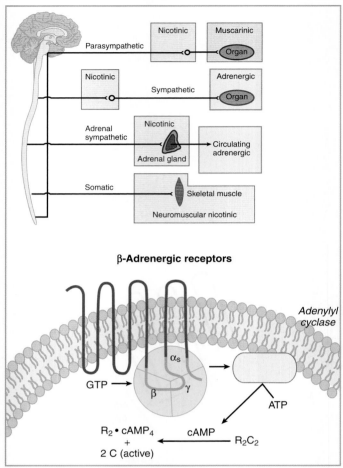

β-Adrenergic receptors

Figure 6-11. Stimulation of adenylyl cylcase by the β-receptors. All the β-receptors are coupled to a stimulatory G-protein (*G*$_s$) and increase synthesis of cyclic adenosine monophosphate (*cAMP*). Stimulation of β-receptors produces widely different effects depending on downstream effectors present in specific cells. In this case, cAMP triggers dissociation of the inactive protein kinase A holoenzyme (*R*$_2$*C*$_2$) into regulatory subunit dimers (*R*$_2$ • *cAMP*$_4$) and active catalytic subunits (*C*) *GTP*, guanosine triphosphate; *ATP*, adenosine triphosphate.

autoreceptor agonist, is used to lower blood pressure—through agonist actions on autoreceptors located within the CNS as opposed to peripheral receptor activities. Dexmedetomidine is another α$_2$-agonist that has a higher affinity for CNS α$_2$-receptors. Although its use is associated with hypotension and bradycardia, dexmedetomidine is primarily used to provide deep intravenous sedation without causing respiratory depression.

Alpha-Adrenergic Antagonists
Alfuzosin, Doxazosin, Phenoxybenzamine, Phentolamine, Prazosin, Silodosin, Tamsulosin, Terazosin, and Yohimbine

As with the adrenergic agonists, there are selective antagonists for α- and β-receptors (see Fig. 6-12). Phentolamine and phenoxybenzamine are α antagonists but do not

TABLE 6-7. Examples of Selective and Nonselective Adrenergic Agonists and Antagonists

RECEPTOR	AGONIST	ANTAGONIST
α$_1$	Phenylephrine	Prazosin Phentolamine (α$_1$/α$_2$) Phenoxybenzamine (α$_1$/α$_2$) Labetalol (α$_1$ and β)
α$_2$	Clonidine Dexmede-tomidine	Yohimbine Phento-lamine (α$_1$/α$_2$) Phenoxybenzamine (α$_1$/α$_2$)
β$_1$	Dobutamine Isoproterenol (β$_1$/β$_2$/β$_3$)	Metoprolol Acebutolol Atenolol Propranolol (β$_1$/β$_2$) Labetalol (α$_1$ and β)
β$_2$	Terbutaline Albuterol Isoproterenol (β$_1$/β$_2$/β$_3$)	Propranolol (β$_1$/β$_2$) Labetalol (α$_1$ and β)
β$_3$	Isoproterenol	β$_1$/β$_2$/β$_3$

discriminate between α$_1$ and α$_2$. The two drugs differ in that the former is a *reversible* antagonist, whereas the latter is an *irreversible* blocker. Clinically, their primary use is preoperative management of patients with pheochromocytoma (a catecholamine-secreting adrenal medullary tumor). This adrenal tumor releases high concentrations of epinephrine. These drugs prevent the effects of epinephrine on the body and "desensitize" the body to circulating catecholamines. This is particularly important during surgery because surgical manipulations of the tumor also trigger release of epinephrine.

Examples of drugs with α$_1$-selective antagonist actions include prazosin (and related compounds doxazosin and terazosin). These drugs have historically been used to treat hypertension by decreasing total peripheral resistance and preventing sympathetic-mediated vasoconstriction. Recall that in the vasculature, sympathetic tone predominates because there is no parasympathetic innervation. Therefore a major side effect of these drugs is postural hypotension (especially with the first dose).

Recently, α$_1$-receptor antagonists have fallen out of favor as antihypertensives because, as blood pressure falls, the kidneys secrete renin. Renin release counteracts the vasodilation induced by these drugs, and activation of the renin-angiotensin-aldosterone system has been associated with increased incidence of heart failure. However, these drugs are still widely used to treat benign prostatic hypertrophy (see Chapter 12). Adrenergic α$_1$ blockade in prostatic tissue causes relaxation of prostate muscle, allowing better urine

α-Selective	Mixed	β-Selective
Norepinephrine	Epinephrine	Isoproteronol
Methoxamine		Terbutaline (β_2)
Phenylephrine (α_1)		Albuterol (β_2)
Clonidine (α_2)		Dobutamine (β_1)
Dexmedetomidine (α_2)		Dopamine (β_1)

A

α-Selective	Mixed	β-Selective
Phenoxybenzamine	Labetolol	Propranolol
Phentolamine		Timolol
Prazosin (α_1)		Atenolol (β_1)
Yohimbine (α_2)		Metoprolol (β_1)
		Acebutolol (β_1)

B

Figure 6-12. Pharmacologic profiles of adrenergic drugs. **A,** Adrenergic agonists. **B,** Adrenergic antagonists. Selectivity is indicated by the position of the drug on the α-to-β continuum.

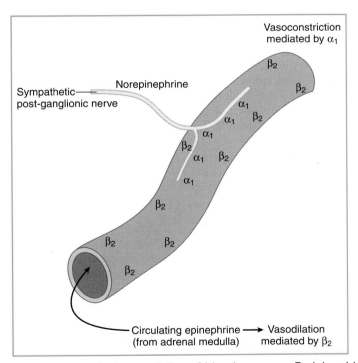

Figure 6-13. Role of noninnervated β-receptors in the regulation of blood pressure. Peripheral blood vessels are innervated by sympathetic nerves that release norepinephrine and stimulate α_1-receptors. In addition, the vessels contain noninnervated β_2-receptors that normally respond to circulating epinephrine. The former receptors produce vasoconstriction (increased blood pressure), whereas the latter produce vasodilation (decreased blood pressure).

flow. Specifically, doxazosin, terazosin, tamsulosin, alfuzosin, and silodosin have been approved for treating benign prostatic hypertrophy. In fact, the latter three are thought to be more selective for those α_1-receptors of the lower urinary tract and so are approved for benign prostatic hypertrophy but not for general hypertension.

Yohimbine is a selective α_2-autoreceptor antagonist (recall that the α_2-receptor is a release-modulating autoreceptor). This drug has a variety of effects and is not widely used in the clinical setting. It has been used as a treatment for erectile dysfunction and as a mydriatic. However, numerous other drugs are effective in these applications, so yohimbine is not widely used.

Beta Drugs

β-Adrenergic Agonists
Albuterol, Dobutamine, Dopamine, Isoproterenol, Ritodrine, Salmeterol, and Terbutaline

Isoproterenol is the prototypical β-agonist. Unfortunately, because of its lack of selectivity (it is equipotent at β_1 and β_2), it is not widely used clinically. It may be used to manage hypovolemia and septic shock. β-Selectivity comes in the form of two important classes of compounds. Dobutamine is a β_1-selective compound and is beneficial for selectively *increasing* cardiac output in patients with congestive heart failure (see Fig. 6-9). β_2-Selective agonists such as albuterol are beneficial for the treatment of asthma. Indeed, inhaled β_2-agonists are drugs of choice for managing acute asthma attacks. A lipophilic version of albuterol (salmeterol) has a long duration of action, making this drug useful in asthma prophylaxis (it is the β_2-agonist component of fluticasone/salmeterol combinations). Because it has a delayed time for onset of action, salmeterol is not to be used in an acute asthma attack. In addition, β_2-selective drugs such as terbutaline and ritodrine are used as tocolytics (medications to inhibit labor), because β_2-agonist activity in the uterus causes relaxation of uterine smooth muscle.

Dopamine deserves consideration at this point. As noted in Figure 6-8, dopamine is the direct chemical precursor to norepinephrine. However, dopamine is also an important neurotransmitter in its own right and plays prominent roles in mental health, substance abuse, and motor function (loss of dopamine neurons in the CNS is the underlying cause of Parkinson disease). At high enough doses, dopamine also binds to adrenergic receptors, with selectivity for β_1-receptors. β_1-Selectivity increases cardiac output. At low doses, dopamine stimulates bona fide dopamine receptors (D_2) in the renal vasculature. This produces vasodilation and increases blood flow to the kidneys. These are important considerations in cases of shock. When dopamine is used to manage cardiogenic shock, activity at β-receptors increases cardiac output, whereas stimulation of renal dopamine receptors may prevent renal failure. At extraordinarily high doses, dopamine acts on α-receptors and causes vasoconstriction (useful in patients in hemorrhagic shock).

Beta-Adrenergic Antagonists (β-Blockers)
Acebutolol, Carvedilol, Labetalol, Metoprolol, Nebivolol, Pindolol, Propranolol, and Timolol

Note that the names of these drugs end in "-lol."

The β-blockers have had extensive clinical use because of their ability to decrease cardiac output, myocardial oxygen demand, and total peripheral resistance without leading to debilitating postural hypotension. This is because they do not affect the α_1 tone that regulates blood pressure (see Fig. 6-9). Propranolol is the prototypical β-blocker. It lacks selectivity and effectively blocks both β_1 and β_2. Clinically, β-blockers are used in a variety of settings. First and foremost, they are used to treat hypertension. They are also effective in angina (by reducing workload and the concomitant oxygen demand) and in the treatment of atrial fibrillation, where they reduce atrioventricular nodal conduction and protect the ventricles. In addition, β-blockers are effective cardioprotectants after a myocardial infarction (and are a standard treatment modality). β-Blockers (timolol, in particular) also reduce intraocular pressure and are beneficial in long-term management of glaucoma (where they decrease aqueous humor production). Finally, certain β-blockers, such as carvedilol and metoprolol, are effective in the treatment of congestive heart failure, where few classes of drugs have been shown to reduce mortality rates.

Acebutolol (as well as pindolol) represents a novel antagonist that has weak intrinsic *agonist* activity—also called *partial agonist activity*, or in the case of the cardiovascular system, *intrinsic sympathomimetic activity*. The best way to understand these dual effects is to remember that these compounds bind to receptors and block endogenous stimulation by epinephrine and norepinephrine yet elicit weak stimulatory effects of their own. This minimizes the bradycardia usually associated with β-blockade.

Labetalol is another drug with a unique mechanism of action: it is a nonselective α_1 and β_1/β_2 blocker. Based on this spectrum of activity, labetalol decreases cardiac output *and* total peripheral resistance (see Fig. 6-9). Similarly, carvedilol has both α_1- and β_1-selective blocking properties. Orthostatic hypotension is a significant side effect of these agents. Nebivolol is the newest β-blocker and displays a preference for the β_1-receptor (cardioselective β-blocker). As a result, it has some value in treating hypertension. However, nebivolol is much more restricted in its use; unlike carvedilol, it is not approved for heart failure or left ventricular dysfunction after myocardial infarction.

●●● CLINICALLY IMPORTANT INDIRECT EFFECTORS OF AUTONOMIC FUNCTION

Discussions up to this point have focused primarily on direct-acting agonists and antagonists. However, many pharmacologic compounds act indirectly. Of immediate and widespread relevance is the ability to block catecholamine reuptake (dopamine, norepinephrine, and epinephrine; Table 6-8). Recall that this is the primary mechanism by which sympathetic signals are terminated. Reuptake is mediated by an Na^+-dependent symporter pump (the norepinephrine/epinephrine transporter and the dopamine transporter). As discussed in Chapter 13, the norepinephrine transporter is a target for tricyclic antidepressants (e.g., imipramine). Contrasting with this therapeutically beneficial approach, the dopamine and norepinephrine transporters (along with the serotonin transporter) are targets of an abused drug, cocaine. Another drug, pseudoephedrine, is commonly used to treat congestion by promoting release of pre-formed catecholamines from nerve terminals. In all cases, the result of transporter blockade or enhanced neurotransmitter release is an increased amount of time that the neurotransmitter spends in the synapse, increasing the apparent sympathetic activity. This leads to the designation of these compounds as indirect-acting sympathomimetics. Through a different mechanism, amphetamines accomplish the same effect. In the case of

TABLE 6-8. Clinically Important Indirect Effectors of Autonomic Function

ACTIVITY	AGENTS	EFFECTS
Block catecholamine reuptake	Cocaine, tricyclic antidepressants	Increase norepinephrine in synapse; have sympathomimetic actions
Facilitate catecholamine release	Amphetamine, pseudoephedrine	Stimulate sympathetic nervous system by releasing norepinephrine; have sympathomimetic actions
Block ACh breakdown	Cholinesterase inhibitors (pesticides and nerve gas agents)	Block ACh degradation; overstimulate cholinergic systems (muscarinic → SLUD syndrome)
Block catecholamine breakdown	MAO inhibitors (pargyline, selegiline) COMT inhibitors (entacapone, tolcapone)	Increase norepinephrine/epinephrine activities without direct stimulation (augment existing activities)

ACh, acetylcholine; *COMT*, catechol-*O*-methyltransferase; *MAO*, monoamine oxidase; *SLUD*, salivation, lacrimation, urination, defecation.

amphetamines, neurotransmitters are released from synaptic vesicles and through a reversal of the symporter pump, catecholamines are released into the synapse via backward flow through the transporter.

Considering the toxicologically relevant inhibition of AChE (see Fig. 6-9), the toxicology profile of AChE inhibitors should be apparent. Any intervention that prevents the cell from terminating a cholinergic response results in heightened stimulation of nearly every branch of the ANS either directly or indirectly (e.g., through ganglionic stimulation of the sympathetic nervous system). This is what makes nerve gas agents, such as sarin, so deadly.

Finally, a number of new approaches increase adrenergic function in the nervous system by modulating the degradation of catecholamines. Most signal termination is accomplished through reuptake transporters. However, a small amount of metabolic degradation occurs via monoamine oxidase and catechol-*O*-methyltransferase, enzymes that are the targets of compounds such as pargyline and selegiline as well as tolcapone and entacapone. Although this approach is more common in the CNS (see Chapter 13), it is interesting to note that interfering with neurotransmitter metabolism does not interfere with tone of the system. That is, molecules are packaged and released in an integrated neuronal fashion. However, the effectiveness of neurotransmitter release can be enhanced by increasing catecholamine levels in the synapse.

●●● TOP FIVE LIST

1. Sympathetic and parasympathetic nerves use essentially two neurotransmitters (norepinephrine and AChE, respectively). They generate pharmacologic diversity through multiple receptor subtypes.
2. nAChRs are poor choices for pharmacologic intervention because they serve too many different functions.
3. Although muscarinic ACh receptors are pharmacologically suitable drug targets, compounds with receptor selectivity are lacking.
4. Adrenergic receptors are strong pharmacologic targets; there is drug selectivity for numerous receptor subtypes.
5. Different adrenergic receptors on the same organ can have opposite effects. At the same time, similar adrenergic receptors on different organs can have opposite effects.

Self-assessment questions can be accessed at www. StudentConsult.com.

Hematology 7

CONTENTS

ANTICOAGULANT DRUGS
  Heparins
  Direct Thrombin Inhibitors
  Vitamin K Antagonists (Orally Active Anticoagulants)
ANTIPLATELET DRUGS
  Salicylates
  Phosphodiesterase Inhibitors
  Adenosine Diphosphate Inhibitors
  Glycoprotein IIb/IIIa Inhibitors
THROMBOLYTIC DRUGS
  First-Generation Thrombolytics
  Second-Generation Thrombolytics: Tissue
    Plasminogen Activators
BLEEDING DISORDERS
ANEMIA
  Agents to Treat Anemias
  Hematopoietic Stimulating Factors
ORPHAN HEMATOLOGIC DISEASES
TOP FIVE LIST

This chapter is all about keeping the plumbing clear. Numerous arterial (e.g., myocardial infarct, stroke, peripheral ischemia) and venous (e.g., deep vein thrombosis, pulmonary embolism) pathologies occur as a result of occlusions (stenotic lesions) within the vasculature. Under normal circumstances, blood clot formation (hemostasis) and breakdown (fibrinolysis) take place along a physiologic continuum. However, when these processes go awry, pathologic consequences such as thrombi arise, leading to potentially severe consequences. Understanding the physiologic and biochemical mechanisms underlying blood clotting offers not only a prospectus on how these processes are altered by aging and in diabetes, inflammation, cardiovascular and renal diseases, but also identifies pharmacologic targets for therapeutic interventions.

In addition to its ability to buffer extracellular pH, blood plays a number of important roles in maintaining internal equilibrium. Among these various functions is hemostasis, or the cessation of bleeding from damaged blood vessels. The process of hemostasis is composed of three major interrelated steps: vessel constriction, platelet plug formation, and clotting. As a result of injury to the vessel, platelets are activated, resulting in release of vasoconstrictors, including thromboxane A_2, serotonin (5 HT; 5-hydroxytryptamine),

and adenosine diphosphate (ADP). Vascular constriction is the initial response to blood vessel injury. Soon after vasoconstriction occurs, collagen—which underlies the vessel endothelium and is exposed as a result of the injury—allows platelet adherence and aggregation to form a platelet plug. Platelet activation and aggregation also expose glycoprotein IIb/IIIa, a receptor site for fibrinogen, the precursor molecule to formation of a fibrin clot (Fig. 7-1).

Clotting, which is the final step in hemostasis, results in a meshwork of fibrin that traps blood cells. Its main function is to reinforce the platelet plug and to provide a relatively strong seal at the site of vascular injury. Fibrin clots are the end result of the proteolytic activation of clotting factors that make up both the intrinsic (blood trauma) and extrinsic (tissue trauma) pathways. Activation of either the intrinsic or the extrinsic pathway ends with activation of thrombin, which then converts fibrinogen to fibrin to form a fibrin clot. Physicians have three major types of drugs to prevent or diminish thrombus formation: anticoagulants, platelet inhibitors, and thrombolytics (Fig. 7-2).

●●● ANTICOAGULANT DRUGS

In hypercoagulable states, the risk of thrombus formation is elevated and pharmacologic management is centered on the prevention of pathologic clot formation. It is important to remember that the liver plays a crucial role in coagulation, because it is a site that produces many clotting factors. The liver is also the site of production of bile salts that facilitate absorption of vitamin K and aid in production of clotting factors II, VII, IX, and X. The following are the major types of anticoagulants:

- Heparins
- Vitamin K cofactor antagonists (warfarin)
- Direct thrombin inhibitors

PATHOLOGY

Lines of Zahn

When thrombi form in the heart or aorta, they may have apparent laminations, referred to as lines of Zahn. These lines are produced by alternating pale layers of platelets and fibrin mixed with darker layers containing red blood cells. The main significance of lines of Zahn is that they imply antemortem thrombus formation at a site of blood flow.

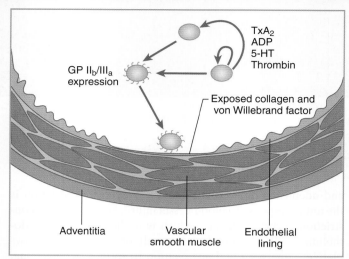

Figure 7-1. Platelet activation. Release of adenosine diphosphate (*ADP*), thromboxane (*TxA₂*), serotonin (*5-HT*), and thrombin from adhered platelets induces additional platelet recruitment and augmented expression of glycoprotein (*GP*) IIb/IIIa receptors. These glycoprotein receptors bind fibrinogen and von Willebrand factor to lead to platelet aggregation at the site of endothelial injury. The anionic phospholipid surface of the aggregated platelet mass helps localize the coagulation cascade factors that ultimately activate thrombin, the enzyme that converts fibrinogen to fibrin.

PATHOLOGY

Transient Protein C Deficiency

Transient protein C (autoprothrombin IIA) deficiency can be induced when initiating treatment with warfarin because factors VII and protein C have the shortest half-lives of the coagulation and anticoagulation factors. Consequently, the extrinsic pathway and protein C system are inactivated, leaving the intrinsic pathway to continue to function for a few days. During this period of transient hypercoagulability, dermal vascular thrombosis and skin necrosis may occur.

Heparins

Unfractionated heparin was, for many years, the clinician's primary option when selecting a parenteral anticoagulant. However, more selective forms of heparins, known as the *fractionated, low-molecular-weight heparins* (LMWHs), can now be administered.

Unfractionated Heparin
Mechanism of action
Heparin is a large, endogenous, sulfated glycosaminoglycan found in mast cells. Under normal circumstances, it is rapidly destroyed and not detected in plasma. The heparin used pharmacologically is extracted from bovine lung or porcine intestinal mucosa.

Heparin's anticoagulant action is derived from its binding to antithrombin III. Antithrombin III inhibits activated coagulation factors, especially thrombin (factor II), Xa, XIIa and IXa. When heparin binds to antithrombin III, a conformational

change is induced that opens the reactive site of antithrombin III, increasing its ability to inhibit coagulation factors by 1000-fold.

Pharmacokinetics
The large molecular size of heparin prevents the drug from crossing membranes; thus heparin must be given parenterally. Heparin has a short half-life (t½) and is both metabolized by heparinase in the liver and degraded in the periphery by endothelial cells. Patient response to heparin is quite variable. In part, this variability occurs because heparin binds nonspecifically to plasma proteins. Because each individual possesses differing amounts of plasma proteins to which heparin may bind, heparin's effects vary greatly between individuals. When heparin is bound to plasma proteins, it is unable to bind to antithrombin III.

Clinical uses
Heparin is a first-line agent for anticoagulation in patients with an acute deep vein thrombosis (DVT), pulmonary embolism, or myocardial infarction (MI). Heparin is also used for preventing postoperative DVT and PE in high-risk patients, including pregnant women. The need for continuous intravenous infusions of heparin or repeated subcutaneous injections significantly reduces its usefulness in long-term outpatient management.

Antidote
In hemorrhagic situations, protamine sulfate can be administered. Protamine sulfate binds to heparin by virtue of positively charged protamine interacting with the sulfates on heparin and interferes with heparin's ability to bind to antithrombin III.

Adverse effects
Aside from hemorrhage, other prominent adverse effects include skin necrosis at the injection site, osteoporosis with long-term use, severe thrombocytopenia, and hypersensitivity reactions.

Contraindications
Because heparin is derived from animal sources, hypersensitivity to bovine or porcine components may cause anaphylactic reactions. Heparin should always be avoided in any situation in which a patient is likely to bleed (Box 7-1).

Monitoring
Activated partial thromboplastin time is used to monitor heparin's efficacy. Typically, the activated partial thromboplastin time goal to manage an anticoagulated patient is 1.5 to 2.5 times baseline (normal adult control values range from 28 to 42 seconds).

Low-Molecular-Weight Heparin
Ardeparin, Dalteparin, Enoxaparin, and Tinzaparin
Mechanism of action. Although similar to unfractionated heparin, LMWHs are more selective in action. As with heparin, LMWHs increase the activity of antithrombin III; however, with LMWHs, factor Xa is preferentially affected over other clotting factors.

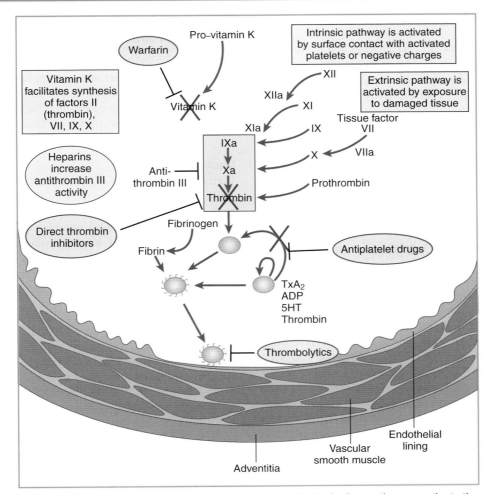

Figure 7-2. A platelet-centric view of coagulation. Both the intrinsic and extrinsic clotting pathways activate thrombin, which converts bound fibrinogen on platelet IIb/IIIa receptors into fibrin. This reinforces the clot and may lead to blood flow occlusion. The major sites of pharmacologic intervention are depicted in purple. As noted in the figure, platelet-triggered clots that are formed can be reversed ("dissolved") by the thrombolytics. TxA_2, thromboxin A_2; *ADP*, adenosine diphosphate; *5HT*, serotonin.

Box 7-1. CONTRAINDICATIONS TO HEPARIN BECAUSE OF BLEEDING RISKS

- Hemophilia and all bleeding disorders
- Gastrointestinal ulcers/bleeding
- Thrombocytopenia
- Recent brain, spinal cord, or eye surgery
- During or before lumbar puncture or regional anesthetic blockade

Box 7-2. ADVANTAGES OF LOW-MOLECULAR-WEIGHT HEPARINS OVER UNFRACTIONATED HEPARIN

- Can be used by patients at home (subcutaneous versus intravenous injection)
- Routine monitoring of coagulation times is unnecessary
- Predictable dose-response relationships
- Improved bioavailability
- Longer half-life ($t_{1/2}$)
- Once or twice daily dosing

Pharmacokinetics. Unlike unfractionated heparin, there is less nonspecific binding to plasma proteins with LMWHs. This results in fewer drug interactions, a more predictable anticoagulant response, and less interpatient variability. Additional advantages of LMWHs over unfractionated heparin are listed in Box 7-2. LMWHs are eliminated renally, and dosage adjustments are needed in patients with renal insufficiency.

Clinical uses. LMWHs can be used to prevent or treat DVT and PE and to prevent ischemic complications associated with unstable angina and non–Q-wave MI. In many situations, LMWHs have replaced unfractionated heparin.

Adverse effects. Although bleeding, osteoporosis, thrombocytopenia, and skin reactions near the injection site may occur with LMWHs, the incidence and severity of these side effects are greatly reduced compared with those for unfractionated heparin.

Monitoring. Routine coagulation monitoring is not required although specific tests are available to monitor factor Xa activity periodically in patients with renal insufficiency or morbid obesity or in pregnant women.

Synthetic Heparin Alternatives
Fondaparinux

Fondaparinux is a synthetic pentasaccharide that is the shortest sequence within heparin that binds to antithrombin III to inactivate factor Xa. Because this is a synthetic compound, there is less potential for hypersensitivity reactions, as compared with unfractionated heparins from bovine or porcine sources. In addition, it has a longer $t_{1/2}$ and requires less monitoring and is less likely to cause heparin-induced thrombocytopenia. Yet, unlike heparin, no antidote is available in the event of bleeding complications.

Direct Thrombin Inhibitors

Argatroban, Bivalirudin, Dabigatran, and Lepirudin
Mechanism of action

These drugs directly bind to the active site of thrombin, inhibiting its effects on fibrinogen. The drug lepirudin is a recombinant form of hirudin, the irreversible thrombin inhibitor derived from leeches—the same leeches that have been used for medicinal purposes for centuries. The Food and Drug Administration in 2004 approved the use of leeches for certain medical purposes, such as removal of pooled blood from under a skin graft to promote healing, restoration of circulation in blocked veins, and surgical reattachment of fingers and ears. Lepirudin, bivalirudin, and argatroban are administered parenterally. One orally active thrombin inhibitor, dabigatran, is also available.

Clinical use

Lepirudin, bivalirudin, and argatroban are used in patients who have experienced heparin-induced thrombocytopenia. These drugs may also be administered to patients undergoing angioplasty. Dabigatran is an alternative to warfarin in patients with atrial fibrillation.

Adverse effects

As with other anticoagulants, bleeding is the most common adverse event.

Vitamin K Antagonists (Orally Active Anticoagulants)

Warfarin

For students who sometimes wonder how drug names are selected, warfarin is derived from the Wisconsin Alumni Research Foundation, the patent-holding arm of the University of Wisconsin, where warfarin was discovered.

Mechanism of action

Warfarin inhibits the synthesis of vitamin K–dependent clotting factors, which are factors II, VII, IX, and X. Specifically, synthesis of these clotting factors requires γ-carboxylation, a process that uses vitamin K. In the process of γ-carboxylation, vitamin K gets oxidized. Oxidized vitamin K must be reduced to regenerate active vitamin K, but warfarin interferes with the reduction step by inhibiting the actions of the enzyme, vitamin K epoxide reductase (see Fig. 7-3).

Pharmacokinetics

Warfarin has a slow onset of action. In fact, warfarin's therapeutic effect is delayed for 4 to 5 days, until all existing activated factors II, VII, IX, and X are depleted from the circulation.

Warfarin binds extensively and nonspecifically to plasma proteins. From 97% to 99.9% of warfarin is protein bound, with only a small percentage of the drug free in circulation to exert its biologic effects. As a result, coadministration of other highly protein-bound drugs may displace warfarin from its binding sites, leading to greater amounts of freely circulating warfarin and increased risks of bleeding. Other drug-drug interactions with warfarin may occur as a result of the inhibition of warfarin's hepatic metabolism or pharmacodynamic actions with other drugs that also alter coagulation (e.g., aspirin, nonsteroidal anti-inflammatory drugs, salicylates). Table 7-1 lists drugs that may increase the risk of bleeding when used with warfarin, and Table 7-2 lists drugs that decrease warfarin's efficacy. Numerous foods that are rich in vitamin K also antagonize warfarin's anticoagulant effects, leading to reduced efficacy (Box 7-3). Furthermore, numerous herbal or natural products alter the effects of warfarin; these interactions can

TABLE 7-1. Drugs That Increase Risk of Bleeding When Used with Warfarin

INHIBIT WARFARIN METABOLISM	INTERFERE WITH VITAMIN K	PLATELET EFFECTS	OTHER
Azole antifungals		NSAIDs	Cephalosporins (parenteral)
HMG-CoA reductase inhibitors	Tetracyclines	Penicillins (parenteral)	Disulfiram
Metronidazole	Vitamin E	Fish oils	Pentoxifylline
Fibric acid		SSRIs	Thrombolytics

HMG-CoA, 3-hydroxy-3-methylglutaryl-coenzyme A; *NSAIDs*, nonsteroidal antiinflammatory drugs; *SSRIs*, selective serotonin reuptake inhibitors.

TABLE 7-2. Drugs That Decrease Anticoagulant Effects of Warfarin

DECREASED ABSORPTION OR INCREASED ELIMINATION	INDUCTION OF HEPATIC MICROSOMAL CYTOCHROME P450 ENZYMES	UNKNOWN MECHANISM
Spironolactone	Barbiturates	Clozapine
Sucralfate	Carbamazepine	Oral contraceptives
	Dicloxacillin	Estrogens
Vitamin K (antagonizes warfarin)	Nafcillin	Griseofulvin
	Rifampin	Haloperidol
		Trazodone

Box 7-3. FOODS RICH IN VITAMIN K THAT CAN DIMINISH WARFARIN'S ANTICOAGULANT ACTIONS

Brussels sprouts	Spinach
Broccoli	Seaweed
Cabbage	Turnip greens
Chickpeas	Bok choy
Lettuce	Kohlrabi

either increase or decrease the risk of bleeding (Boxes 7-4 and 7-5). Of note are the "3 Gs": garlic, ginger, and ginkgo biloba—three commonly used supplements that increase warfarin's anticoagulant actions. More food, drug, and herbal interactions occur with warfarin than with any other drug.

It is worth noting that resistance to warfarin therapy is usually due to excessive vitamin K intake from diet or supplements. However, hereditary warfarin resistance because of mutations in vitamin K epoxide reductase complex subunit

Box 7-4. NATURAL PRODUCTS THAT INCREASE THE RISK OF BLEEDING WHEN USED WITH WARFARIN

Black cohosh	Ginkgo biloba
Fenugreek	Horseradish
Feverfew	Licorice
Fish oils	Red clover
Garlic	Sweet clover
Ginger	Vitamin E

Box 7-5. NATURAL PRODUCTS THAT DIMINISH THE ANTICOAGULANT EFFECTS OF WARFARIN

Agrimony	Mistletoe
Ginseng	Yarrow
Goldenseal	

1, have also been reported. Conversely, variant CYP2C9 alleles (one of the P450 hepatic microsomal enzymes that inactivate warfarin) may enhance sensitivity to warfarin.

Clinical use

Warfarin is used for long-term prophylaxis and treatment of DVT and PE. Other uses for warfarin include prophylactic treatment of patients with atrial fibrillation to prevent mural thrombi (although some recent literature indicates aspirin may be a suitable alternative in appropriate patients), rheumatic heart disease, and patients with prosthetic heart valves. Warfarin may also be used as an adjunctive treatment when coronary arteries are occluded.

Adverse effects

The major factor limiting the use of warfarin is the risk of hemorrhage. Warfarin should be discontinued if skin necrosis or nonhemorrhagic purple-toe syndrome occurs. Teratogenicity (including hemorrhagic disorders and abnormal bone formation) prohibits warfarin use during pregnancy. Other contraindications to warfarin use are listed in Box 7-6. It is worth noting that while there is an increased risk of bleeding when warfarin is combined with aspirin, this combination is frequently used for synergistic anticoagulation.

Antidote

For minor bleeding, warfarin therapy may simply be interrupted. However, for major bleeding, vitamin K may be administered. In emergency situations, clotting factors may be replenished via administration of fresh-frozen plasma or by administration of commercially available recombinant factor VIIa.

Box 7-6. CONTRAINDICATIONS TO WARFARIN THERAPY

Bleeding tendency of any type
Severe hepatic or renal disease
Chronic alcoholism
Vitamin K deficiency
Malignant hypertension

Monitoring

Historically, prothrombin time (PT) has been used to monitor a patient's response to warfarin therapy. However, because PT is variable depending on the type of thromboplastin used in laboratory assays, the International Normalized Ratio (INR) is currently the recognized gold standard for monitoring warfarin (see Clinical Medicine box). The INR standardizes PT times so that they are consistent no matter which type of thromboplastin is used. For most indications, an INR of 2.0 to 3.0 is sufficient, although in patients with prosthetic (metallic) heart valves or patients with recurrent systemic emboli, an INR of 2.5 to 3.5 may be desired.

In summary, Table 7-3 describes the key points that distinguish unfractionated heparin from warfarin. Remember that heparins inhibit activated coagulation factors via activation of antithrombin III, in contrast to warfarin, which inhibits vitamin K–dependent synthesis of coagulation factors (see Fig. 7-2). Figure 7-3 describes the mechanism of action of warfarin.

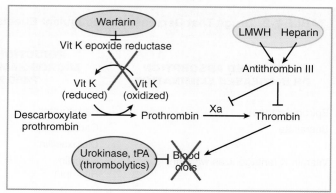

Figure 7-3. Overview of the pharmacologic regulation of blood clots. Clotting can be reduced in two ways. First, heparin-like molecules can directly activate anti-thrombin III to inhibit the activities of factor X and thrombin (and to a lesser extent factors IX, XII, and XI). Alternatively, warfarin inhibits the reductase responsible for regenerating vitamin (Vit) K. As a result, the ability to make new *active* thrombin is inhibited and, after depletion of clotting factors II, VII, IX, and X, clotting activity is decreased. Finally, after clots are formed, they can be "dissolved" with thrombolytics. *LMWH*, low-molecular weight heparin; *tPA*, tissue plasminogen activator.

●●● ANTIPLATELET DRUGS

While interfering with clotting factors is a good approach for preventing thrombosis, the risk of hemorrhage associated with anticoagulants has necessitated the use of drugs that work through alternative mechanisms. As previously mentioned, platelet adhesion and activation occur at sites of vascular injury where factors such as thromboxane A_2, ADP, collagen, serotonin, and thrombin facilitate increased expression of glycoprotein IIb/IIIa receptors. This, in turn, leads to platelet adhesion by cross-linking reactions, which occurs after an initial fibrinogen-glycoprotein IIb/IIIa bond. Antiplatelet drugs work on one or more of these targets. Table 7-4 lists endogenous factors and drugs that affect platelet aggregation. Platelet inhibitors include (Fig. 7-4):

- Salicylates
- Phosphodiesterase inhibitors
- ADP inhibitors
- Glycoprotein IIb/IIIa inhibitors

TABLE 7-3. Warfarin Versus Heparin

PARAMETER	HEPARIN	WARFARIN
Molecular structure	Large polysaccharide, water-soluble	Small molecule, lipid-soluble
Pharmacokinetics	Given parenterally (intravenous/subcutaneous), hepatic and endothelial elimination, $t_{1/2} = 2$ hours, no placental access	Given orally, >98% protein bound, liver metabolism, $t_{1/2} = 30+$ hours, placental access
Mechanism of action	↑ Binding of antithrombin III to factors IIa and Xa	↓ Hepatic synthesis of vitamin K–dependent factors II, VII, IX, X→ warfarin prevents γ-carboxylation No effect on factors already present in vivo
Laboratory tests	Activated partial thromboplastin time for unfractionated heparin	Prothrombin time/international normalized ratio
Overdose treatment	Protamine sulfate–chemical antagonism, fast onset	Vitamin K ↑ cofactor synthesis = slow onset; fresh-frozen plasma = fast onset
Clinical utility	Rapid anticoagulation (intensive) for thromboses, emboli, unstable angina, disseminated intravascular coagulation, open-heart surgery	Longer term anticoagulation (controlled) for thromboses, emboli, post-myocardial infarction, heart valve damage, atrial arrhythmias, cerebrovascular accidents
Adverse effects	Bleeding, osteoporosis, heparin-induced thrombocytopenia, hypersensitivity	Bleeding, skin necrosis (if low Protein C), purple toe syndrome, drug interactions, teratogenicity (bone dysmorphogenesis)

CLINICAL MEDICINE

International Normalized Ratio

Coagulation of whole blood can be completely prevented in vitro by adding a Ca^{++} chelator such as citrate or ethylenediaminetetraacetic acid (EDTA) (calcium is required at a variety of different stages of blood clotting in both the extrinsic pathway and the intrinsic pathway). By adding a variety of factors back to citrated platelet-poor plasma, such as phospholipids, kaolin, and thromboplastin, bleeding times can be altered (see the table below).

	Clotting Time
Whole blood	4–8 min
Whole blood + EDTA or citrate	Infinite
Citrated platelet-poor plasma + Ca^{++}	2–4 min
Citrated platelet-poor plasma + phospholipids + Ca^{++}	60–85 sec
Citrated platelet-poor plasma + kaolin + phospholipids + Ca^{++}	21–32 sec (aPTT)
Citrated platelet-poor plasma + thromboplastin + Ca^{++}	11–12 sec PT)

The activated partial thromboplastin time is used to monitor coagulation status of the intrinsic pathway when heparin is administered, whereas the PT provides an estimate of the coagulation status of the extrinsic pathway when warfarin is given. Because numerous companies manufacture their own thromboplastin (protein + phospholipids) and concentrations of various components tend to vary by manufacturer, a need for standardization was apparent. In fact, patients' bleeding times were variable depending on the laboratory where their blood was drawn. As a result, each batch of thromboplastin is now required to be "standardized." Today, that standardization is taken into account when the PT is measured and PTs are converted to an INR. As a result of thromboplastin standardization, a patient's INR will be consistent regardless of which laboratory is used.

TABLE 7-4. Endogenous Factors and Drugs Affecting Platelet Aggregation

INCREASED AGGREGATION	DECREASED AGGREGATION
ADP	PGI_2
5-HT	cAMP
Thromboxane A_2	Aspirin
Thrombin	Dipyridamole
	Ticlopidine
	Clopidogrel

ADP, adenosine diphosphate; *cAMP*, cyclic adenosine monophosphate; *5-HT*, serotonin; *PGI₂*, prostaglandin I₂.

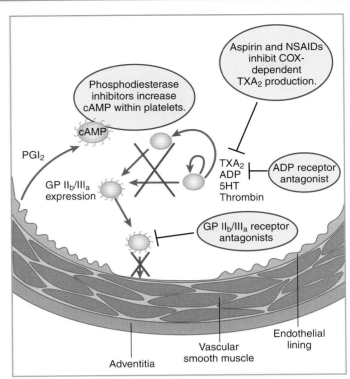

Figure 7-4. Sites of action for antiplatelet drugs. Prostaglandin I_2 (*PGI₂*) is the natural signal from endothelial cells for inactivating platelet responses through generation of cyclic adenosine monophosphate. *NSAIDs*, nonsteroidal antiinflammatory drugs; *COX*, cyclooxygenase; *TXA₂*, thromboxane A_2; *ADP*, adenosine diphosphate; *5HT*, serotonin; *cAMP*, cyclic adenosine monophosphate; *GP*, glycoprotein.

Salicylates

Aspirin

Mechanism of action

Aspirin's main effect is blockade of thromboxane A_2 production from arachidonic acid (Fig. 7-5; see also Fig. 7-4) in platelets, by irreversibly acetylating the enzyme cyclooxygenase, the rate-limiting step in thromboxane synthesis. Remember that aspirin is acetylsalicylic acid and that acetylation of cyclooxygenase leads to inactivation of this enzyme. Platelets lack nuclei, so once aspirin inactivates cyclooxygenase, additional enzyme cannot be resynthesized, which limits most of the actions of aspirin to platelets. Aspirin also inhibits production of prostacyclin from endothelial cells, a prostaglandin that inhibits platelet aggregation (see Fig. 7-4). However, this endothelium-specific effect is short lived because endothelial cells, unlike platelets, can resynthesize cyclooxygenase.

Clinical use

The most common uses of aspirin are preventing and treating myocardial infarctions and cerebrovascular accidents. Aspirin may also be used in atrial fibrillation and transient ischemic attacks. Of course, aspirin is also used for its analgesic, antipyretic, and antiinflammatory effects as well.

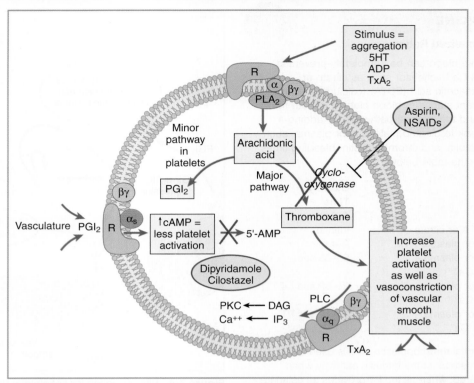

Figure 7-5. Aspirin inhibits cyclooxygenase to prevent thromboxane (TxA_2) synthesis. The phosphodiesterase inhibitors (dipyridamole, cilostazol) increase cyclic adenosine monophosphate ($cAMP$), which in turn decreases platelet activation. *DAG*, diacylglycerol; *IP₃*, inositol trisphosphate; *NSAIDs*, nonsteroidal antiinflammatory drugs; *PKC*, protein kinase C; *PLA₂*, phospholipase A₂; *PLC*, phospholipase C; *R*, receptor.

Adverse effects

Children younger than 12 years may develop Reye syndrome if given aspirin products. Aspirin is known to induce bronchospasm and gastrointestinal hemorrhage, thereby limiting its utility in patients with asthma or peptic ulcer disease.

Phosphodiesterase Inhibitors

Cilostazol and Dipyridamole
Mechanism of action

These phosphodiesterase inhibitors prevent breakdown of cyclic adenosine monophosphate (cAMP) within platelets, and the resultant increase in intracellular cAMP levels leads to diminished platelet activity. Dipyridamole may also inhibit platelet aggregation via inhibiting adenosine uptake by red blood cells (RBCs) or by inhibiting thromboxane A₂ formation.

Clinical use

Dipyridamole may be used adjunctively with warfarin for preventing postoperative thromboembolic complications associated with prosthetic cardiac valves or in combination with aspirin to prevent cerebrovascular ischemia. Cilostazol is used to treat intermittent claudication (exercise-induced pain in legs because of advanced peripheral vascular disease).

Adverse effects

Side effects are mainly limited to hypotension and accompanying dizziness, abdominal distress, headache, and rash.

Adenosine Diphosphate Inhibitors

Clopidogrel, Prasugrel and Ticlopidine
Mechanism of action

These agents irreversibly block the ADP receptor on platelets, thus reducing platelet aggregation. Antiplatelet effects persist for the life of the platelet.

Clinical use

Currently, ADP inhibitors are considered the main alternatives to aspirin for preventing thrombotic events in atherogenic patients with recent myocardial infarctions, strokes, transient ischemic attack, and unstable angina.

Adverse effects

Similar to other antiplatelet agents, ADP inhibitors increase the risk of bleeding. Clopidogrel is preferred over ticlopidine because of life-threatening hematologic reactions associated with ticlopidine, including neutropenia/agranulocytosis and thrombotic thrombocytopenic purpura. Clopidogrel is a prodrug that must be activated by cytochrome P450 ZC19. Genetic polymorphisms in ZC19 or drugs that inhibit its activity can decrease clopidogrel's efficacy. Prasugrel has the advantage that it is not a prodrug and its antiplatelet effects are independent of CYP450 activity.

Glycoprotein IIb/IIIa Inhibitors

Abciximab, Eptifibatide, and Tirofiban
Mechanism of action

Eptifibatide and tirofiban are small-molecule antagonists of the glycoprotein IIb/IIIa receptor on platelets, and abciximab is a monoclonal antibody that targets the same receptor. (Note that abciximab ends in "-mab," denoting that it is a monoclonal antibody.) Activation of this receptor causes fibrinogen and von Willebrand factor to bind to platelets, which subsequently leads to platelet aggregation. These drugs prevent fibrinogen from interacting with platelet glycoprotein IIb/IIIa receptors, thereby inhibiting platelet aggregation.

Clinical use

Glycoprotein IIb/IIIa receptor antagonists are primarily used to manage acute coronary syndromes and to prevent acute cardiac ischemia in patients undergoing percutaneous coronary intervention.

Adverse effects

In addition to the possibility of hypersensitivity reactions with abciximab, the major adverse effect associated with glycoprotein IIb/IIIa receptor antagonists is bleeding.

●●● THROMBOLYTIC DRUGS

Thrombolytics are the only drugs that actually lyse thrombi. These drugs act by facilitating conversion of plasminogen to plasmin. Plasmin is a nonspecific protease that digests fibrin clots (as well as other clotting factors). These drugs play important roles during acute ischemic events (transmural MI, PE, DVT, and arterial thrombosis and emboli) by not only dissolving clots but also by restoring hemodynamic flow and promoting faster recovery. Of note, there may be greater than a 60% decrease in mortality rate if thrombolytics are used within 3 hours of an acute MI.

First-Generation Thrombolytics

Streptokinase and Urokinase
Mechanism of action

Streptokinase is a protein (but, despite its name, not an enzyme) synthesized by β-hemolytic streptococci that forms a stable 1:1 complex with plasminogen, altering its conformation to facilitate its conversion to plasmin. Because of its antigenic nature, streptokinase is quickly removed from circulation. Urokinase is an enzyme produced by human kidney cells that directly converts plasminogen to active plasmin. Both streptokinase and urokinase act on clot-bound plasminogen and free plasminogen. Thus these thrombolytics not only dissolve pathologic thrombi but also may digest fibrin deposits at other body sites. As such, these drugs tend to be hemorrhagic, creating a lytic state throughout the body, which can result in major bleeding events. With the advent of tissue plasminogen activators (and their favorable side effect profiles; see next section), streptokinase is now infrequently used.

Clinical use

These pharmacologic agents are indicated during treatment of acute events such as evolving transmural MI, PE, DVT, and other arterial thrombosis and emboli.

Adverse effects

Because of their biologic origins, streptokinase and urokinase are highly antigenic and can cause hypersensitivity reactions, including anaphylaxis. Patients with antistreptococcal antibodies can develop fever or allergic reactions and demonstrate therapeutic resistance. Of course, bleeding events are among the most frequent adverse effects and can be fatal.

Second-Generation Thrombolytics: Tissue Plasminogen Activators

Alteplase, Reteplase, and Tenecteplase
Drug names end in "-plase."

Mechanism of action

Recombinant plasminogen activator (tPA) is released by endothelial cells in response to stasis produced by vascular occlusion. tPA is colocalized to fibrin. Therefore exogenous tPA will preferentially activate plasminogen that is in close proximity to fibrin clots, making these drugs somewhat clot specific. However, no empiric evidence indicates that the incidence of bleeding events is actually lower with these drugs. In contrast to alteplase or reteplase, tenecteplase may offer an advantage because it is administered as a bolus rather than a 90-minute infusion.

Clinical use

Similar to streptokinase and urokinase, tPA is used during management of acute MI, acute ischemic strokes, and acute PE. Yet, in contrast to streptokinase, hypersensitivity reactions are not problematic with recombinant tPA.

Adverse effects

Again, bleeding is the most common adverse effect, with a threefold higher risk with these agents compared with heparin. Although relatively rare, hemorrhagic stroke is a major concern. Thrombocytopenia may also occur with tPA. Contraindications are listed in Table 7-5.

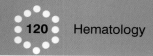

TABLE 7-5. Contraindications to Thrombolytic Therapy

MAJOR CONTRAINDICATIONS	RELATIVE CONTRAINDICATIONS
Recent surgery or internal biopsy	Paracentesis
Recent cerebrovascular process or neurosurgical procedure	Thoracentesis
Recent needle puncture of noncompressible vessels	Prolonged CPR
Active bleeding	Septic thrombophlebitis
Uncontrolled hypertension	Any other condition deemed to be a bleeding risk
Intracranial malignancy	
Pregnancy	
Recent trauma with possible internal injury	
CPR with rib fractures	

CPR, cardiopulmonary resuscitation.

●●● BLEEDING DISORDERS

The flip side to drugs that dissolve clots is the class that induces clotting. The cause of bleeding disorders can generally be classified into one of three groups: genetic, acquired, or iatrogenic (treatment-associated). Hereditary bleeding disorders are rare and typically present as either hemophilia A (factor VIII deficiency), hemophilia B (factor IX deficiency), or von Willebrand disease (abnormal bruising and mucosal bleeding as a result of a qualitative defect in platelet activity). Acquired causes primarily result from liver disease or vitamin K deficiency. The most important iatrogenic causes for bleeding disorders are the use of anticoagulant therapy and the administration of fibrinolytics. Therapeutic interventions to correct bleeding disorders include administration of clotting factors (fresh-frozen plasma [factor VIIa, factor VIII, and factor IX concentrates], cofactors [vitamin K], heparin antidotes [protamine], clotting factor stimulators [desmopressin], and antifibrinolytic agents [aminocaproic acid, tranexamic acid]). Of note, vitamin K should be infused slowly to prevent adverse reactions. In addition to its use as an antidote to reverse the effects of oral anticoagulation with warfarin, maternal therapy with vitamin K is used prophylactically to manage drug-induced hypoprothrombinemia as well as hemorrhagic diseases in newborns. Aminocaproic acid and tranexamic acid prevent activation of plasminogen and therefore prevent fibrinolysis. These drugs are especially useful in hemophiliac patients who have undergone surgical procedures or during surgical procedures where large blood losses may be expected.

●●● ANEMIA

Anemia is a common problem worldwide. Anemia is defined as a hematocrit or hemoglobin value below a normal reference range for specific populations. It is a serious disease in its own right but frequently is a symptom of some other underlying disease. It is further histologically characterized as being microcytic hypochromic (RBCs are small in size and pale) or macrocytic hyperchromic (RBCs are large in size and dark). The most common types of anemias usually result from either blood loss or a deficiency of vitamin B_{12}, folate, and/or iron (the most common cause worldwide) (Table 7-6). The best indicator of iron deficiency is decreased serum ferritin (a storage form of iron) in conjunction with an elevated total iron-binding capacity. Causes of iron deficiency typically include inadequate gastrointestinal absorption, blood loss (slow gastrointestinal bleeds), and increased demands for iron (pregnancy, adolescence).

Agents to Treat Anemias

Supplementation with Iron, Vitamin B_{12}, and Folate

Mechanism of action

Dietary supplementation with iron increases serum iron as well as amount of iron stored in liver and bone. Iron is crucial for normal erythropoiesis as well as for the formation of numerous iron-containing proteins (such as hemoglobin). Both vitamin B_{12} and folate are crucial for DNA synthesis and vital for effective erythropoiesis (generation of new RBCs). Megaloblastic anemias result when folic acid-dependent or vitamin B_{12}–dependent nucleic acid synthesis—is impaired in immature erythrocytes, since a series of reactions catalyzed by vitamin B_{12} and folate are necessary for both DNA and RNA synthesis. With inadequate amounts of these vitamins, DNA and RNA synthesis is slowed and mitotic divisions are skipped, thus producing abnormally large cells.

Pharmacokinetics

The preferred method of iron supplementation is via the oral route. However, only approximately 40% to 60% of orally administered iron is absorbed. Foods that are rich in iron, as well as foods that aid gastrointestinal iron absorption or inhibit iron absorption, are listed in Box 7-7. As a general rule, iron is best absorbed on an empty stomach, but gastrointestinal intolerance may render this impossible. Doses of iron should be based on the elemental dose of iron. Table 7-7 shows the amount of elemental iron obtained from different ferrous salts. Parenteral iron is an option for patients who are intolerant of or noncompliant with oral iron therapy; who continue to

TABLE 7-6. Comparing Three Common Anemias

ANEMIA	MICROSCOPIC APPEARANCE	CLINICAL FEATURES	LABORATORY FINDINGS
Iron deficiency	Microcytic	Pallor Tachycardia Lightheadedness Breathlessness Fatigue Headache Sensitivity to cold Loss of skin tone	Decreased hematocrit Decreased hemoglobin Low or normal reticulocyte count Decreased serum iron Decreased serum ferritin Elevated total iron-binding capacity Decreased transferrin saturation ratio Mean corpuscular volume decreased
Vitamin B$_{12}$ deficiency	Macrocytic	Weakness Painful, enlarged tongue Paresthesias Nausea Anorexia Ataxia Dementia	Low or normal reticulocyte count Decreased vitamin B$_{12}$ Mean corpuscular volume typically elevated
Folate deficiency	Macrocytic	Pallor Fatigue Cardiac symptoms	Low or normal reticulocyte count Decreased serum folate Decreased hematocrit Decreased hemoglobin Mean corpuscular volume elevated

Box 7-7. FOODS THAT AFFECT IRON ABSORPTION

Good Dietary Sources of Iron

Red meats
Raisins
Fish
Eggs
Legumes
Potatoes
Rice

Foods/Drugs That Impair Iron Absorption

Milk
Tea
Phytates
Antacids
Tetracyclines
Fluoroquinolones

Foods That Aid Iron Absorption

Vitamin C
Meat
Orange juice

TABLE 7-7. Elemental Iron in Various Iron Salts

IRON SALT	AMOUNT OF ELEMENTAL IRON
Ferrous sulfate 300 mg	60 mg
Ferrous gluconate 300 mg	35 mg
Ferrous fumarate 100 mg	33 mg

experience blood loss, perhaps via gastrointestinal bleeding; and who have malabsorptive disorders, perhaps because of bowel removal. Iron can form complexes with other medications, impairing the absorption of iron or the target drug. Iron interferes with absorption of tetracyclines and fluoroquinolone antibiotics.

Oral vitamin B$_{12}$ may be used for nutritional deficiencies; however, parenteral B$_{12}$ (cyanocobalamin or hydroxycobalamin) should be used if a lack of intrinsic factor causes inadequate B$_{12}$ absorption.

Clinical use

Iron is helpful for treating certain types of microcytic anemias. Hematologic responses begin within 3 days of initiation of iron replacement therapy. Vitamin B$_{12}$ and folate are used to treat macrocytic anemias that are caused by B$_{12}$ and folate deficiency, respectively (Box 7-8). It is also recommended

Box 7-8. RISK FACTORS FOR FOLATE DEFICIENCY

Decreased Absorption Caused by

Celiac disease
Crohn disease

Inadequate Intake Caused by

Alcoholism
Advanced age
Malnutrition/poverty

Hyperutilization Caused by

Pregnancy
Growth spurts

that all women of child-bearing age take folate to prevent neural tube defects in their offspring. Although recent data show that folate lowers homocysteine levels, it may not offer protection against atherosclerosis.

Adverse effects

Iron causes gastrointestinal upset including nausea, vomiting, constipation, a metallic taste, and darkened stools. Patients who experience constipation may be supplied with a stool softener. Iron may also discolor the urine. Iron tablets are the most common cause of accidental overdose (and death) for children younger than 6 years of age. Parenterally administered iron may cause anaphylactic hypersensitivity reactions, serum sickness, and pain at the site of injection. Parenterally administered vitamin B_{12} may be associated with anaphylaxis. Hyperuricemia, hypokalemia, and Na retention may also occur, and these laboratory parameters should be monitored.

Hematopoietic Stimulating Factors

Erythropoietins (Epoetin-α, Darbepoetin-α), Granulocyte Colony-Stimulating Factor (Filgrastim, Pegfilgrastim), Granulocyte-Macrophage Colony-Stimulating Factor (Sargramostim), and Plerixafor

The drugs in parentheses are recombinant forms of natural hormones.

Mechanism of action

Erythropoietin is normally produced by the kidneys in response to a decrease in blood O_2 tension. Erythropoietin stimulates erythropoiesis (RBC production) and increases the hematocrit. Recombinant erythropoietin is the predominant form available for use in patients. Filgrastim and pegfilgrastim stimulate proliferation, differentiation, migration, and functional activity of neutrophils. Sargramostim stimulates proliferation, differentiation, and functional activity of neutrophils, monocytes, and macrophages. Unlike the filgrastims, sargramostim inhibits neutrophil migration. Plerixafor inhibits the CXCR4 chemokine receptors that are involved in anchoring hematopoietic stem cells in the bone marrow matrix. Inhibition mobilizes these stem cells into the circulation, where they differentiate into blood cells.

Pharmacokinetics

Compared with epoetin-α, darbepoetin-α has a threefold longer $t_{1/2}$, thus requiring fewer infusions per month. Pegfilgrastim (administered subcutaneously) has the advantage of a longer duration of activity over filgrastim (administered intravenously); thus it can be administered once per chemotherapy cycle.

Clinical use

Erythropoietin has demonstrated clear benefits in patients with anemia as a result of chronic renal failure and in patients after chemotherapy. It can also be helpful before allogenic blood transfusions. Filgrastims are used to decrease the duration and extent of neutropenia. Sargramostim also decreases the duration and extent of neutropenia and is used for myeloid reconstitution after bone marrow transplantation and after chemotherapy (see Chapter 5 for review). Plerixafor and granulocyte colony-stimulating factor are used to mobilize hematopoietic stem cells for collection and subsequent autologous transplantation (for treatment of non-Hodgkin lymphoma and multiple myeloma). These types of drugs can be misused by athletes for performance enhancement (no 'juicing' allowed).

Adverse effects

With erythropoietin, there have been reports of dose-dependent increases in blood pressure and platelet counts. With all of the recombinant biologics, some people experience influenza-like symptoms and hypersensitivities. Leukocytosis, accompanied by risk of splenic rupture, may occur if the neutrophil count rises too high with the filgrastims or sargramostims. Sargramostim and plerixafor may cause local reactions at the injection site. This is minimized when the drug is given intravenously or very slowly by the subcutaneous route. Bone pain and anaphylaxis may occur with filgrastims or sargramostim.

●●● ORPHAN HEMATOLOGIC DISEASES

C1 Inhibitor, Eculizumab, Eltombopag, Nitisonone, Romiprostim, and Seropterin

In the years since the first edition of *Elsevier's Integrated Pharmacology* (2007), there has been a significant surge in availability of new drugs and biologics. In addition to the new drug entities described within the body of this chapter, hematology has seen the introduction of several fundamentally different drugs that either work via novel mechanisms or are the "first in class" to address orphan hematologic diseases that heretofore lacked effective therapies. These new compounds are briefly addressed in this section.

Hereditary Tyrosinemia

Nitisinone is the first drug approved for the treatment of hereditary tyrosinemia type 1. This is a rare disorder arising from a genetic deficiency in fumarylacetoacetase—the enzyme that catalyzes the final step in tyrosine metabolism. The resulting accumulation of metabolic precursors and toxic by-products leads to significant organ toxicity (liver, kidney). Nitisinone inhibits an earlier step in the pathway and prevents the accumulation of toxic metabolites. Unfortunately, as a side effect, it produces an accumulation of tyrosine, and so dietary intake of tyrosine and its precursor amino acid, phenylalanine must be restricted.

Paroxysmal Nocturnal Hemoglobinuria

Eculizumab is the first agent approved for the treatment of paroxysmal nocturnal hemoglobinuria, which is a rare disease that results from a genetic mutation that produces red cells that lack complement inhibitors and are susceptible to complement-mediated destruction. The disease is mis named, because the cell destruction occurs throughout the day, but is manifested at night when the urine is concentrated. The mutation is in an X-linked gene responsible for providing lipid (glycosyl-phosphatidylinositol) membrane anchors for a number of blood cell surface proteins (see Chapter 2 for an introduction to this concept). Currently, patients with paroxysmal nocturnal hemoglobinuria are treated with transfusions and immunosuppression. Eculizumab is a monoclonal antibody against complement that alleviates the hemolysis and improves symptoms and quality of life without addressing the underlying genetic defect. Because it inhibits aspects of the immune response, however, eculizumab increases the risk of infection (especially risk of meningococcal infections). Therefore this drug bears a black box warning that patients must be prophylactically treated with a meningococcal vaccine before treatment. As a biologic, this drug also causes side effects resembling influenza.

Phenylketonuria

Seropterin is the first drug to be approved for the *reduction* of phenylalanine concentrations in patients with phenylketonuria (PKU)—as opposed to merely restricting dietary intake of the amino acid. PKU is the manifestation of genetic defects in phenylalanine hydroxylase the enzyme that converts phenylalanine to tyrosine and is the rate-limiting step in phenylalanine metabolism. There are more than 600 documented mutations in phenylalanine hydroxylase and some result in a reduced activity that is responsive to increasing the levels of the rate-limiting substrate tetrahydrobiopterin (BH_4) (this disease is also known as BH_4-responsive PKU). In 2007, seropterin (a synthetic version of BH_4) was approved for treatment of BH_4-responsive PKU. Unfortunately, we are unable to predict BH_4-responsiveness at this time, so treatment efficacy is based on trial and error. Seropterin has a very favorable side effect profile, however, headache is a most common complaint.

Immune Thrombocytopenic Purpura

Eltrombopag (small molecule receptor antagonist) and romiplostim (biologic) are two new drugs—with fundamentally different approaches to the same problem—for treatment of immune thrombocytopenic purpura. Interestingly, the two drugs were approved within months of each other in 2008. Immune thrombocytopenic purpura is an autoimmune disorder in which the body produces antibodies against platelets resulting in serious bleeding disorders (heavy menstruation, petechial rash, bruising, nosebleeds). Romiplostim is a chimeric recombinant biologic (thrombopoietin receptor agonist fused to Fc-peptide) that increases platelet production. As a biologic, romiplostim bears significant influenza side effects. Moreover, it can be *too* effective (producing too many platelets) with resulting thrombotic/thromboembolic complications. It has also been shown to increase reticulin deposition in the bone marrow (with subsequent risk of fibrosis of the marrow). Eltrombopag is a new small molecule thrombopoietin

receptor antagonist that also stimulates platelet production. It bears the advantage of oral administration (as opposed to subcutaneously). The major problem is that it has a black box warning for potential hepatotoxicity so liver enzymes should be carefully monitored. As with romiplostim, eltrombopag also has a risk of increasing reticulin deposition in marrow, as well as producing too robust a stimulation of platelets.

Hereditary Angioedema

Hereditary angioedema is a genetic deficiency of the C1-esterase inhibitor, a naturally occurring plasma regulator of the complement system. This deficiency produces potentially life-threatening inflammatory responses. Human C1 inhibitor is purified from human plasma and is approved to temporarily increase C1 inhibitor activity after intravenous administration. Current therapies (steroids and danazol) are relatively ineffective and display significant side effects. The C1 inhibitor, being a natural human protein, has a favorable side effect profile.

CLINICAL MEDICINE

Vitamin B_{12} and Folate Demand

Because all animal products contain vitamin B_{12}, only strict vegetarians are at risk of B_{12} dietary deficiencies. Other risk factors for vitamin B_{12} deficiencies include decreased gastrointestinal absorption (possibly from removal of the bowel) and inadequate utilization because of transcobalamin (a transport protein) deficiency in the gastrointestinal tract. Folate deficiency is more common than vitamin B_{12} deficiency. Humans must obtain folate through their diet, and the most common cause of folate deficiency is lack of dietary green vegetables. In addition to inadequate intake, other risk factors include decreased absorption and hyperutilization. Folate demand increases during pregnancy. Evidence now shows that periconceptional folate supplementation in normal women reduces the incidence of fetal neuronal tube defects (spina bifida, meningocele, anencephaly). Folate is absolutely necessary for the developing fetal nervous system. Newborns with congenital folate malabsorption syndrome are born with mental retardation, cerebral calcifications, seizures, and peripheral neuropathies.

●●● TOP FIVE LIST

1. Heparin inhibits coagulation by combining with and activating antithrombin III, resulting in more efficient inactivation of clotting factors IIa, IXa, Xa, and XIIa. Activated partial thromboplastin time is used to monitor the effects of heparin on the intrinsic coagulation pathway, and protamine is an antidote if excessive bleeding occurs.
2. LMWHs inhibit coagulation by combining with and activating antithrombin III, resulting in efficient inactivation primarily of factor Xa. LMWHs have a predictable dose response; routine anticoagulation monitoring is not usually necessary.

3. Warfarin derives its anticoagulant actions through inhibition of hepatic carboxylation of vitamin K–dependent clotting factors (i.e., clotting factors II, VII, IX, and X). Warfarin's effects are monitored by PT (or more reliably by INR). The therapeutic onset takes time (up to 1 week) as the existing active clotting factors must be degraded. In the event of excessive bleeding, vitamin K, fresh-frozen plasma, or concentrated clotting factors may be administered. More food, drug, and herb interactions occur with warfarin than any other drug.

4. A variety of drugs—cyclooxygenase inhibitors, phosphodiesterase inhibitors, ADP inhibitors, and glycoprotein IIb/IIIa inhibitors—inhibit coagulation by inhibiting platelets through different signal transduction mechanisms.

5. Unlike other drugs used in anticoagulation, thrombolytics actually lyse existing clots rather than simply preventing additional clot formation.

Self-assessment questions can be accessed at www. StudentConsult.com.

Cardiovascular System

8

CONTENTS

PHARMACOLOGIC MANAGEMENT OF HYPERTENSION
  Diuretics
  β-Blockers
  Angiotensin-Converting Enzyme Inhibitors
  Angiotensin Receptor Blockers
  Aldosterone Receptor Antagonists
  Renin Inhibitors
  α_1-Receptor Blockers
  Calcium Channel Blockers
  Centrally Acting α_2-Agonists
  Vasodilators
  Summary
PHARMACOLOGIC MANAGEMENT OF PULMONARY ARTERIAL HYPERTENSION
PHARMACOLOGIC MANAGEMENT OF STABLE ANGINA
  Nitrates:
  Partial Fatty Acid Oxidation Inhibitor
  Summary
PHARMACOLOGIC MANAGEMENT OF HEART FAILURE
  Positive Inotropes
  Summary
PHARMACOTHERAPY OF ANTIARRHYTHMICS
  Class I: Sodium Channel Blockers
  Class II: β-Blockers
  Class III: Potassium Channel Blockers
  Class IV: Calcium Channel Blockers
  Other Antiarrhythmics
  Summary
HYPERLIPIDEMIAS
  Statins
  Fibrates
  Ezetimibe
  Bile Acid Sequestrants (Resins)
  Niacin
  Omega-3-Acid Ethyl Esters (Fish Oil)
  Summary
COMPLEMENTARY AND ALTERNATIVE MEDICINE
TOP FIVE LIST

The cardiovascular system is more than just the curve, that is, the Frank-Starling curve—which states that the left ventricular end-diastolic pressure is proportional to cardiac output. In more clinical terms, pathologies that result in altered cardiac output, because of changes in stroke volume or heart rate, can be treated with drugs that affect hemodynamic parameters that control left ventricular end-diastolic pressure, such as preload and afterload. However, drugs that regulate hemodynamic parameters are often ineffective and do not prolong life in patients with failing hearts. In reality, with the cardiovascular system it is all about making the failing heart more effective (i.e., moving the Frank-Starling curve upward and to the left). This can be accomplished pharmacologically by increasing myocardial contractility through positive inotropes as well as by reducing inefficient cardiac hypertrophy via angiotensin-converting enzyme (ACE) inhibitors and angiotensin II receptor blockers (ARBs).

Pathologies that compromise cardiac output include hypertension, coronary artery disease, heart failure, (HF) cardiac arrhythmias, and hypercholesterolemia. Because these conditions affect multiple parameters associated with cardiac output and total peripheral resistance, it should not be surprising that there is considerable overlap in the drugs used to treat these five medical conditions, and the drugs frequently are used in combination.

In many ways, cardiovascular pharmacology fits hand in hand with autonomic pharmacology. Many drugs used for treatment of cardiovascular disease act as agonists or antagonists of the α- or β-adrenergic receptors in the heart and the vasculature. Regulation of these receptors modulates preload and afterload pressures, total peripheral resistance, and myocardial contractility, culminating in control of cardiac output.

●●● PHARMACOLOGIC MANAGEMENT OF HYPERTENSION

Regulation of blood pressure is all about exquisite wireless communication between organ systems. Receptors that assess pressure and solute concentrations regulate interconnected neuronal, cardiovascular, and renal networks. The interplay among the renal, neuronal, and cardiovascular systems ultimately controls blood pressure (*total peripheral resistance* and *cardiac output*) through tight control of fluid and solute load as well as endogenous regulators of vasoconstriction. Disturbances in these feed-forward and feed-back pathways lead to exacerbations of cardiovascular disease and identify targets for pharmacologic intervention.

Identifiable causes of hypertension (and methods for controlling it) are summarized in Box 8-1 and Figure 8-1. In patients with hypertension, baroreceptors acquire a new set point that is higher than normal, resulting in central stimulation of the sympathetic nervous system. This heightened sympathetic tone increases norepinephrine release.

Box 8-1. IDENTIFIABLE CAUSES OF HYPERTENSION

Sleep apnea	Long-term steroid therapy
Illicit drug use (e.g., cocaine, amphetamines)	Cushing syndrome
	Pheochromocytoma
Chronic kidney disease	Coarctation of the aorta
Primary aldosteronism	Thyroid disease
Renovascular disease	Parathyroid disease

In the heart, norepinephrine increases myocardial contractility and heart rate via actions at β_1-receptors, thereby increasing cardiac output. Increased noradrenergic activity in the vasculature directly stimulates vasoconstriction via actions at α_1-receptors, which increases total peripheral resistance.

Norepinephrine also stimulates renal β_1-receptor–mediated release of renin, which activates the renin-angiotensin-aldosterone (RAA) pathway. Renin is the enzyme that cleaves angiotensinogen to form angiotensin I, which is then hydrolyzed by ACE into angiotensin II. Angiotensin II is a potent vasoconstrictor. Angiotensin II also stimulates the release of aldosterone from the adrenal gland, which leads to sodium reabsorption. Ultimately, activation of the RAA system increases total peripheral resistance via vasoconstriction and increases cardiac output via sodium (and water) retention.

Identifying the mechanisms that underlie hypertension helps define targets or pathways suitable for pharmacologic intervention (Fig. 8-2). In brief, centrally acting α_2-agonists inhibit norepinephrine release. β-Blockers decrease cardiac output by slowing heart rate and decreasing myocardial contractility. β-Blockers also antagonize renal β_1-receptors to block renin release, thereby preventing activation of the RAA system. ACE inhibitors, ARBs, aldosterone receptor antagonists, and renin inhibitors block various steps within the RAA pathway. Diuretics reduce cardiac output by increasing excretion of Na^+ and H_2O. Direct-acting vasodilators may be used to directly vasodilate the vasculature to reduce total peripheral resistance. In addition, calcium channel blockers, which inhibit the actions of Ca^{++} in the myocardium or the periphery, may also be used to decrease myocardial contractility and heart rate and reduce total peripheral resistance.

The Joint National Committee on Prevention, Detection, Evaluation, and Treatment of High Blood Pressure published its seventh set of guidelines for managing hypertension in 2003 (JNC-VII). JNC-VIII is expected in 2012. These guidelines are summarized in Figure 8-3. Although these guidelines are currently the gold standard for hypertension management, some hypertension specialists prefer to treat patients according to whether they exhibit high plasma renin activity, have a volumetric (sodium) excess, or vessel vasoconstriction. Drug choices for each of these types of hypertension are listed in Table 8-1.

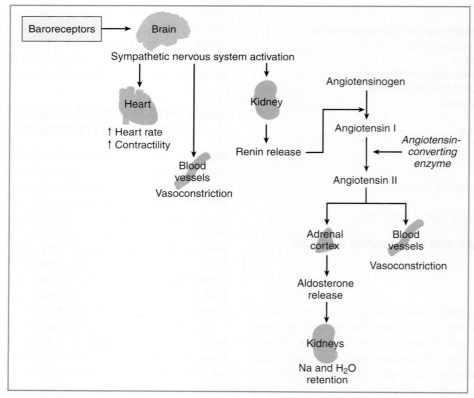

Figure 8-1. Network control of blood pressure.

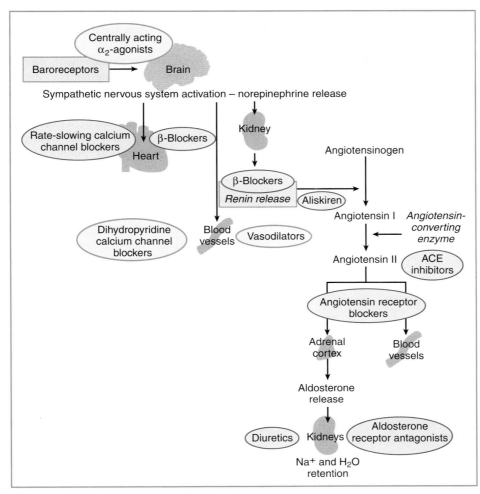

Figure 8-2. Site of action for antihypertensive drugs. *ACE*, anglotensin-converting enzyme.

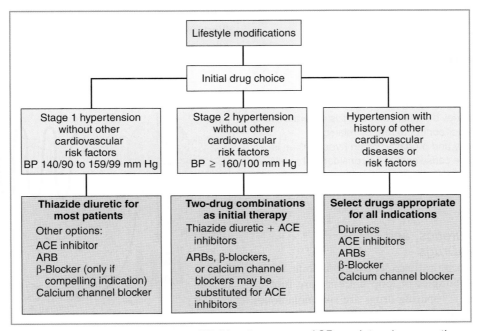

Figure 8-3. Algorithm for initial hypertension treatment. *BP*, blood pressure; *ACE*, angiotensin-converting enzyme inhibitor; *ARB*, angiotensin receptor blocker. (Data from the Seventh Report of the Joint National Committee on Prevention, Evaluation, and Treatment of High Blood Pressure [JNC-VII], December 2003. Available at www.nhlbi.nih.gov/guidelines/hypertension/index.htm).

TABLE 8-1. Antihypertensive Treatment Options*

VOLUMETRIC EXCESS	HIGH RENIN ACTIVITY
Thiazide or loop diuretics	Angiotensin-converting enzyme inhibitors
Spironolactone	Angiotensin II receptor blockers
Ca^{++} channel blockers α-Blockers	β-Blockers

*Based on volumetric excess or high renin activity.

The following classes of drugs are used to treat hypertension:

1. Diuretics
2. β-Blockers
3. ACE inhibitors
4. ARBs
5. Aldosterone-receptor antagonists
6. Renin inhibitors
7. $α_1$-Blockers
8. Ca^{++} channel blockers
9. Centrally acting $α_2$-blockers
10. Vasodilators

PHYSIOLOGY

Defining Blood Pressure

Blood pressure is the product of cardiac output × total peripheral resistance ($BP = CO \times TPR$). Cardiac output is a product of heart rate × stroke volume ($CO = HR \times SV$). Stroke volume is a function of preload (the amount of blood returning to the heart), afterload (the pressure that the heart must pump against), and contractility. Antihypertensives either lower cardiac output or lower total peripheral resistance.

CLINICAL MEDICINE

Controlling Blood Pressure

As blood pressure rises, there is a greater risk of coronary artery disease, stroke, and kidney disease. Therefore it is imperative to get blood pressure under control to reduce related cardiovascular morbidity and mortality. When hypertension is first noted, an identifiable cause should be considered, but 95% of the time an obvious cause cannot be found.

Diuretics

Thiazides, Loop Diuretics, and Potassium-Sparing Drugs

Thiazides include hydrochlorothiazide, chlorthalidone, metolazone, indapamide. Examples of loop diuretics are furosemide and bumetanide. K^+-sparing drugs are spironolactone, triamterene, and amiloride.

An initial strategy for managing hypertension is often to alter volumetric excess through dietary restriction of Na^+. Diuretics (see Chapter 9) essentially capitalize on sodium restriction because these drugs facilitate sodium excretion. Diuretics are often included in antihypertensive treatment regimens.

In hypertension management, diuretics initially decrease blood volume by facilitating Na^+ excretion, hence reducing extracellular fluid volume; however, antihypertensive effects are maintained even after excess Na^+ has been diuresed. It has been speculated that high plasma sodium concentrations increase vessel rigidity; thus antihypertensive effects are maintained because low plasma sodium indirectly induces vasodilation.

According to JNC-VII, thiazide diuretics are the first-line antihypertensive for most patients. These drugs are particularly effective antihypertensives for patients of African ancestry and the elderly. Note, however, that with the exception of metolazone, thiazides are not effective at low glomerular filtration rates; therefore loop diuretics are preferred when kidney function is compromised. In addition, thiazides are often not first-line choices for diabetic patients or patients with hyperlipidemia because the drugs may exacerbate these conditions. Often, K^+-sparing diuretics (amiloride and triamterene) are used in combination with thiazides to offset K^+ loss.

β-Blockers

β₁ Selective: Acebutolol, Atenolol, Betaxolol, Bisoprolol, Esmolol, Metoprolol, Nebivolol

Nonselective: Carteolol, Carvedilol, Labetalol, Nadolol, Penbutolol, Pindolol, Propranolol, Sotalol, and Timolol

Note that the drug names all end in "-olol" or "-alol."

Mechanism of action

β-Blockers are antagonists of β-adrenergic receptors. Figure 8-4 illustrates how β-blockade *prevents* accumulation of cyclic adeonsine monophosphate (cAMP) and activation of protein

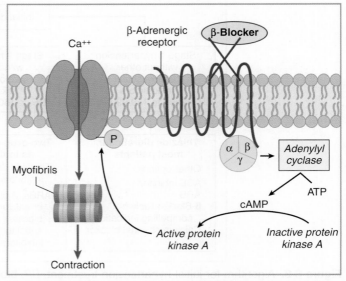

Figure 8-4. Mechanism of β-blocker action on heart. *cAMP*, cyclic adenosine triphosphate; *ATP*, adenosine triphosphate.

kinase A, thereby reducing Ca^{++} entry into myocardial cells, decreasing heart rate, and reducing myocardial contractility. These combined effects reduce cardiac output and are responsible for initial antihypertensive effects. In addition, β-blockers exert sustained antihypertensive actions by antagonizing β_1-receptors in the kidneys, an effect that reduces renin release and decreases total peripheral resistance.

All β-blockers are not created equal. For the most part, selective β_1-receptor blockers, such as metoprolol and atenolol, are the preferred β-blockers to treat hypertension, especially for patients with peripheral vascular disease or airway diseases such as asthma. Remember that nonselective blockade of β_2-receptors in the lung can aggravate pulmonary bronchoconstriction and airway resistance. Therefore, propranolol may aggravate asthma because it blocks both β_1- and β_2-receptor subtypes.

Other nonselective β-antagonists, such as pindolol, possess intrinsic sympathomimetic activity because they exhibit partial agonist activity. A partial agonist weakly stimulates the receptor to which it is bound but simultaneously blocks the activity of stronger endogenous agonists (epinephrine or norepinephrine). It is difficult to define pindolol as a β-antagonist when, in fact, it is really a poor agonist. This partial β-agonist activity decreases blood pressure, but it does not induce bradycardia. β-Blockers that possess intrinsic sympathomimetic activity should not be used in patients with angina or those who have had a myocardial infarction. The newest β-blocker, nebivolol, is selective for antagonizing β_1-receptors and also increases nitric oxide–mediated vasodilation.

β-Blockers such as labetalol and carvedilol also are not selective β_1-blockers, but these drugs antagonize both α- and β-adrenergic receptors. By antagonizing α-adrenergic receptors in the vasculature, these drugs preferentially reduce total peripheral resistance in the periphery without causing significant effects on heart rate or cardiac output. Thus these drugs are especially useful to manage special hypertensive situations such as pheochromocytoma (an epinephrine-secreting tumor of the adrenal medulla) and hypertensive crisis. Clinically relevant pharmacologic differences among various β-blockers are highlighted in Table 8-2.

Clinical use

In addition to their use as antihypertensives, β-blockers are used as antiarrhythmics and for management of angina and treatment of HF, and they should be included in most post–myocardial infarction therapeutic regimens. β-Blockers also are used prophylactically to prevent migraine headaches and may be administered ocularly to reduce intraocular pressure. Timolol decreases intraocular pressure by preventing production of aqueous humor. Some unique indications for β-blockers are listed in Table 8-3.

Adverse effects

Because β-blockers depress myocardial contractility and excitability, they may cause hypotension, may precipitate cardiac conduction abnormalities (second- or third-degree atrioventricular block), may worsen acutely decompensatedHF, and may cause bradycardia. β-Blockers are *absolutely contraindicated* in patients who have profound sinus bradycardia and greater than first-degree heart block or signs of bronchoconstriction. Therapy with β-blockers should not be stopped abruptly because rebound hypertension may occur. β-Blockers commonly cause fatigue, malaise, sedation, depression, and sexual dysfunction. These drugs may also impair the ability to exercise because they lower the maximal exercise-induced heart rate. In addition, β-blockers inhibit sympathetically stimulated lipolysis, inhibit hepatic glycogenolysis, mask symptoms of hypoglycemia (e.g., tremor, cardiac palpitations), mask symptoms of hyperthyroidism,

TABLE 8-3. Unique Uses for Commonly Used β-Blockers

β-BLOCKER	USE
Esmolol	Hypertensive emergencies (intravenous)
Timolol	Ocular hypotensive effects in glaucoma
Labetalol	Hypertensive crisis
Propranolol	Migraine prophylaxis
Carvedilol	Heart failure

TABLE 8-2. Pharmacologic Differences Among β-Blockers (Commonly Used Drugs)

β_1-/β_2-NONSELECTIVE ANTAGONISTS	β_1-SELECTIVE ANTAGONISTS	NONSELECTIVE AGENTS WITH INTRINSIC SYMPATHOMIMETIC ACTIVITY	α- AND β-ANTAGONISTS
Carteolol	Acebutolol	Acebutolol	Carvedilol
Nadolol	Atenolol	Carteolol	Labetalol
Penbutolol	Betaxolol	Pindolol	
Pindolol	Bisoprolol		
Propranolol	Esmolol		
Sotalol	Metoprolol		
Timolol	Nebivolol		

adversely affect cholesterol levels, and increase the risk of developing diabetes. Because of their myriad side effects, β-blockers are no longer recommended as first-line antihypertensive treatment unless comorbidities exist that would simultaneously benefit from this drug class. Overall, relative contraindications for β-blockers are listed in Box 8-2.

Angiotensin-Converting Enzyme Inhibitors

Enalapril, Lisinopril, Captopril, Benazepril, Fosinopril, Quinapril, Ramipril, Moexipril, and Perindopril

Note that the drug names all end in "-pril."

Mechanism of action

ACE inhibitors reduce total peripheral resistance by blocking the actions of ACE, the enzyme that converts angiotensin I to angiotensin II (Fig. 8-5). Recall that angiotensin II is a potent vasoconstrictor and stimulates release of aldosterone from the adrenal cortex, which causes sodium and water retention. ACE inhibitors are balanced vasodilators, meaning that they cause vasodilation of both arteries and veins. Unlike other vasodilators, this class of drugs does not exert reflex actions on the sympathetic nervous system (tachycardia, increased

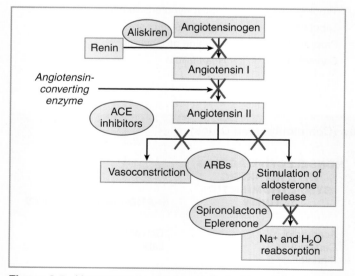

Figure 8-5. Hypertension can be controlled by pharmacologically regulating the renin-angiotensin-aldosterone system. *ACE*, angiotensin-converting enzyme inhibitors; *ARBs*, angiotensin receptor blockers.

cardiac output, fluid retention). Finally, as angiotensin II also possesses mitogenic activity in the myocardium, inhibition of angiotensin II may lead to diminished myocardial hypertrophy or remodeling, situations often seen in patients with hypertension or HF.

Pharmacokinetics

As a class, ACE inhibitors can be subdivided into three subclasses. Captopril is the prototype. With captopril, the parent compound is pharmacologically active, but it is also converted to active metabolites. This drug possesses a sulfhydryl moiety that is thought to be responsible for some side effects that are more likely with this drug compared to the others (rash, loss of taste, neutropenia, oral lesions). Most of the ACE inhibitors fall into the second subclass. These drugs are administered as inactive pro-drugs that require activation by hepatic conversion (e.g., inactive enalapril is converted to active enalaprilat). Most of these drugs are excreted only via renal mechanisms. Lisinopril falls into the third ACE inhibitor subclass. Lisinopril is not a prodrug, it is the active form. It does not undergo hepatic metabolism and is excreted unchanged in the urine.

Clinical use

ACE inhibitors are especially useful antihypertensives in young and middle-aged whites. Elderly and black patients are relatively resistant to the antihypertensive effects of ACE inhibitors, but resistance can be overcome by adding diuretics to the regimen. Some of this resistance has been linked to a high-salt diet, which induces hypertension despite a low renin state. ACE inhibitors have beneficial actions in HF and reduce the risk of strokes, even in patients with well-controlled blood pressure. ACE inhibitors also slow progression of kidney disease in patients with diabetic nephropathies. Renal benefits are probably a result of improved renal hemodynamics from decreased glomerular arteriolar resistance.

Adverse effects

As many as 40% of patients cannot tolerate ACE inhibitors because of induction of a dry cough. This cough is thought to occur as a result of accumulation of bradykinin. Normally, ACE converts bradykinin to inactive metabolites. However, when ACE is inhibited, bradykinin concentration rises. Bradykinin causes tissue edema and bronchospasm, so bradykinin accumulation is thought to be responsible for causing the cough (Fig. 8-6). Bradykinin accumulation may also induce angioedema of the lips and tongue, even after patients have used ACE inhibitors for many years. Dysgeusia (unpleasant taste in the mouth) and rashes are possible. Severe hypotension may occur in patients who are volume depleted. Hyperkalemia may also occur because of inhibition of aldosterone, especially in patients using potassium supplements and potassium-sparing diuretics. ACE inhibitors are contraindicated during the second and third trimesters of pregnancy because of adverse effects on the fetus (fetal hypotension, anuria, renal failure, fetal malformation). ACE inhibitors are also contraindicated in patients with bilateral renal artery stenosis, in whom the drugs can cause acute renal failure. In patients

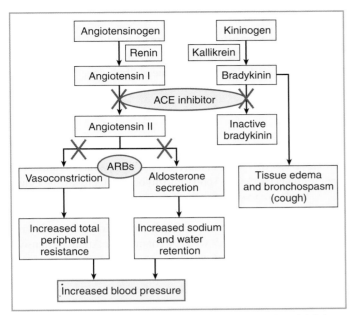

Figure 8-6. Angiotensin-converting enzyme (*ACE*) inhibitors cause bradykinin accumulation. *ARBs*, angiotensin receptor blockers.

with bilateral renal artery stenosis, glomerular filtration is maintained by angiotensin II–mediated vasoconstriction of the efferent arteriole. By blocking formation of angiotensin II, ACE inhibitors decrease glomerular filtration (a rise in serum creatinine is observed in nearly all patients), which can lead to renal failure in those with bilateral renal artery stenosis (Fig. 8-7).

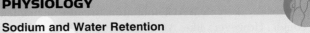

PHYSIOLOGY

Sodium and Water Retention

Diminished renal perfusion pressure causes the kidney to release renin, which then converts angiotensinogen to angiotensin I. ACE removes two terminal amino acids from angiotensin I to form angiotensin II. Angiotensin II stimulates aldosterone secretion from the adrenal cortex. Aldosterone release increases expression of renal Na^+ channels, facilitating Na^+ reabsorption and water retention.

Angiotensin Receptor Blockers

Losartan, Candesartan, Eprosartan, Irbesartan, Olmesartan, Telmisartan, and Valsartan

Note that all drugs end in "-sartan."

Mechanism of action
In contrast to ACE inhibitors, which inhibit production of angiotensin II, ARBs block the effects of angiotensin II by acting as antagonists at angiotensin II receptors. This action results in decreased vasoconstriction and decreased release of aldosterone and antidiuretic hormone.

Clinical use
ARBs are used for treating the same conditions as ACE inhibitors. However, ARBs may be better tolerated than ACE inhibitors because of the lack of bradykinin-induced bronchospasm.

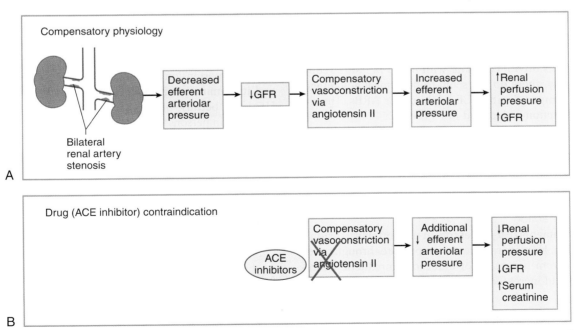

Figure 8-7. A, To compensate for the decrease in glomerular filtration rate (*GFR*) that occurs in individuals with bilateral renal artery stenosis, the renal vasculature relies on angiotensin II. In individuals affected by bilateral renal artery stenosis, renal function is preserved by an angiotensin II–induced vasoconstriction of the efferent arterioles, which increases renal perfusion pressure and maintains GFR. **B,** Angiotensin-converting enzyme (*ACE*) inhibitors are contraindicated in patients with bilateral renal artery stenosis because the drugs cause dilation of the efferent arterioles, which decreases renal perfusion pressure. As a result, these drugs can precipitate acute renal failure as GFR to declines and serum creatinine increases. Indeed, any patient in whom ACE inhibitors are initiated will have a rise in serum creatinine.

Adverse effects

ARBs are less likely than ACE inhibitors to cause angioedema or cough. However, like ACE inhibitors, ARBs can cause hyperkalemia and are contraindicated during pregnancy and in those with bilateral renal artery stenosis.

Aldosterone Receptor Antagonists

Spironolactone and Eplerenone
Mechanism of action

These drugs bind to cytosolic mineralocorticoid receptors and block aldosterone from binding its receptors and inducing nuclear localization. Thus the action of aldosterone to increase blood pressure, by reabsorbing Na^+, is inhibited. When aldosterone receptors are blocked, Na^+ is excreted but K^+ is retained. Thus, as discussed in Chapter 9, spironolactone is known as a K^+-sparing diuretic. Spironolactone also antagonizes other steroid receptor subtypes, explaining its adverse endocrine effects (gynecomastia, decreased libido, hirsutism, menstrual disturbances). Eplerenone is a specific antagonist of aldosterone receptors.

Adverse effects

Spironolactone and eplerenone can cause hyperkalemia. Eplerenone is contraindicated in patients with poor renal function or patients using potent P450 3A4 inhibitors (e.g., azole antifungals, clarithromycin, ritonavir) because eplerenone is metabolized by hepatic P450 enzymes.

Renin Inhibitors

Aliskiren

Aliskiren is the first direct renin inhibitor. It is less likely than ACE inhibitors to cause a cough as an adverse effect. However, although plasma renin activity is reduced with aliskiren, these reductions do not correlate with blood pressure reductions. Presently, there do not seem to be clinical advantages to aliskiren compared with ACE inhibitors or ARBs. The site of aliskiren's action is depicted in Figure 8-2.

α_1-Receptor Blockers

Prazosin, Doxazosin, and Terazosin
Note that all drugs end in "-zosin."

Mechanism of action

These drugs antagonize α_1-receptors in the periphery, leading to vasodilation. However, patients compensate through reflex tachycardia (from baroreceptor-induced sympathetic neuronal activity) and increased release of renin.

Clinical use

Unfortunately, these compensatory mechanisms have been shown to contribute to HF. As a result, α_1-receptor blockers are not routinely recommended for treating hypertension and are reserved as last-line agents. Another use for these drugs is in management of benign prostatic hypertrophy. In the prostate and the neck of the bladder, α_1-antagonists reduce smooth muscle tone, thus relieving urinary symptoms.

Calcium Channel Blockers

Myocardial Specific: Verapamil and Diltiazem

Vascular-Acting Dihydropyridines: Amlodipine, Clevidipine, Felodipine, Isradipine, Nicardipine, Nifedipine, Nimodipine, and Nisoldipine. Note that the dihydropyridines all end in "-dipine."

Mechanism of action

All calcium channel blockers prevent Ca^{++} from entering either cardiac or vascular smooth muscle cells. Verapamil and diltiazem preferentially block Ca^{++} entry into myocardial cells. In myocytes, Ca^{++} binds to troponin, which relieves troponin's inhibitory effects, thus allowing actin and myosin to interact (Fig. 8-8A). The actions of verapamil or diltiazem result in bradycardia, reduced contractility, and slowed AV conduction. Antihypertensive effects occur as a result of decreased cardiac output.

Dihydropyridines interfere with vasoconstriction by blocking Ca^{++} entry into vascular smooth muscle cells. In vascular smooth muscle cells, Ca^{++} binds to calmodulin. This calcium-calmodulin complex activates myosin light chain kinase, which phosphorylates myosin, thus stimulating contraction (Fig. 8-8B). Antihypertensive effects occur as a result of diminished vascular smooth muscle contraction and reduced total peripheral resistance.

Nifedipine is unique in that it blocks Ca^{++} influx in both myocardial tissues and the vasculature, exhibiting properties of both verapamil and the dihydropyridines; however, the effects on the myocardium are much less than those in the periphery. Clevidipine also has distinctive properties. Like nicardipine, clevidipine is administered intravenously; however, clevidipine is a milky white oil-in-water emulsion that is sensitive to temperature (must be stored refrigerated) and light (undergoes photodegradation). It has a rapid onset of action (2 to 4 minutes) and a short duration of action (15 minutes), thus providing minute-to-minute control of blood pressure when oral drugs cannot be used to treat hypertension. It is metabolized by esterases in the blood, and its elimination is independent of liver or renal function. However, because of components in the emulsion, it is contraindicated in persons with egg or soy allergies.

Clinical use

Calcium channel blockers are especially useful antihypertensives in patients who have low renin hypertension. Heart rate–slowing Ca^{++} channel blockers, such as verapamil and diltiazem, are also used as antiarrhythmics. Additional uses for Ca^{++} channel blockers include angina, migraine prophylaxis, and preterm labor.

Adverse effects

Calcium channel blockers that cause bradycardia HF (verapamil and diltiazem) should be avoided in patients with HF or cardiac conduction defects, especially if patients are also prescribed β-blockers. Dihydropyridines cause peripheral edema, hypotension, dizziness, flushing, and headaches because of their vasodilatory effects. All Ca^{++} channel blockers may cause or worsen gastroesophageal reflux disease by lowering lower esophageal sphincter tone. Many Ca^{++} channel blockers are highly protein bound and capable of inhibiting

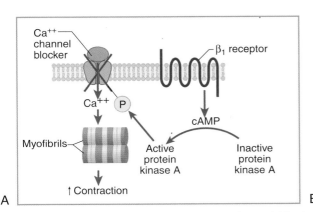

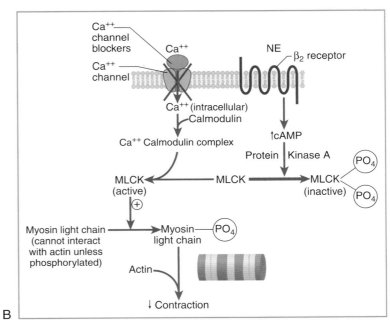

Figure 8-8. Mechanism by which calcium channel blockers affect myocardial contractility (**A**) and vascular tone (**B**). The cross-talk and interplay between Ca^{++} (and Ca^{++} channel blockers) and norepinephrine at β_1 and β_2 receptors is also depicted. *NE*, norepinephrine; *cAMP*, cyclic adenosine monophosphate; *MLCK*, myosin light chain kinase.

the P-glycoprotein transporter. These mechanisms are believed to account for some of the drug interactions involving Ca^{++} channel blockers. One particularly serious interaction involves combination of the non-dihydropyridines (verapamil or diltiazem) and digoxin; digoxin levels have increased 25% to 70% with these Ca^{++} channel blockers. If these drugs must be used simultaneously, careful monitoring and dosage adjustments are necessary.

Centrally acting α_2-Agonists

Methyldopa and Clonidine

Mechanism of action. These drugs act as agonists of synaptic α_2-receptors in the central nervous system (Fig. 8-9). Essentially, these receptors are autoreceptors; when stimulated, they feed-back to negatively inhibit adrenergic tone and decrease norepinephrine release in the periphery. Ultimately, antihypertensive effects result from (1) decreased total peripheral resistance, (2) blunted baroreceptor reflexes (these drugs cause very little tachycardia), (3) decreased heart rate, and (4) reduced renin activity.

Pharmacokinetics

Clonidine exerts its actions directly on α_2-receptors. In contrast, methyldopa acts indirectly. Methyldopa is converted to α-methylnorepinephrine by the same enzymes involved in the biosynthesis of dopamine and is released as a false neurotransmitter (Fig. 8-10). Methylnorepinephrine is the "active" drug that stimulates presynaptic α_2-receptors centrally. Clonidine is available as an oral tablet and as a transdermal patch that is applied once weekly.

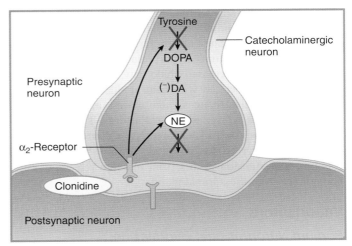

Figure 8-9. Mechanism of centrally acting α_2-agonists. Clonidine binds to α_2-autoreceptors and, by feedback inhibition, prevents neurotransmitter synthesis and release. *DA*, dopamine; *DOPA*, dihydroxyphenylalanine; *NE*, norepinephrine.

Clinical use

Methyldopa is often used to manage eclampsia during pregnancy. In addition to its antihypertensive actions, clonidine is used off-label to manage numerous conditions, including alcohol withdrawal, attention deficit–hyperactivity disorder, mania, psychosis, and restless legs syndrome. Clonidine is useful in combination with vasodilators to blunt reflex tachycardia.

Adverse effects

The adverse effects associated with these two drugs are quite different from each other. Prolonged use of methyldopa causes sodium and water retention; therefore it is best used in combination with diuretics. Orthostatic hypotension may occur and is

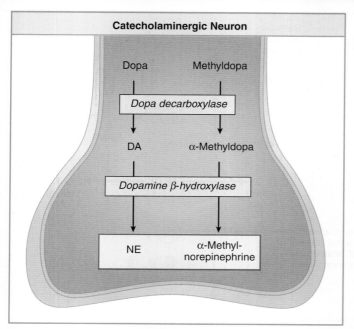

Figure 8-10. Central activation of methyldopa. *DOPA*, dihydroxyphenylalanine; *NE*, norepinephrine.

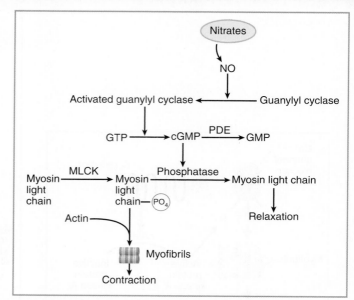

Figure 8-11. Mechanism of nitrate-induced vasodilation, *GTP*, guanosine triphosphate; *GMP*; guanosine monophosphate; *cGMP*, cyclic GMP, *PDE*, phosphodiesterase; *MLCK*, myosin light chain kinase; *NO*, nitric oxide

more likely in patients who are volume depleted. Methyldopa can cause hepatitis, so liver function tests should be monitored regularly during therapy, and methyldopa may also cause hemolytic anemia. Because of structural similarities with dopamine, Parkinson symptoms, hyperprolactinemia, galactorrhea, gynecomastia, and decreased libido may also occur.

Clonidine is associated with central side effects including sedation, sleep disturbances, nightmares, and restlessness. These effects are worsened when the drug is used simultaneously with other central nervous system depressants. Clonidine should never be discontinued abruptly because severe rebound hypertension occurs from massive release of catecholamines from the adrenal gland.

Vasodilators

Sodium Nitroprusside, Hydralazine, and Minoxidil

Mechanism of action

These drugs directly relax vascular smooth muscle, decreasing total peripheral resistance. Nitroprusside is metabolized in vascular endothelial cells to nitric oxide. Nitric oxide activates guanylyl cyclase to form cyclic guanosine monophosphate (cGMP). cGMP exerts vasodilatory actions in both arteries and veins, presumably by activating an as of yet unidentified phosphatase that de-phosphorylates myosin light chain, preventing myosin's interaction with actin. This makes nitroprusside a useful intravenous option for managing hypertensive crisis (Fig. 8-11). (Additional nitric oxide–producing drugs are discussed later in more detail as treatments for stable angina.) At this time, the astute reader will notice that smooth muscle relaxation is intricately regulated cellularly by a number of mechanisms that all achieve the same end point, including nitric oxide (Fig. 8-11), Ca^{++} channel blockade (Fig. 8-8B), and β_2-adrenergic receptor stimulation (see Chapter 6 and

Figs. 6-11 and 6-13). The mechanism of hydralazine is unknown, but it directly relaxes smooth muscle only in the arteries. Minoxidil stimulates adenosine triphosphate (ATP)–activated potassium channels in smooth muscle. Increased intracellular potassium stabilizes the membrane at resting potential and makes vasoconstriction less likely. As with hydralazine, minoxidil vasodilates only arteries.

Pharmacokinetics

Metabolism of hydralazine is by acetylation and is genetically determined. Roughly half the population are rapid acetylators and half are slow acetylators. Hydralazine has a plasma half-life ($t_{1/2}$) of only 1 hour, yet its hypotensive effects persist for 12 hours—a phenomenon for which there is no explanation, in part because the mechanism of this drug is unknown.

Nitroprusside has a rapid onset of action and a short $t_{1/2}$. Typically, the effects of this drug subside within 1 to 2 minutes of discontinuing infusions. The drug is metabolized to cyanide and nitrite ions, both of which are responsible for adverse effects.

Clinical use

Typically hydralazine and minoxidil are reserved for treatment-resistant hypertension. Because compensatory mechanisms tend to counteract the actions of vasodilators, these drugs are most effective when combined with a diuretic (to counteract sodium retention) and a β-blocker (to counteract reflex sympathetic activation that causes reflex tachycardia and renin release). As mentioned, nitroprusside is usually reserved for hypertensive crisis (Box 8-3 lists other drugs that are also used to manage hypertensive crisis). Topically, minoxidil is used to treat male-pattern baldness.

Adverse effects

Tachycardia and fluid retention occur to compensate for drug-induced vasodilation. In addition, flushing, headache, and hypotension occur because of vasodilation. Because arterial

Box 8-3. EXAMPLES OF INTRAVENOUS DRUGS USED TO MANAGE HYPERTENSIVE CRISIS

Clevidipine	Nicardipine
Enalaprilat	Nitroglycerin
Esmolol	Nitroprusside
Hydralazine	Trimethaphan
Labetalol	

vasodilators cause reflex tachycardia, these drugs can exacerbate angina or myocardial ischemia.

Hydralazine can cause lupuslike syndromes; therefore arthralgias, myalgias, rash, fever, anemia, antinuclear antibodies, and complete blood counts should be monitored regularly. Hypertrichosis, or hair growth, may be an unwanted adverse effect associated with oral minoxidil. Cyanide toxicity may occur when sodium nitroprusside is administered rapidly or for longer than 2 days. Methemoglobinemia may also occur as a result of nitroprusside metabolism to nitrite ions. Nitrite ions complex with hemoglobin, forming methemoglobin, which has a low affinity for binding to O_2.

Summary

The bottom-line approach to hypertension management is to make sure it is treated. Guidelines are in place to select appropriate therapy. Patients with comorbidities may respond better to one class of medications than another. Table 8-4, a special populations pocket guide, lists preferred drugs, as well as those to avoid, in some special situations.

● ● ● PHARMACOLOGIC MANAGEMENT OF PULMONARY ARTERIAL HYPERTENSION

Pulmonary arterial hypertension involves abnormally high blood pressures in the arteries of the lungs. It makes the right side of the heart work harder than normal. There is no known cure, so the goal of treatment is to control symptoms of chest pain, dizziness during exercise, shortness of breath during exercise, and fainting. Medicines used to treat pulmonary arterial hypertension are found in Table 8.5. The drugs used to treat pulmonary arterial hypertension are drugs that induce vasodilation, including calcium channel blockers; sildenafil, which is typically used to treat erectile dysfunction; prostaglandin analogs; and endothelin receptor antagonists. Prostaglandin analogs such as epoprostenol, also known as *prostacyclin* or *PGI₂*, are strong vasodilators of all vascular beds. Endothelin antagonists block endothelin receptors on vascular endothelium and smooth muscle. Stimulation of these receptors by endothelin is associated with intense vasoconstriction because endothelin is one of the most potent vasoconstrictors known. Although bosentan blocks both ET_A and ET_B receptors, its affinity is higher for the A subtype

TABLE 8-4. Drug Considerations for Special Populations and Comorbidities with Hypertension

POPULATION OR COMORBIDITY	COMMENT
Blacks	Tend to respond well to diuretics. Diuretics improve responsiveness to ACE inhibitors. Also respond well to Ca⁺⁺ channel blockers.
Children	Often managed with ACE inhibitors or Ca⁺⁺ channel blockers.
Elderly	Tend to respond well to diuretics. The elderly are especially sensitive to volume depletion. Ca⁺⁺ channel blockers or ACE inhibitors are also reasonable choices. On the other hand, β-blockers can precipitate heart failure.
Angina	β-blockers (without ISA) and rate-slowing Ca⁺⁺ channel blockers are good choices. Dihydropyridine Ca⁺⁺ channel blockers may cause reflex tachycardia because of their vasodilatory effects, which will worsen angina.
Status post myocardial infarction	Good choices are β-blockers without ISA (sympathetic stimulation is unwanted post-MI) and ACE inhibitors or ARBs. Optimally, after myocardial infarction every patient will receive a β-blocker and an ACE inhibitor or ARB.
Diabetes mellitus	Good choices are ACE inhibitors, Ca⁺⁺ channel blockers, and α₂-agonists. β-blockers should be used with caution because they can mask hypoglycemia and increase the risk of developing type 2 diabetes mellitus.
Gout	Avoid diuretics because thiazides and loops can worsen uric acid control.
Bilateral renal artery stenosis	Avoid ACE inhibitors, ARBs, and renin inhibitors because these drugs can precipitate acute renal failure in this population.
Advanced renal insufficiency	Select a loop diuretic over a thiazide diuretic. Select other antihypertensives on the basis of which ones are not excreted renally.
Heart failure	Good choices are loop diuretics (which will also reduce edema and congestive symptoms), β-blockers, ACE inhibitors, ARBs, and aldosterone antagonists.
Asthma	Do not use β-blockers in patients who are actively wheezing. β₁-selective agents are preferred in this population.

ACE, angiotensin-converting enzyme; *ARB*, angiotensin II receptor blocker; *ISA*, intrinsic sympathomimetic activity.

TABLE 8-5. Drugs Used to Manage Pulmonary Arterial Hypertension

DRUG	NOTES
Prostaglandin analogues	Prostaglandins cause direction vasodilation of vascular beds and inhibit platelet aggregation.
Epoprostenol	Administered by continuous IV infusion.
Iloprost	Administered by inhalation.
Treprostinil	Administered by continuous SQ or IV infusion (if SQ is not tolerated).
Endothelin receptor antagonists	Endothelins are a group of peptide hormones released by endothelial cells that have potent vasoconstrictive actions. The drugs are administered orally; there is a risk of hepatotoxicity and teratogenicity.
Ambrisentan	Is more selective for ET_A receptors.
Bosentan	Antagonizes both ET_A and ET_B receptors.
Phosphodiesterase-5 inhibitors	
Sildenafil	Prevents reduction in cGMP levels.
Ca^{++} channel blockers	Fewer than 10% of patients respond.

IV, intravenous; *SQ*, subcutaneous; *cGMP*, cyclic guanine monophosphate.

(found in vascular smooth muscle) than the B subtype (found primarily in endothelial cells).

PHARMACOLOGIC MANAGEMENT OF STABLE ANGINA

Angina is a symptom of ischemic heart disease. Angina pectoris (pain in the chest) is an example of poor O_2 economics—there is an imbalance of O_2 supply and O_2 demand. The goal of therapy is to (1) increase blood flow to ischemic tissues and/or (2) reduce the O_2 demand of the heart.

To reduce myocardial O_2 demand, treatments include reducing heart rate and contractility, reducing afterload and arterial pressure, and reducing preload and cardiac filling. Treatment strategies for managing stable angina are listed in Box 8-4. For the most part, β-blockers are the primary agents to manage chronic stable angina prophylactically (Box 8-5), although Ca^{++} channel blockers may also be used in patients with stable angina or patients with spasmodic, non-exercise–induced Prinzmetal's angina (Table 8-6). Note, however, that appropriate caution

Box 8-4. TREATMENT OF STABLE ANGINA

Reduction of risk factors through lifestyle modifications	Weight loss
	β-Blockers
	Nitrates
Smoking cessation	Low-dose aspirin
Low-density lipoprotein cholesterol reduction	Ca^{++} channel blockers

Box 8-5. RATIONALE FOR USE OF β-BLOCKERS IN ANGINA MANAGEMENT

Antagonize actions of norepinephrine in cardiac tissue
Decrease heart rate
Increase diastolic perfusion
Decrease contractility
Decrease blood pressure
Decrease total peripheral resistance by preventing renin release
Reduce O_2 demand and increase O_2 supply

TABLE 8-6. Rationale for Use of Ca^{++} Channel Blockers in Angina

TYPE OF Ca^{++} CHANNEL BLOCKER	RATIONALE
Verapamil and diltiazem	Reduce myocardial contractility and conduction velocity
Dihydropyridines	Vasodilate systemic arterioles and coronary arteries Decrease arterial pressure Decrease coronary artery vasculature resistance Prevent coronary artery vasospasm

must be used if heart rate-slowing Ca^{++} channel blockers are combined with β-blockers because atrioventricular blockade can occur. Because these agents were previously reviewed for hypertension control, focus will be on another class of drugs, the nitrates, that reduce myocardial O_2 demand by reducing preload via venous vasodilation. See Chapter 7 for treatments for unstable angina (e.g., thrombus-causing myocardial infarction).

Nitrates

Nitroglycerin, Isosorbide Mononitrate, and Isosorbide Dinitrate
Mechanism of action

As discussed earlier, nitrates induce vasodilation by direct activation of guanylyl cyclase by nitric oxide and the resultant increase in cGMP. All nonintravenous forms of nitrates predominantly vasodilate veins, thereby reducing preload. In contrast, intravenous nitrates are balanced vasodilators, with vasodilatory actions in both veins and arteries.

Pharmacokinetics

Nitrates are available as oral tablets, transdermal patches, sublingual tablets, translingual sprays, topical ointments, and intravenous infusions. The onset of action of sublingual forms of nitroglycerin occurs within 1 to 3 minutes, but effects are terminated in less than an hour because of rapid metabolism. Nitroglycerin sublingual tablets must be kept in their original glass container because the medication adsorbs onto standard plastic prescription vials. The benefits provided by nitrates for patients with angina are featured in Box 8-6.

Clinical use

Nitrates are used to treat acute anginal attacks and as prophylaxis against recurrent attacks. They may also be used during a myocardial infarction and to manage perioperative hypertension. Box 8-7 lists additional situations in which nitrates may be useful.

Adverse effects

Tolerance, termed *tachyphylaxis*, develops quickly to the effects of nitrates. To prevent tolerance from occurring there should be a nitrate-free interval (at least 12 hours) during each 24-hour period (typically overnight). Headaches, flushing, and postural hypotension accompanied by reflex tachycardia may occur as a result of vasodilation. Nitrates are contraindicated with phosphodiesterase-5 inhibitors, which are used for erectile dysfunction (e.g., sildenafil, vardenafil, tadalafil), because these drugs inhibit the breakdown of cGMP. Fatal hypotension has occurred when phosphodiesterase-5 inhibitors have been combined with nitrates.

Partial Fatty Acid Oxidation Inhibitor

Ranolazine

Mechanism of action

This is the newest drug added to the armamentarium of treatments for angina. Specifically, ranolazine inhibits late Na^+ currents, an action that modulates myocardial metabolic pathways, resulting in partial inhibition of fatty acid oxidation. This, in turn, increases glucose oxidation, an action that results in more ATP generated for each molecule of O_2 consumed. This shift in energy utilization helps decrease myocardial O_2 demand, reduces the rise in lactic acid and acidosis, and helps the heart make its energy (ATP) more efficiently. Specifically, ranolazine decreases the activity of fatty acid oxidase (decreasing β-oxidation of fatty acids) and upregulates pyruvate dehydrogenase (producing a shift to glucose metabolism).

Clinical use

Ranolazine is used only as an add-on drug, added to other anti-anginal therapies in people who are still symptomatic in spite of adequately dosed β-blockers, Ca^{++} channel blockers, and nitrates. On average, it only reduces anginal episodes by one incidence per week.

Adverse effects

The chief complaints with ranolazine are dizziness and headaches, with other minor gastrointestinal disturbances also reported. Ranolazine prolongs the QT interval on electrocardiograms and should be used cautiously in patients taking other QT-prolonging drugs. Because ranolazine is metabolized by CYP3A4, drug interactions occur when it is combined with strong inhibitors (e.g., clarithromycin) or inducers (e.g., rifampin) of CYP3A4.

Summary

Combinations of drugs are often used to manage stable angina. Nitrates are frequently given in concert with β-blockers and Ca^{++} channel inhibitors. Rationales for these combinations are given in Table 8-7. Because some unstable angina symptoms may be caused by acute coronary syndrome, a review of the drugs used to restore coronary flow (antiplatelet agents, anticoagulants, antithrombin agents) is suggested.

TABLE 8-7. Rationale for Use of Drug Combinations in Angina

DRUG COMBINATION	RATIONALE
Nitrates and β-blockers	Nitrates decrease preload and cause venous pooling. β-Blockers prevent nitrate-induced reflex tachycardia.
Nitrates and Ca^{++} channel blockers	Nitrates reduce preload. Dihydropyridines decrease afterload or rate-slowing Ca^{++} channel blockers reduce heart rate.
Ca^{++} channel blockers and β-blockers	β-Blockers prevent reflex tachycardia associated with dihydropyridine-induced blood pressure decrease.
Nitrates, Ca^{++} channel blockers, and β-blockers	Dihydropyridines reduce afterload. Nitrates reduce preload. β-Blockers decrease heart rate and contractility to blunt nitrate-induced and dihydropyridine-induced reflex tachycardia.

●●● PHARMACOLOGIC MANAGEMENT OF HEART FAILURE

Essentially, HF occurs when myocardial dysfunction (myocardial hypertrophy and fibrosis) is so severe that the cardiac output is no longer adequate to provide O_2 for the tissues. Signs and symptoms of HF include decreased exercise tolerance, shortness of breath, tachycardia, cardiomegaly, fatigue, as well as peripheral and pulmonary edema. In the subset of patients with HF in whom congestive symptoms develop, the condition is commonly referred to as *congestive heart failure*. Precipitating factors are listed in Table 8-8.

With the Frank-Starling curve (Fig. 8-12), note that patients with HF have reduced cardiac output for any end-diastolic pressure on the curve. As myocardial activity worsens, congestive symptoms such as pulmonary edema occur, as do low-output symptoms such as fatigue and oliguria (producing abnormally small volumes of urine). Initially, the baroreceptors attempt to compensate for reduced cardiac output through activation of compensatory reflexes such as heightened sympathetic tone and activation of the RAA system. However, these compensatory mechanisms only worsen myocardial function by increasing total peripheral resistance and increasing afterload (Fig. 8-13). This only makes the failing heart work more inefficiently, leading to further maladaptive myocardial hypertrophy and remodeling (an example of a deadly feed-forward mechanism, the vicious cycle).

The primary goal of pharmacotherapeutic management of HF is to slow ventricular remodeling and the maladaptive ventricular changes (e.g., apoptosis, abnormal gene expression) associated with it. Diuretics move the depressed Frank-Starling cardiac output curve only to the left, providing symptomatic relief from edema, but diuretics do not increase cardiac output. In contrast, vasodilators, ACE inhibitors, ARBs, spironolactone, eplerenone, β-blockers, and positive inotropes (e.g., digoxin) shift the depressed cardiac output curve upward. As with most cardiovascular diseases, a combination of therapies is used to manage HF symptoms. Rationale for each of the pharmacotherapies is listed in Table 8-9. The "ABCDs" for managing patients

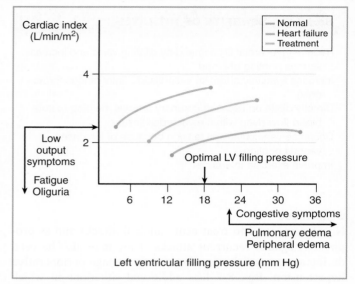

Figure 8-12. Frank-Starling curve. *LV,* left ventricular.

with worsening HF are listed in Table 8-10. Note that pharmacologic interventions can be beneficial in high-risk patients even before symptoms begin.

For the most part, the first-line therapeutics are the previously described drugs that blunt the RAA system. Drugs that block the formation (ACE inhibitors) or the actions (ARBs) of angiotensin II are balanced vasodilators and will reduce preload and afterload (Box 8-8). In addition, because angiotensin II is a potent stimulus for myocardial hypertrophy, inhibiting its actions with either ACE inhibitors or ARBs will diminish or reverse myocardial remodeling and disease progression. Spironolactone and the selective aldosterone receptor antagonist eplerenone can decrease HF mortality rates by 30% by blocking the effects of elevated aldosterone in HF patients (Box 8-9). It is also believed that aldosterone receptor blockers diminish the maladaptive cardiofibrosis associated with HF. In clinical trials, spironolactone improved survival in patients with HF. However, life-threatening complications resulting from hyperkalemia are common. Patients taking spironolactone need to have their K^+ levels closely monitored. When congestive symptoms of HF are evident, loop diuretics are used to manage fluid retention.

In patients with HF, β-blockers are often prescribed. This should appear counterintuitive. In fact, β-blockers are contraindicated in patients with acutely decompensated congestive HF owing to diminished myocardial contractility. Yet, surprisingly, three β-blockers—metoprolol XL, bisoprolol, and carvedilol—are approved for managing HF. As summarized in Box 8-10, these β-blockers slow progression of HF by diminishing oxidative damage and myocardial remodeling or hypertrophy by blocking the adverse effects of norepinephrine on myocardial tissues. Because β-blockers can worsen symptoms in the short term, patients should be stabilized with ACE inhibitors and diuretics before adding the β-adrenergic receptor blockade.

Another class of drugs used to manage symptomatic HF is composed of the positive inotropes (digoxin, milrinone, dobutamine, dopamine, and nesiritide), which improve myocardial contractility. These drugs are introduced below.

TABLE 8-8. Factors That May Precipitate Heart Failure

FACTOR	DRUG EXAMPLES
Uncontrolled hypertension	
Cardiac arrhythmias	
Myocardial infarction	
Negative inotropes	Antiarrhythmics
	β-Blockers
Heart rate–slowing Ca^{++} channel blockers	Verapamil
	Diltiazem
Cardiotoxic chemotherapies	Daunorubicin
	Doxorubicin
Drugs that cause sodium/ water retention	Carbenicillin/ticarcillin
	Glucocorticoids
	Nonsteroidal antiinflammatory drugs

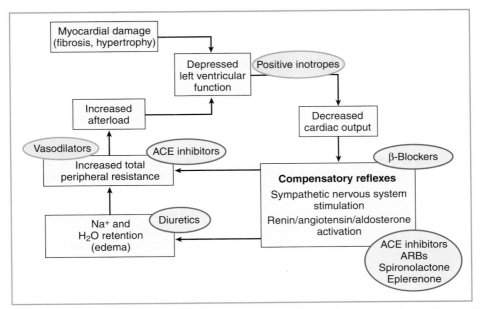

Figure 8-13. Drug therapies to break the vicious cycle of heart failure. The primary pharmacologic goal in heart failure treatment is to reduce symptoms. The secondary goal is to reduce myocardial fibrosis and hypertrophy in the failing heart. *ACE*, angiotensin-converting enzyme inhibitor; *ARBs*, angiotensin receptor blocker.

TABLE 8-9. Rationale for Pharmacotherapies Used in Managing Heart Failure

GOAL	RATIONALE AND PHARMACOTHERAPY
Improve heart function	Decrease myocardial remodeling and fibrosis (by blocking effects of aldosterone) ACE inhibitors ARBs Spironolactone Eplerenone Enhance contractility Positive inotropes Improve ventricular function β-Blockers
Decrease preload	Loop diuretics
Decrease afterload	Vasodilators ACE inhibitors, ARBs
Other	Correct arrhythmias Warfarin anticoagulation

ACE, angiotensin-converting enzyme; *ARB*, angiotensin II receptor blocker.

Positive Inotropes

Digoxin

Mechanism of action

There are two schools of thought regarding the exact mechanism of action of digoxin. What is agreed upon is that digoxin inhibits the Na^+/K^+-ATPase pump by binding to the potassium-binding site. Initially, it was believed that after inhibiting the Na^+/K^+-ATPase pump, the resulting increase in intracellular Na^+ drives the Na^+/Ca^{++} exchanger, which increases intracellular Ca^{++} in exchange for Na^+. Furthermore, this elevation in intracellular Ca^{++} was thought to facilitate Ca^{++} release from the sarcoplasmic reticulum. More recently, it has been suggested that after inhibiting the Na^+/K^+-ATPase pump, the resultant increase in intracellular Na^+ levels reduces the transmembrane Na^+ gradient; thus the Na^+/Ca^{++} exchanger drives less Ca^{++} out of the cell. The increased Ca^{++} is stored in the sarcoplasmic reticulum, such that with subsequent action potentials, a greater than normal amount of Ca^{++} is released into the cytoplasm to intensify the force of contraction. Regardless of the exact intermediate step, the end result of digoxin's binding to myocardial Na^+/K^+-ATPase is more intracellular Ca^{++} that ultimately facilitates interactions between actin and myosin. In this way, digoxin increases the force of myocardial contractility to improve efficiency of the failing heart (Fig. 8-14).

As digoxin increases cardiac stroke volume and cardiac output, baroreceptor-regulated compensatory sympathetic neuronal pathways are diminished. This leads to predominance of parasympathetic tone, which slows heart rate and vasodilates the vasculature. Improved renal hemodynamics also allows edematous fluid to be excreted, which reduces preload. However, despite all the beneficial contractile and hemodynamic effects of digoxin, the drug has never been shown to improve survival. For this reason, digoxin is usually not a first-line drug for the treatment of HF and is reserved for patients who remain symptomatic despite other pharmacologic interventions. However, digoxin also possesses antiarrhythmic activity, and it is sometimes a first-line choice for patients with both heart failure and atrial fibrillation.

Pharmacokinetics

Digoxin has a narrow therapeutic index of 1 to 2 ng/mL and a J-shaped mortality curve, meaning that when mortality is plotted on the *y*-axis and dose is plotted on the *x*-axis, at low concentrations digoxin decreases mortality, but at higher concentrations mortality increases because of drug toxicity (resulting in a J-shaped curve). In general, clinicians should

TABLE 8-10. ABCDs of Managing Heart Failure

SYMPTOMS	MANAGEMENT
A: Patient does not have heart failure but is at high risk because of uncontrolled hypertension, coronary artery disease, or diabetes.	Encourage blood pressure control. 　Encourage lipid control. 　ACE inhibitors or ARBs are recommended.
B: Patient does not have symptoms of heart failure but has structural damage or recently had a myocardial infarction.	ACE inhibitors or ARBs and β-blockers are recommended.
C: Patient has structural disease and symptoms of heart failure (these are the patients usually thought of as having heart failure).	Diuretics are recommended for fluid retention. 　ACE inhibitors or ARBs are recommended unless contraindicated. 　β-Blockers are recommended if patient is stable. 　Digoxin is recommended if patient is symptomatic.
D: Patient has refractory symptoms even at rest.	Ventricular assistance devices. 　Continuous inotropic infusions. 　Heart transplantation.

ACE, angiotensin-converting enzyme; *ARB*, angiotensin II receptor blocker.

Box 8-8. ADVANTAGES OF ANGIOTENSIN-CONVERTING ENZYME INHIBITORS AND ANGIOTENSIN II RECEPTOR BLOCKERS IN HEART FAILURE MANAGEMENT

Provide balanced vasodilation (arteries and veins)
Improve myocardial function
Improve cardiac workload and stroke volume
Reduce blood pressure
Improve exercise tolerance
Slow disease progression (decrease myocardial fibrosis and hypertrophy)
Improve survival

Box 8-9. ADVANTAGES OF SPIRONOLACTONE IN HEART FAILURE

Assist in sodium/fluid excretion
Prevent myocardial remodeling, which improves heart function
Prevent myocardial fibrosis, which reduces the likelihood of arrhythmias
Reduce vascular fibrosis

Box 8-10. ADVANTAGES OF β-BLOCKERS IN COMPENSATED HEART FAILURE MANAGEMENT

Prevent adverse effects of norepinephrine on the heart
Prevent myocardial remodeling (fibrosis and hypertrophy)
Improve ventricular function
Improve exercise tolerance
Decrease renin release
Decrease oxidative damage
Prolong survival
Slow progression of heart failure

aim for plasma levels of 0.5 to 1.5 ng/mL because greater than 2.0 ng/mL is always toxic.

Bioavailability of digoxin varies among various formulations (tablet, gel cap, oral elixir, intravenous injection) and from patient to patient. One reason for interpatient variability is altered metabolism within the gut. Roughly 10% of the population carries *Eubacterium* as a part of the normal gastrointestinal flora. This microorganism inactivates digoxin. In these patients, treatment with antibiotics (which eliminates *Eubacterium*) may suddenly increase digoxin's toxicologic potential. Digoxin binds nonspecifically to plasma proteins and especially to proteins of the skeletal muscle. This can make plasma concentrations of "free" drug variable from person to person, depending on muscle mass. Approximately 70% of digoxin is excreted renally. Renal function should be monitored because failure to reduce digoxin dose in the presence of declining renal function often underlies digoxin toxicity.

Adverse effects

Digoxin toxicity, if untreated, can be fatal. The first symptoms of digoxin toxicity are gastrointestinal (abdominal cramps, vomiting, diarrhea) and visual disturbances (green or yellow halos, "fuzzy shadows"—like driving at night with dirty glasses). Confusion and yellow vision may occur with chronic toxicity, followed by atrioventricular blockade, bradycardia, and ventricular arrhythmias. Digoxin toxicity is managed according to the information presented in Box 8-11. Digoxin toxicity is also worsened by hypokalemia. Because digoxin binds to the K^+ site of the Na^+/K^+-ATPase pump, low serum potassium levels increase the risk of digoxin toxicity. Conversely, hyperkalemia diminishes digoxin's effectiveness. Because the typical patient taking digoxin is elderly, often with K^+ imbalances and poor renal function, toxicities are not uncommon. A number of other cardiovascular drugs predispose patients to digoxin toxicity, including verapamil, diltiazem, quinidine, and amiodarone. The dosage of digoxin must be substantially reduced if given concomitantly with these drugs. The presumed mechanism underlying this interaction involves the ability of these drugs to inhibit the P-glycoprotein transporter.

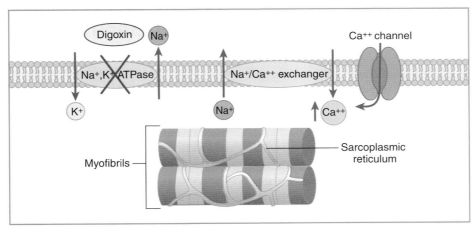

Figure 8-14. Mechanism of digoxin.

Adverse effects

Because milrinone is a positive inotrope, it can also be pro-arrhythmogenic. It is used only in cases of acute HF because prolonged use results in increased mortality.

Dobutamine
Mechanism of action

Dobutamine is a β_1-adrenergic receptor agonist. Exactly opposite to β-blockers, dobutamine increases stroke volume in the failing heart. At low doses, cardiac output increases with little change in heart rate.

Milrinone
Mechanism of action

Milrinone is a phosphodiesterase inhibitor. Phosphodiesterases degrade cyclic nucleotides, such as cAMP. Inhibiting phosphodiesterase in myocardial cells increases cAMP concentration, so milrinone acts as a positive inotrope (Fig. 8-15).

Pharmacokinetics

Dobutamine is administered as a continuous intravenous infusion. As such, it is used only in cases of acute HF.

Adverse effects

As a positive inotrope, dobutamine may cause hypertension, tachycardia, arrhythmias, or angina. Tachyphylaxis develops quickly, probably because of β_1 receptor downregulation.

Pharmacokinetics

Milrinone is given as a continuous intravenous infusion.

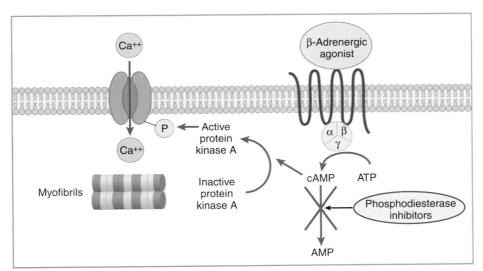

Figure 8-15. Mechanism of phosphodiesterase inhibitors (milrinone) in heart failure. *ATP*, adenosine triphosphate; *AMP*, adenosine monophosphate; *cAMP*, cyclic AMP.

Dopamine
Mechanism of action

Dopamine is primarily a dopamine receptor agonist; however, at higher doses, dopamine activates α- and β-adrenergic receptors, too. Dopamine is administered as a continuous intravenous infusion. At low doses, dopamine preferentially stimulates D_1 and D_2 receptors in the renal vasculature, which leads to vasodilation and promotes renal blood flow to preserve glomerular filtration. At intermediate doses, dopamine also stimulates $β_1$-receptors on the heart. At high doses, dopamine stimulates α-adrenergic receptors in the vasculature, which exacerbates HF by increasing afterload. (However, this may be a desired effect in patients who are in hemorrhagic shock.)

Clinical use

Dopamine is especially useful in situations of cardiogenic shock, in which there is inadequate perfusion of vital organs.

Adverse effects

Same as for dobutamine.

Nesiritide
Mechanism of action

Nesiritide is a B-type natriuretic peptide. Like endogenous atrial natriuretic factor produced by the heart, this drug activates guanylyl cyclase to form the potent vasodilator cGMP. Administration of the drug leads to balanced vasodilation in the arteries and veins, diuretic effects (via enhanced Na^+ excretion), suppression of the RAA system, and suppression of the sympathetic nervous system. As a result, not only does circulation improve, but symptoms of HF improve as well.

Pharmacokinetics

Nesiritide is administered as a continuous intravenous infusion.

Adverse effects

Although less likely than dobutamine to cause tachycardia or arrhythmias and better tolerated than intravenous nitroglycerin, nesiritide has been associated with prolonged hypotension. In addition, there is new concern with respect to the potential of this drug to increase the risk of renal impairment and mortality. Even though nesiritide has been shown to be hemodynamically beneficial in the short term, it may not be beneficial in the long term. Use of nesiritide should be reserved for patients who do not respond to other therapies.

Summary

The bottom line for HF management is preventing it from happening in the first place. However, once the heart begins to fail, drug combinations may be indicated, including diuretics to decrease congestive symptoms; ACE inhibitors, ARBs, or aldosterone receptor antagonists to decrease myocardial fibrosis and remodeling; β-blockers to block effects of sympathetic nervous stimulation; and positive inotropes to improve myocardial contractility.

●●● PHARMACOTHERAPY OF ANTIARRHYTHMICS

One of the most serious complications of congestive HF and other cardiovascular diseases is cardiac arrhythmia (Box 8-12). Whether from an ectopic focus or a reentrant circus rhythm, abnormal electrical conductance pathways can be life-threatening. Antiarrhythmic drugs work by several different mechanisms (Box 8-13). Because these drugs alter electrical conduction, all antiarrhythmics can potentially worsen conduction. There is a narrow margin of safety between obtaining the desired antiarrhythmic effect and provoking a new arrhythmia.

Antiarrhythmics are classified according to their predominant pharmacologic effects into class I, II, III, or IV agents (Table 8-11).

Although a given drug may fall into a particular class, many of the antiarrhythmics used today have activities that fall into more than one class.

Class I: Sodium Channel Blockers

Class IA, IB, and IC Drugs
Class IA: Quinidine, Procainamide, and Disopyramide
Class IB: Lidocaine, Tocainide, and Mexiletine
Class IC: Propafenone and Flecainide
Mechanism of action

All class I antiarrhythmics block Na^+ channels, but the pharmacokinetics of this blockade differ among individual drugs, producing action potential differences (Table 8-12 and Fig. 8-16). Class IA drugs increase the refractory period

---

Box 8-12.   CONDITIONS THAT PROVOKE ARRHYTHMIAS

- Ischemic damage
- Heart failure
- Hypovolemia
- Hypercapnia
- Hypotension
- Electrolyte disturbances (K^+, Mg^{++}, Ca^{++})
- Drug toxicities (digoxin, antiarrhythmics, caffeine, alcohol)

Box 8-13.   MECHANISMS OF ANTIARRHYTHMIC DRUGS

Decrease the slope of phase 4 depolarization
Elevate the threshold potential for phase 0 upward shoot
Shorten refractoriness in area of unidirectional block to allow anterograde conduction to proceed
Prolong refractoriness in area of unidirectional block to cause bidirectional block so that the impulse cannot proceed in a retrograde fashion

TABLE 8-11. Predominant Pharmacologic Effects of Antiarrhythmics

CLASS	CONDUCTION VELOCITY	REFRACTORY PERIOD	AUTOMATICITY	ION BLOCK
IA	↓	↑	↓	Na^+
IB	−/↓	↓	↓	Na^+
IC	↓↓	−	↓	Na^+
II	↓	↑	↓	Ca^{++} (indirectly)
III	−	↑↑	−	K^+
IV	↓	↑	↓	Ca^{++}

Most antiarrhythmics decrease automaticity and conduction velocity by altering movement of specific ions (Na^+, Ca^{++}, K^+).

TABLE 8-12. Class I Na^+ Channel Blockers

ANTIARRHYTHMIC DRUG	KINETICS WITH Na^+ CHANNEL	EFFECT
Class IA	Intermediate rate of association	Slows rate of rise (phase 0) of action potential. Prolongs action potential (increases refractory period).
Class IB	Rapid rate of association	Shortens refractory period (phase 3 repolarization). Decreases duration of action potential.
Class IC	Slow rate of association	Markedly slows phase 0 depolarization. No effect on refractory period.

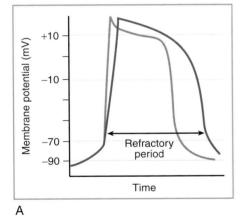
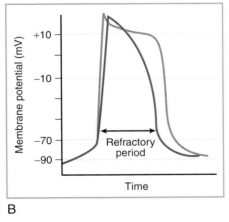
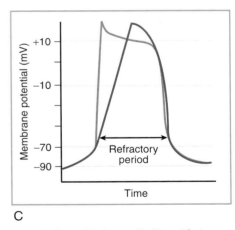

Figure 8-16. Actions of class I antiarrhythmics on ventricular action potential. **A,** Class IA drugs. **B,** Class IB drugs. **C,** Class IC drugs. The *gray line* represents a normal action potential. The *red line* represents the pharmacologic effect of the antiarrhythmic. Note that the refractory period is lengthened by class IA agents, shortened for class IB drugs, and relatively unchanged for class IC therapies.

(see Fig. 8-16A), whereas class IB antiarrhythmics decrease the refractory period (see Fig. 8-16B). Drugs falling into class IC markedly slow phase 0 depolarization (see Fig. 8-16C).

The unique ability of class IB antiarrhythmics to block Na^+ channels when activated or inactivated (especially if those channels remain in a polarized state) provides certain advantages. For example, lidocaine (an example of a class IB antiarrhythmic) preferentially affects diseased, as opposed to normal, tissue. As a result, with lidocaine treatment there is

a loss of excitability and conduction blockade in ischemically damaged tissues, whereas normal, healthy tissues are relatively unaffected by the drug.

Clinical use

Class IB antiarrhythmics are used to manage ventricular arrhythmias, especially during cardiac procedures or after myocardial infarction. Drugs in this class shorten phase 3 repolarization and decrease the duration of the action potential (see Fig. 8-16B). Class IB antiarrhythmics have accentuated effects for turning areas of unidirectional block into "no block at all." With these drugs, anterograde conduction is allowed to proceed because the refractory period of damaged tissue has been reduced.

Class IA and IC drugs are not first-line agents because therapeutic approaches currently focus on heart *rate* control rather than *rhythm* control. Quinidine and procainamide (class IA drugs) were historically used to chemically convert atrial fibrillation back to a normal sinus rhythm and to maintain normal sinus rhythms after direct current conversions. Class IA antiarrhythmics prolong the refractory period and turn areas of unidirectional block into bidirectional block (see Fig. 8-16). Similarly, class IC antiarrhythmics are not usually first-choice antiarrhythmics because they are quite proarrhythmogenic and increase mortality.

Pharmacokinetics

Numerous drug interactions are likely with many of the class I antiarrhythmics. For example, quinidine is a P450 substrate for some CYP450s enzymes, is an inhibitor of other P450s, and is also an inhibitor of P-glycoprotein. Lidocaine (a class IB drug) is administered parenterally to avoid first-pass hepatic metabolism. Tocainide and mexiletine can be thought of as "oral lidocaine."

Adverse effects

As a class, these drugs have an extremely narrow therapeutic window. Many are proarrhythmogenic or possess negative inotropic properties.

ANATOMY

Normal Conduction Pathway of the Heart

The electrical activity in the heart is generated by the SA node. Normally, the SA node has the highest degree of spontaneous firing. The impulse produced by the SA node spreads throughout the atria and then is slightly delayed at the AV node. This delay allows time for the atria to contract. The electrical impulse propagates to the bundle of His and then bifurcates to travel down the Purkinje fibers, exciting the cardiac muscle of both ventricles.

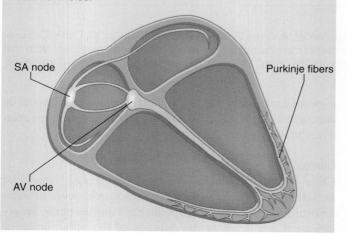

Class IA antiarrhythmics are proarrhythmogenic because they cause QT prolongation, which can lead to potentially fatal torsades de pointes, a life-threatening ventricular arrhythmia. Quinidine is also associated with a conglomeration of symptoms termed *cinchonism*, in which patients may experience tinnitus, blurred vision, headache, nausea, delirium, and psychosis. Both quinidine, and to a greater extent, procainamide, cause a drug-induced lupus syndrome. In addition, quinidine and disopyramide possess severe anticholinergic adverse effects.

Because of lipid solubility, central nervous system adverse effects are likely with lidocaine. Tocainide is associated with adverse hematologic effects and pulmonary fibrosis.

Although class IC drugs do not prolong the QT interval, these drugs are also quite prone to inducing new arrhythmias.

PHYSIOLOGY

Phases of Ventricular Membrane Depolarization

The electrical properties of the heart are often described as *ventricular membrane depolarizations*. Ventricular action potentials have four phases. Before excitation, an electrical gradient exists in which the inside of the myocytes are −80 to −90 mV more negative with respect to the outside of the cell. Electrical stimulation (or depolarization) occurs when ions begin entering the cell. Phase 4 is unique to pacemaker cells. Other cell types lack this slow, inward, positive current seen during diastole. During phase 4, there is a slow leak of Na^+ ions into the cell and a slow K^+ efflux. Over time, K^+ efflux diminishes but Na^+ influx continues. After a critical threshold potential is reached, voltage-gated Na^+ channels open and Na ions rapidly rush into the cell. This is known as *phase 0*, or *depolarization*. During phase 1, there is passive chloride ion influx and potassium efflux. The hallmark features of phase 2, or the plateau phase, are Ca^{++} influx and K^+ efflux. During phase 3, the cell repolarizes as potassium efflux continues. Recall that depolarization cannot occur again until the cell has completely repolarized. Note: the Na^+/K^+-ATPase pump is constantly working to reestablish Na^+ and K^+ homeostasis.

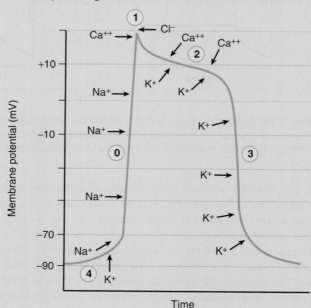

Ectopic Foci and Reentrant Circus Rhythms

Ectopic foci occur when myocardial cells located outside the SA node take over the normal pacemaker function of the SA node by becoming unusually "automatic." Reentrant circus rhythms occur when an impulse is propagated indefinitely. When a premature impulse encounters refractory tissue (tissue that has not yet repolarized), the impulse is simply terminated. If, however, the impulse proceeds in a different direction and "reenters" the area, which has now repolarized, the impulse may proceed in a retrograde (i.e., backward) manner. Thus the impulse may continue to propagate itself indefinitely in a circular fashion.

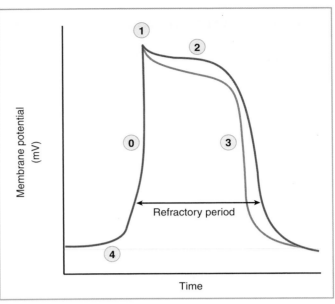

Figure 8-17. Actions of class III antiarrhythmics on ventricular action potential.

Class II: β-Blockers

Propranolol and Esmolol
Mechanism of action

β-blockers (class II antiarrhythmics) also have antiarrhythmic actions. β-Blockers indirectly prevent calcium entry into myocardial cells; therefore β-blockers slow conduction velocity, slow automaticity, and prolong the refractory period.

Clinical use

Because certain exercise-induced arrhythmias are produced by heightened sympathetic tone, β-blockers are often effective therapies. As another example, the sinoatrial (SA) and atrioventricular (AV) nodes are heavily innervated by the adrenergic system, making β-blockers useful for managing tachyarrhythmias in which these nodes are abnormally automatic or involved in a reentrant circus rhythm. β-blockers should be included in the therapeutic regimens of all patients after myocardial infarction to prevent ventricular tachycardia and to slow the ventricular rate in response to atrial fibrillation or atrial flutter. β-Blockers have been shown to reduce arrhythmia-related mortality, making them a common first choice for treatment of atrial tachyarrhythmias.

Class III: Potassium Channel Blockers

Amiodarone, Bretylium, Dofetilide, Dronedarone, Ibutilide, and Sotalol
Mechanism of action

As a generalization, class III antiarrhythmics prolong cardiac action potentials, resulting in an increase in the effective refractory period. With the exception of ibutilide, which slows outward Na^+ currents during repolarization, the class III drugs block potassium channels. However, properties of individual drugs in this class vary considerably. For example, bretylium initially causes catecholamine release which can be proarrhythmogenic, and although amiodarone is usually considered a K^+ channel blocker, it also blocks Na^+ channels, Ca^{++} channels, and β-adrenergic receptors. What is consistent among class III antiarrhythmics is that they prolong phase III repolarization without changing phase 0 depolarization

(Fig. 8-17). This reduces myocardial automaticity, prolongs action potentials, increases the refractory period, and increases the QT interval. Prolongation of the QT interval is one mechanism by which class III antiarrhythmics can induce secondary arrhythmias (these drugs are proarrhythmogenic).

Pharmacokinetics

Bretylium and ibutilide are poorly absorbed from the gastrointestinal tract and are administered only intravenously. Amiodarone has a long $t_{1/2}$, roughly 40 to 60 days; therefore it takes a long time for the drug to reach a steady state. In addition, when adverse effects occur, they are slow to resolve because it takes a long time for the drug to be eliminated from the body. More than 96% of amiodarone is nonspecifically bound to plasma proteins. Amiodarone is metabolized by hepatic P450 microsomal enzymes and inhibits these metabolic enzymes and P-glycoprotein. As a result, numerous drug interactions occur because amiodarone increases plasma drug concentrations of digoxin, quinidine, phenytoin, flecainide, and warfarin.

Clinical use

Bretylium is reserved primarily for treating life-threatening ventricular arrhythmias and for attempts to resuscitate patients from ventricular fibrillation. Amiodarone is used to manage recurrent ventricular fibrillation or ventricular tachycardia. Its use has been shown to decrease mortality after myocardial infarction and in HF patients. Dronedarone is approved for managing persistent atrial fibrillation. Sotalol decreases the fibrillation threshold and is used to prevent atrial and ventricular fibrillation. Dofetilide is used to convert atrial fibrillation or flutter to normal sinus rhythm and to maintain normal sinus rhythm after cardioversion. Ibutilide is used for rapid conversion of atrial fibrillation or atrial flutter of recent onset (<90 days) to sinus rhythm. Patients with atrial arrhythmias of a longer duration are less likely to respond to ibutilide.

Box 8-14. ADVERSE EFFECTS OF AMIODARONE

Serious pulmonary toxicity (interstitial lung disease)	Optic neuritis
	"Smurfism"
Liver damage	Hypothyroidism or
Heart block	hyperthyroidism
Bradycardia	Photosensitivity
Hypotension	Neuropathy
Corneal deposits	Muscle weakness

Adverse effects

For the most part, class III agents can induce life-threatening QT prolongation. Patients require close monitoring for life-threatening ventricular arrhythmias. In fact, amiodarone should be prescribed only by physicians who are thoroughly familiar with its risks. A substantial number of patients experience adverse effects with high doses of amiodarone, often necessitating that the drug be discontinued because adverse effects are sometimes fatal. A partial listing of adverse effects is located in Box 8-14. The chemical structure of amiodarone contains iodine and is structurally related to thyroid hormone. This accounts for amiodarone's adverse effects on the thyroid gland and for "smurfism," which is a blue-gray skin discoloration resulting from iodine accumulation. Because of the numerous adverse effects, patients should regularly have their visual function, cardiac function (electrocardiogram), thyroid function, pulmonary function, and liver function checked. Dronedarone was developed to overcome some of amiodarone's adverse effects. Dronedarone has a more predictable dose-response curve and has fewer side effects, but costs four times as much, has numerous drug interactions from P450 effects, and is contraindicated in patients with decompensated HF because of higher mortality rates. Because of the risk for QT prolongation, prescriptions for dofetilide may only be written by physicians who have completed specialized training.

Class IV: Calcium Channel Blockers

Rate-Slowing Calcium Channel Blockers
Verapamil and Diltiazem

Mechanism of action. Some Ca^{++} channel blockers are also antiarrhythmics. Rate-slowing Ca^{++} channel blockers directly block slow inward Ca^{++} currents from entering myocardial cells. This action decreases and prolongs phase 4 spontaneous depolarization. These effects are most prominent in tissues that (1) fire frequently, (2) are less polarized at rest, and (3) depend on Ca^{++} for activation.

Clinical use. As with β-blockers, rate-slowing Ca^{++} channel blockers are most useful for managing tachyarrhythmias in which the SA node or the AV node are abnormally automatic or involved in a reentrant circus rhythm. These Ca^{++} channel blockers slow AV conductance in atrial fibrillation, thus protecting the ventricles.

Other Antiarrhythmics

Digoxin
Mechanism of action
As previously discussed, by enhancing vagal activity, digoxin may terminate atrial arrhythmias.

Adenosine
Mechanism of action
Adenosine is a naturally occurring nucleoside that slows conduction through the AV node by opening acetylcholine-sensitive K^+ channels and blocking Ca^{++} influx in the atrium and nodal tissues.

Pharmacokinetics
Because the drug has an extremely short $t_{1/2}$ (15 seconds), it is administered only intravenously.

Clinical use
Adenosine may be used to convert acute reentrant supraventricular tachycardias at the AV node back to normal sinus rhythm.

Adverse effects
Adverse effects associated with adenosine include bronchospasm, flushing, sweating, chest pain, and hypotension.

Summary

Because all antiarrhythmics alter ionic conductances in myocardial tissue—thereby slowing automaticity and conduction velocity—caution must be used when prescribing these drugs because of their ability to induce new arrhythmias.

●●● HYPERLIPIDEMIAS

Hyperlipidemia is defined as an elevation of cholesterol or triglycerides. Cholesterol is, of course, essential for synthesis of plasma membranes, steroid hormones, and bile acids. Likewise, triglycerides play essential roles in transporting and storing fatty acids for energy. However, these lipids may contribute to disease processes. Elevated levels of cholesterol can lead to atherosclerosis and coronary artery disease; elevated triglycerides can lead to pancreatitis. Classic therapy is directed at lowering low-density lipoprotein (LDL), lowering triglycerides, or raising high-density lipoprotein (HDL).

Cholesterol and triglycerides are synthesized by the liver or obtained from dietary sources (Fig. 8-18). As lipids, cholesterol and triglycerides are insoluble in blood; therefore they must be transported within lipoproteins, which differ from each other in composition and mission. Key points about the drugs used to manage hypercholesterolemia are summarized in Table 8-13.

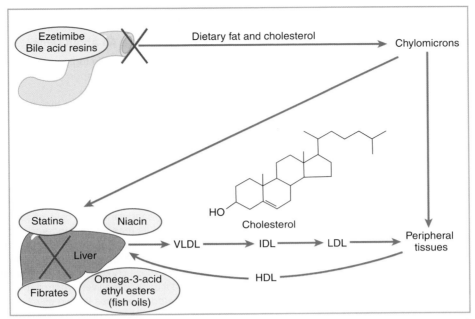

Figure 8-18. Cholesterol transport. In contrast to statins, fibrates, niacin, and fish oils (which work at the level of the liver), ezetimibe and bile acid resins work by blocking absorption. *VLDL*, very-low-density lipoprotein; *IDL*, intermediate-density lipoprotein; *LDL*, low-density lipoprotein; *HDL*, high-density lipoprotein.

TABLE 8-13. Pharmacotherapy of Hyperlipidemia

DRUGS	CLINICAL UTILITY	CLINICAL DRAWBACKS
Statins	Effective for lowering LDL and increasing HDL	Only mildly effective for lowering triglycerides
Fibrates	Effective for lowering triglycerides	Only minimally effective for lowering LDL or increasing HDL
Niacin	Effective for lowering triglycerides, lowering LDL, and increasing HDL	Adverse effects may limit utility
Omega-3-acid ethyl esters	Effective for lowering triglycerides	Prescription form only approved for those with triglycerides >500 mg/dL Purity and dosage of dietary supplements may vary
Bile acid resins	Moderately effective for lowering LDL	Increase triglycerides
Ezetimibe	Moderately effective for lowering LDL	Only minimally effective for increasing HDL

HDL, high-density lipoprotein; *LDL*, low-density lipoprotein.

Statins

Lovastatin, Pravastatin, Simvastatin, Atorvastatin, Fluvastatin, and Rosuvastatin

Note that all these drug names end in "-statin."

Mechanism of action

Statins inhibit 3-hydroxy-3-methyl-glutaryl-coenzyme A (HMG-CoA) reductase. This enzyme catalyzes the rate-limiting step in hepatic cholesterol synthesis (Fig. 8-19). Reduced hepatic cholesterol synthesis decreases hepatocyte cholesterol concentration, leading to increased hepatic expression of LDL receptors, which is the primary mechanism by which LDL is internalized and degraded.

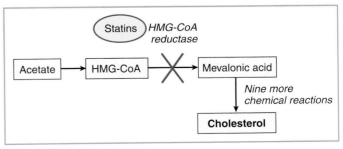

Figure 8-19. Statins inhibit 3-hydroxy-3-methyl-glutaryl-coenzyme A reductase, the rate-limiting step in cholesterol synthesis.

Pharmacokinetics

With the exception of pravastatin and rosuvastatin, most statins are metabolized by the hepatic P450 microsomal enzymes and are contraindicated with drugs that inhibit the P450s. Grapefruit juice also decreases P450 activity and is contraindicated with most statins. Lovastatin should be taken with food to increase its bioavailability; other statins may be taken without regard to meals.

Clinical use

Statins lower LDL by 15% to 60%, lower triglycerides by 25% to 40%, and raise HDL by 6% to 10%.

Adverse effects

Statins are usually well tolerated. Predictable side effects associated with statins are listed in Box 8-15. Major adverse side effects are myopathy and hepatotoxicity. Baseline liver transaminase levels should be obtained before beginning therapy unless using the lowest dosages. Rosuvastatin is the only statin that may cause renal toxicity, which is more likely to occur when the drug is administered at high doses. The risk of myopathy or rhabdomyolysis increases when statins are administered with P450 inhibitors, gemfibrozil, or niacin. (Note: rhabdomyolysis involves breakdown of muscle fibers and release of myoglobin into the circulation; myoglobin and its metabolites may be toxic to the kidneys and can result in kidney failure. Creatinine kinase levels may be checked to monitor for muscle breakdown.) Patients should be queried for muscle pain or weakness. Although some patients may take coenzyme Q10 supplements to combat muscle pains (coenzyme Q10 synthesis occurs downstream of HMG-CoA reductase activity, so statins inhibit formation of coenzyme Q10), there is no evidence that this dietary supplement improves statin-induced muscle pain. On the other hand, low levels of vitamin D are known to cause muscle pain and weakness. Because statins decrease the cholesterol pool available to synthesize vitamin D, a current line of thinking is that vitamin D deficiency (or insufficiency) may underlie statin-induced myopathies.

Box 8-15. ADVERSE EFFECTS ASSOCIATED WITH STATINS

Muscle aches, myopathy, muscle inflammation, rhabdomyolysis
Peripheral neuropathies
Hepatotoxicity (increase in transaminase)
Gastrointestinal upset
Headache
Rash
Itching

PHYSIOLOGY

Lipoproteins Are All About Density

Chylomicrons are rich in triglycerides. They are formed from dietary fat, and they transport lipids from the gastrointestinal tract to the liver.

VLDL contains triglycerides that are synthesized in the liver but are converted to LDLs in the bloodstream. The role of VLDL is to transport triglycerides and cholesterol synthesized hepatically to the tissues.

LDL is formed after VLDL has donated triglycerides and fatty acids to the tissues. LDL is the major cholesterol transport mechanism, but cholesterol is loosely bound and can be deposited in the vasculature. Receptors for LDL exist in the liver, the adrenal gland, and cells of peripheral tissues. When LDL binds to its receptors, it undergoes endocytosis and is broken down intracellularly. (LDL is the "bad" cholesterol.)

HDL is synthesized in the liver and gut. The role of HDL is to scavenge excess cholesterol from peripheral tissues and transport it back to the liver, where it may be secreted into bile and excreted, a process known as *reverse cholesterol transport*. (HDL is the "good" cholesterol.)

PATHOLOGY

Atherosclerotic Lesions

Atherosclerotic lesions may occur after injury to the endothelium. If low-density lipoprotein cholesterol is retained in arterial walls, it may get oxidized, which recruits monocytes and macrophages (foam cells) to the area, provoking an inflammatory response. This process is exacerbated by high levels of cholesterol. Hypercholesterolemia may occur because of genetic disturbances in cholesterol synthesis, transport, or catabolism. Secondary causes of hypercholesterolemia include the use of certain drugs (progestins, glucocorticoids, or anabolic steroids) as well as nephrotic syndrome, diabetes, systemic lupus erythematosus, and hypothyroidism. Pharmacotherapy is useful to lower cholesterol and triglyceride levels when dietary changes are not successful.

Fibrates

Gemfibrozil and Fenofibrate
Mechanism of action

Fibrates reduce hepatic triglyceride levels by inhibiting hepatic extraction of free fatty acids and thus hepatic triglyceride production. These drugs may also lower cholesterol by increasing endothelial lipoprotein lipase activity.

Clinical use

Fibrates are most commonly prescribed to reduce triglyceride levels. Fibrates lower triglyceride levels by approximately 40%, have only a marginal effect on LDL and increase HDL by approximately 5%.

Box 8-16. ADVERSE EFFECTS ASSOCIATED WITH FIBRATES

Myopathy/rhabdomyolysis	Infections/influenza
Elevated liver function tests	Pain
Fatigue	Headache

Adverse effects

Patients should be monitored for elevated liver enzymes. A decrease in white blood cells may also occur. Adverse effects associated with fibrates are listed in Box 8-16. Patients should be warned to report unusual muscle pain, tenderness, or weakness, especially if accompanied by malaise or fever. Fenofibrate is contraindicated in patients with liver disease, gallbladder disease, or severe renal disease. Fibrates may cause cholelithiasis (gallstones) resulting from increased cholesterol excretion into bile. Several severe drug interactions may occur with fibrates, including increased risk of bleeding when fenofibrate is given with warfarin, myopathy or rhabdomyolysis when it is administered with HMG-CoA reductase inhibitors (statins), and hypoglycemia when it is given with sulfonylureas.

Ezetimibe

Mechanism of action

Ezetimibe inhibits intestinal absorption of cholesterol originating from dietary or biliary sources. This decreases the amount of cholesterol that is transported to the liver; thus hepatic stores of cholesterol are decreased and clearance of plasma cholesterol increases.

Clinical use

Ezetimibe lowers LDL by 20% and triglycerides by 10%. It is often combined with statins.

Adverse effects

In general, ezetimibe is well tolerated. It has been associated with allergic responses, respiratory infections, back pain, arthralgias, and gastrointestinal upset. Rarely, liver function tests may be elevated, but this resolves when the drug is discontinued.

Bile Acid Sequestrants (Resins)

Cholestyramine, Colestipol, and Colesevelam

Mechanism of action

Bile acid resins are positively charged, nonabsorbable resins that bind to negatively charged bile acids in the intestinal tract and prevent their reabsorption. This results in fecal elimination of bile acids. As the bile acid pool is depleted, hepatic enzymes increase conversion of cholesterol to bile acids. This increased hepatic demand for cholesterol causes increased synthesis of hepatic LDL receptors and ultimately lowers LDL in the plasma.

Pharmacokinetics

These positively charged resins are not bile specific and therefore bind to all negatively charged materials in the gut. As a result, drug interactions occur when acidic drugs are given

Box 8-17. EXAMPLES OF DRUGS WITH REDUCED BIOAVAILABILITY WHEN ADMINISTERED CONCURRENTLY WITH BILE ACID RESINS

Aspirin (nonsteroidal antiinflammatory drugs)	Furosemide
	Glipizide
Clindamycin	Hydrochlorothiazide
Digoxin	Hydrocortisone
Fat-soluble vitamins (A, D, E, K)	Phenytoin
	Thyroxine

concurrently. Absorption of fat-soluble vitamins (vitamins A, D, E, and K) may be impaired with bile acid resins, and bioavailability of acidic drugs is reduced (Box 8-17).

Clinical use

Bile acid resins decrease total cholesterol by 15% to 25%. These drugs are also used off-label to reduce diarrhea.

Adverse effects

Bile acid resins may actually increase triglyceride levels by 15%; therefore, they are best used in combination with drugs that lower triglyceride levels. Bile acid resins frequently cause constipation, bloating, and flatulence, which can be managed by increasing fluid intake or using stool softeners.

Niacin

Mechanism of action

The mechanisms of niacin are not completely understood but may involve inhibition of a putative lipid translocase that normally liberates free fatty acids from adipose tissue to the liver. Ultimately, synthesis of triglycerides is reduced, which translates to reduced synthesis of very low density lipoprotein (VLDL), which subsequently reduces LDL levels as well. Niacin also increases HDL levels.

Clinical use

Niacin reduces LDL and triglycerides by 15%. Niacin also decreases uptake of HDL by the liver, resulting in a 25% increase in HDL at relatively low doses. Niacin is frequently combined with bile acid resins for additive effects.

Adverse effects

Niacin often causes flushing and itching from release of prostaglandins. These adverse effects may be prevented by preadministration of aspirin. Hepatitis may occur, and as dosages are increased, liver function tests must be monitored. Immediate-release formulations are associated with substantial flushing. Sustained-release niacin formulations are associated with less flushing but a higher incidence of hepatotoxicity. Intermediate-acting formulations are a compromise between the adverse effects. Niacin is teratogenic in pregnancy. Additional adverse effects associated with niacin are listed in Box 8-18.

Box 8-18. ADVERSE EFFECTS ASSOCIATED WITH NIACIN

Flushing
Itching
Hyperuricemia (elevated uric acid; can precipitate gout)
Hyperglycemia (worsens diabetes control)
Gastrointestinal disturbances
Myopathy
Hepatitis
Peptic ulcer reactivation

Omega-3-Acid Ethyl Esters (Fish Oil)

Mechanism of action

The mechanisms of omega-3 fatty acids, eicosapentaenoic acid (20 carbons, 5 double bonds), and docosahexaenoic acid (22 carbons, 6 double bonds) in lowering triglycerides are unclear but may involve decreased hepatic synthesis of triglycerides or an increase in plasma lipoprotein lipase activity. As a biochemical reminder, polyunsaturated omega-3 fatty acids are defined has having three carbon units separating the first double bond from the terminal methyl group. This is in contrast to omega-6 polyunsaturated fatty acids, such as arachidonic acid, where 6 carbon units separate the first double bond from the terminal methyl. It has been speculated that differences in the biochemical actions between omega-3 and omega-6 fatty acids might reflect different bioactive metabolites of these "essential" lipid classes, whose precursors must be obtained from the diet and include plant-based foods and fatty fish.

Clinical use

Omega-3 fatty acids may reduce triglycerides by as much as 50%. The drug is approved for patients whose triglyceride levels are greater than 500 mg/dL.

Adverse effects

Eructation (burping) and a fishy taste in the mouth are commonly reported by patients taking fish oils. There is also an increased risk of bleeding.

Summary

In essence, drugs that reduce cholesterol synthesis (by the liver) or block cholesterol or bile acid absorption through the gastrointestinal tract are effective therapies. Many patients who consume low-fat diets still require pharmacotherapy because of genetic predispositions for hyperlipidemia ("It's not just the frank you eat, but also your Uncle Frank").

●●● COMPLEMENTARY AND ALTERNATIVE MEDICINE

Patients use a variety of natural products to lower their cholesterol. Some of these alternatives are probably safe and effective; others, however, may not be.

Plant sterols and stanols are being added to foods such as orange juice and margarine. They prevent cholesterol from being absorbed. Regular use of these health foods may decrease LDL by 5% to 17%.

Fibrous foods that contain at least 51% whole grains (e.g., whole wheat, whole oats, corn, barley) may help reduce cholesterol. It is the fiber content in whole grains that seems to reduce cholesterol and the risk of heart disease. Oat bran can reduce LDL cholesterol by as much as 26% by increasing the viscosity of food in the stomach and delaying absorption. Psyllium, another source of fiber, can decrease LDL cholesterol by 6% by absorbing dietary fats in the gastrointestinal tract, preventing cholesterol absorption, and increasing cholesterol elimination in fecal bile acids. Adding soy to the diet may also decrease LDL cholesterol by as much 10%.

In addition to its use in treating hypertriglyceridemia, fish oils as dietary supplements are also being used for other cardiovascular purposes. Evidence suggests that these essential fatty acids may decrease the incidence of cardiac arrhythmias, decrease the risk of sudden cardiac death, and lower blood pressure. Although patients commonly complain of eructation and a fishy aftertaste, there is evidence that these side effects are a result of using low-quality fish oils in which the oils have already become oxidized and are rancid. Better quality fish oils do not cause this problem. Antiplatelet activities (bleeding) may occur with fish oil dietary supplements and can increase the International Normalized Ratio in patients taking warfarin. Products that contain red yeast rice are extracts of rice that has been fermented with red yeast. The natural fermentation process yields several different HMG-CoA reductase inhibitors (including lovastatin). These natural products are essentially statins in disguise. Because the natural substances produced via the fermentation process are statins, hepatotoxicity and myopathy can occur as adverse effects. That these natural products are unregulated means that they may contain too much or too little of the active ingredients.

CLINICAL MEDICINE

Lowering "Bad" Cholesterol

Statins are usually the best choice for initial therapy to lower LDL. Patients typically get the most benefits at low to mid-range doses. Doubling the statin dose usually provides only a modest additional reduction in LDL cholesterol and makes adverse effects more likely. It is often more effective to add a second drug. Adding a bile acid sequestrant provides an additional 10% to 20% reduction in LDL, adding ezetimibe lowers LDL an additional 15%, and adding niacin lowers LDL 10% to 15% and can increase HDL and lower triglycerides as well.

●●● **TOP FIVE LIST**

1. Antihypertensives lower blood pressure by reducing cardiac output (β-blockers) or lowering total peripheral resistance (the rest of the drugs).
2. Drugs used to manage angina reduce myocardial O_2 demand or increase O_2 supply.
3. HF therapies focus on preventing additional hypertrophy or remodeling damage; positive inotropes should be reserved for patients who are symptomatic after other therapies have been tried.
4. Antiarrhythmics possess a variety of different mechanisms that target ion channels; however, these drugs may also induce secondary arrhythmias by perturbing these ion channels (proarrhythmogenic).
5. Antihyperlipidemics lower cholesterol or triglyceride levels, but many are associated with muscle aches and elevations of liver function tests.

Self-assessment questions can be accessed at www. StudentConsult.com.

Renal System

9

CONTENTS

ELIMINATION
OSMOTIC DIURETICS
   Mannitol and Urea
CARBONIC ANHYDRASE INHIBITORS
   Acetazolamide and Methazolamide (Oral) and Dorzolamide
    (Ocular)
LOOP DIURETICS
   Furosemide, Bumetanide, Ethacrynic Acid, and Torsemide
THIAZIDES
   Hydrochlorothiazide, Indapamide, Metolazone, and
    Chlorthalidone
POTASSIUM-SPARING AGENTS
   Spironolactone, Amiloride, and Triamterene
HYPONATREMIA
   Tolvaptan, Conivaptan
COMPLEMENTARY AND ALTERNATIVE MEDICINE
TOP FIVE LIST

The renal system is all about osmotic balance. Essentially, renal physiology can be reduced to one simple equation: what goes in must equal what comes out. Despite a variable load of solute and solvent ingestion, the kidney is capable of finely regulating osmotic balance. Multiple Na^+ cotransporters, antiporters, and channels serve to reabsorb Na^+ along the nephron to create the osmotic gradient necessary for water reabsorption. Physicians have at their disposal a vast arsenal of drugs to circumvent Na^+ and water retention, especially in diseases such as congestive heart failure in which retained fluid must be eliminated. The administration of these drugs (diuretics) leads to both diuresis (water loss) as well as natriuresis (Na^+ loss). Diuretics increase the rate of urine formation. By increasing urine volume, there is a net loss of water and accompanying solute. The net loss of electrolytes varies among diuretic agents depending on the drug's site of action. Figure 9-1 provides an overview of the site of action for six classes of diuretic agents.

Given their role in the regulation of water and salts, diuretics are used to manage diseases such as hypertension, congestive heart failure, edema, hypercalciuria, and, historically, glaucoma.

ANATOMY

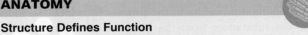

Structure Defines Function

To fully understand the actions of diuretics, practitioners must appreciate the exquisite anatomy of the nephron that underlies renal physiology. In other words, structure (anatomy) drives function (physiology), which can be exploited (pharmacology). The nephron, the functional unit of the kidney, is composed of the glomerulus (the filtration unit) and a series of downstream tubules (proximal, loop of Henle, distal and collecting ducts) that serve to reabsorb solutes and fluid into the peritubular capillary network. Three examples of structure-function relationships within the nephron are described here.

1. The process of selective filtering or sieving within a glomerulus is mediated by the fenestrated endothelial cells of the capillary lumen in juxtaposition to the foot processes of the epithelial cells of the tubule network. The mesenchymal cells within the capillary network of the glomerulus, known as *mesangial cells*, provide the mechanical constrictive force to regulate glomerular filtration rate by changing the surface area available for filtration.

2. The distal tubule of the nephron winds its way between both the afferent and efferent arterioles as well as the glomerulus. This anatomic feature, known as the *macula densa*, allows for cross-talk between nephron elements. Cells within the afferent arteriole (juxtaglomerular cells) release renin, the enzyme that converts angiotensinogen to angiotensin I, by integrating signals from the afferent arteriole (perfusion pressure), renal sympathetic nerves, and distal tubule (solute load). In a similar scenario, the process of tubuloglomerular feedback is mediated by sensing solute load within the distal tubule and turning that information into intracellular signals that modify glomerular filtration rate via mesangial cell contractility.

3. Based on the anatomic hairpin loop of Henle as well as the discrete localization of $Na^+/K^+/2Cl^-$ cotransporters in the thick ascending loop of Henle, an osmotic gradient is generated in the renal medulla that provides the driving force to reabsorb greater than 99% of filtered water.

PHYSIOLOGY

Role of the Glomerulus

During glomerular filtration, the plasma is filtered through the capillary endothelium, a basement membrane, and the epithelium of Bowman's capsule. The most important barriers to prevent substances from freely leaking through the glomerulus are negatively charged heparin sulfates in the basement membrane and the podocytes, which are specialized epithelial cells that stabilize the glomerulus.

● ● ● ELIMINATION

Renal elimination refers to the process by which the kidney removes substances from the body and is the net result of three interrelated processes: glomerular filtration, secretion, and reabsorption (Box 9-1). Filtration is a passive, nonsaturable, linear process by which small ionized and un-ionized molecules are filtered from the plasma via the glomerulus. It is important to remember that only free, unbound drug is filtered. Protein-bound drugs do not enter the filtrate as long as renal function is normal.

Unlike filtration, secretion is an active, saturable process (Fig. 9-2). The kidney has developed multiple mechanisms to actively secrete both un-ionized and charged substances by way of energy-dependent transporters.

CLINICAL MEDICINE

Competition for Renal Secretion

Sometimes drugs compete for renal active transport protein carriers. For example, under normal circumstances, penicillins are actively secreted into the renal tubules from the peritubular capillary network. In certain situations, it is desirable to slow penicillin's elimination from the body and increase the drug's concentration in the plasma. Probenecid, an antiinflammatory drug typically prescribed for gout, can compete with penicillin for the same active transport protein carrier in the renal tubules. When probenecid competes with penicillin for the active transport carrier protein, elimination of penicillin from the body is slowed.

Not all drugs that are passively filtered at the glomerulus or actively secreted into the renal filtrate are immediately eliminated from the body. Drugs that are nonpolar and un-ionized may be reabsorbed from the renal filtrate and reenter the bloodstream. On the other hand, drugs that are polar or ionized become "trapped" in the filtrate and are eliminated from the body in the urine. As should be remembered, the ultimate consequence of drug metabolism is to generate polar hydrophilic metabolites that are not reabsorbed in the tubule network and remain in the urine.

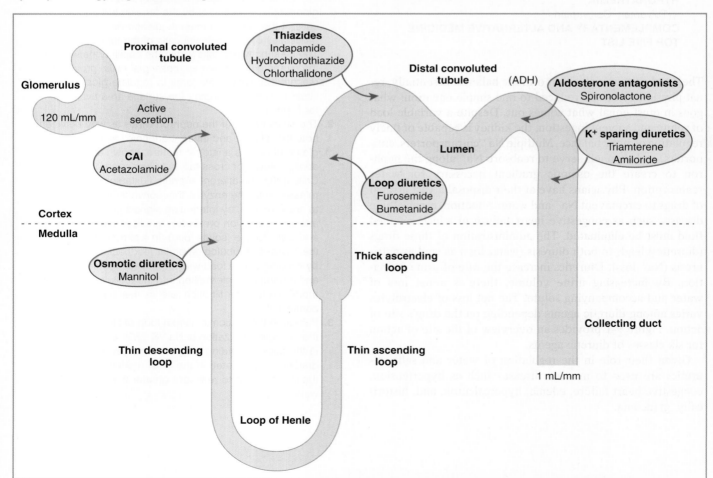

Figure 9-1. Overview of site of action for diuretic drugs. *CAI,* carbonic anhydrase inhibitor; *ADH,* antidiuretic hormone.

Box 9-1. CALCULATING RENAL CLEARANCE

Any discussion of renal elimination warrants a review of the concept of clearance (see Chapter 1). Clearance is defined as the volume of blood cleared of drug per unit time. Although this chapter is primarily about renal elimination, recall that there are other routes of elimination as well, including hepatic, fecal, and pulmonary routes as well as through lactation. In such cases, total body clearance (CL_T) may be represented as

$$CL_T = CL_R \text{(renal clearance)} + CL_{NR} \text{(nonrenal clearance)}$$

Drugs that undergo first-order elimination have a constant clearance because their rate of elimination is directly proportional to plasma levels. Also, when no active secretion or reabsorption occurs, renal clearance is the same as GFR. Because only "free" drugs are filtered at the glomerulus, when a drug is protein bound the renal clearance is represented as follows:

$$CL_{Renal} = GFR \times \text{Free fraction of drug}$$

Kidney function is most commonly quantified in terms of creatinine clearance (CrCl). CrCl is a direct measure of renal function. This value is estimated by using what is known as the *Cockcroft-Gault method*. The formula for males is

$$CrCl (mL/min) = \frac{(140 - Age)(\text{Body weight [kg]})}{(\text{Serum creatinine [mg/dL]})(72)}$$

The formula for females is

$$CrCl (mL/min) = \frac{(140 - Age)(\text{Body weight [kg]}) \times 0.85}{(\text{Serum creatinine [mg/dL]})(72)}$$

These equations are useful unless the patient's weight is excessive. If patients weigh more than 30% over ideal body weight (IBW), this is accounted for by using the following equation for weight, where *TBW* stands for total body weight (in kilograms) and *IBW* is ideal body weight (in kilograms).

$$\text{Corrected body weight} = IBW + [0.4(TBW - IBW)]$$

Ideal body weight is calculated as follows:

For men: $IBW = 50 \text{ kg} + 2.3(\text{number of inches} > 60)$
For women: $IBW = 45 \text{ kg} + 2.3(\text{number of inches} > 60)$

Knowledge of a patient's kidney function is imperative when prescribing any medications that are eliminated renally. For a healthy young adult, CrCl should be approximately 100 to 120 mL/min or 20 mg/kg/day. Because CrCl declines with declining renal function, doses of medication handled by the kidneys will need to be decreased accordingly to prevent adverse effects resulting from drug accumulation. Although not a 1:1 correlation, drug doses are decreased proportionately to diminished CrCl.

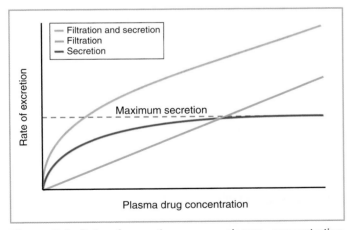

Figure 9-2. Rate of excretion versus plasma concentration for drugs. Excretion is a combination of filtration and active secretion.

●●● OSMOTIC DIURETICS

Mannitol and Urea

Osmotic diuretics are freely filtered at the glomerulus, undergo minimal reabsorption by the renal tubules, and are relatively pharmacologically and metabolically inert. Examples of osmotic diuretics are intravenous mannitol and urea.

Mechanism of Action

Osmotic diuretics primarily inhibit water reabsorption in the proximal convoluted tubule and the thin descending loop of Henle and collecting duct, regions of the kidney that are highly permeable to water. As Na^+ is reabsorbed in the proximal tubule, water normally follows and is reabsorbed by passive diffusion. In the presence of an osmotic diuretic, reabsorption of water is reduced relative to Na^+. In other words, despite the actions of transporters to generate a Na^+ concentration gradient favorable for osmosis, mannitol and urea negate this driving force. Osmotic diuretics also extract water from intracellular compartments, increasing extracellular fluid volume. Overall, urine flow increases with a relatively small loss of Na^+. In fact, urine osmolarity actually decreases.

Clinical Uses

Osmotic diuretics are used to increase water excretion in preference to Na^+ excretion. Urine volume can be maintained even when the glomerular filtration (GFR) rate is low. Osmotic diuretics are particularly effective in preventing anuria (cessation of urine production) accompanying the presentation of large pigment loads to the kidney such as in hemolysis as well as rhabdomyolysis. Osmotic diuretics are used to lower intracranial pressure and for short-term reduction of intraocular pressure. These drugs also promote excretion of nephrotoxic substances such as cisplatin.

Adverse Effects

Acutely, extracellular fluid volume expansion may occur, which is particularly undesirable for patients with cardiac decompensation. As mannitol is cleared by the kidneys, water follows, leading to dehydration and hypernatremia; nausea and vomiting, chest pain, and chills may occur.

CARBONIC ANHYDRASE INHIBITORS

Acetazolamide and Methazolamide (Oral) and Dorzolamide (Ocular)

Mechanism of Action

Carbonic anhydrase (CA) inhibitors block CA on the luminal membrane and inside proximal tubule cells (Fig. 9-3). Inhibition of CA in the cytoplasm of proximal tubule cells causes a decrease in secretion of H^+ through the Na^+/H^+ antiporter. In this way, the driving force to reabsorb Na^+ in the proximal tubule is dissipated, necessitating natriuresis and diuresis. With CA on the luminal membrane also inhibited, the formation of bicarbonate from carbonic acid in the lumen is slowed, as is the diffusion of CO_2 into the tubular cells. Overall, bicarbonate reabsorption in the proximal tubule decreases by 80%, leading

to the possibility of acidosis. As a consequence of less Na^+ reabsorption via Na^+/H^+ exchange in the proximal tubule, more Na^+ is delivered to distal segments of the nephron. Sodium reabsorption in the distal tubule provides the electrogenic driving force to facilitate K^+ secretion into the tubule lumen. This is the mechanism by which most diuretics cause hypokalemia (loss of K^+). To counteract this loss of K^+, patients are often given K^+ supplements or encouraged to eat bananas or drink orange juice. Overall, the enhanced urinary excretion of Na^+ and K^+ leads to increased urine flow.

Clinical Uses

As diuretics, these agents have limited utility because of a rapid depletion of body bicarbonate stores and metabolic acidosis. Because CA inhibitors rapidly reduce total body bicarbonate stores, they are useful for treating chronic metabolic alkalosis. The lack of proton secretion into the tubules as a consequence of CA inhibition may be used to alkalinize the urine to enhance elimination of weak acids, such as uric acid and cystine. CA inhibitors are also useful in treating acute mountain sickness (they rapidly reduce pulmonary and cerebral edema). There is also a role for these agents in treating glaucoma because CA inhibitors reduce intraocular pressure by inhibiting the formation of aqueous humor.

Adverse Effects

Acetazolamide is a nonbacteriostatic sulfonamide. Sulfonamide-type adverse reactions may occur including urticaria, pruritus, rash, Stevens-Johnson syndrome, photosensitivity, bone marrow depression, and blood dyscrasias. The drug is contraindicated in those with sulfonamide hypersensitivity. Other adverse effects include hyperchloremic metabolic acidosis, renal calculi (calcium is insoluble at alkaline pH), hypokalemia, and paresthesias.

Ocular use of dorzolamide can be associated with adverse ocular reactions, dysgeusia (an unpleasant taste in the mouth), and superficial punctate keratitis (corneal disease).

Drug Interactions

Concurrent use of CA inhibitors and salicylates may result in accumulation and toxicity of CA inhibitors, leading to central nervous system toxicity as well as severe metabolic acidosis.

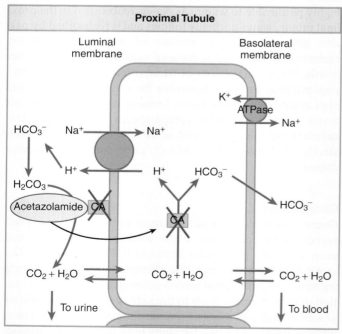

Figure 9-3. Mechanism of action for carbonic anhydrase inhibitors. ATPase, adenosine triphosphatase.

●●● LOOP DIURETICS

Furosemide, Bumetanide, Ethacrynic Acid, and Torsemide

Mechanism of Action

The primary mode of action of loop diuretics is inhibition of the $Na^+/K^+/2Cl^-$ cotransporter on the luminal membrane of the thick ascending limb of the loop of Henle (Fig. 9-4). Inhibition of the $Na^+/K^+/2Cl^-$ cotransporter dissipates the Na^+ gradient generated in the renal medulla, which drives water reabsorption in the water-permeable descending limb of the loop of Henle. Inhibition of $Na^+/K^+/2Cl^-$ cotransport decreases intracellular K^+, which decreases the positive electrogenic potential and hence decreases reabsorption of Ca^{++} and Mg^{++}. Uric acid excretion is also reduced. In a nutshell, loop diuretics decrease reabsorption of Na^+, K^+, Ca^{++}, Mg^{++}, and Cl^-. Because of the large NaCl absorptive capacity of the loop of Henle, loop diuretics cause a large Na^+ load to remain in the tubule system and exert a powerful diuretic action.

Loop diuretics such as ethacrynic acid, furosemide, and bumetanide are both passively filtered at the glomerulus and actively secreted by cells of the proximal tubule. Acidic drugs such as probenecid compete for this secretory transport process and can thus reduce the diuretic action of loop diuretics by reducing their concentration at the loop of Henle.

Clinical Uses

Loop diuretics are useful to reduce edema associated with cardiac, hepatic, or renal disease. They are also helpful in managing acute pulmonary edema and congestive heart failure.

In acute renal failure, loop diuretics may be used in an attempt to convert oliguric (small volume of urine) failure to nonoliguric failure. Loop diuretics have also been used to manage hypercalcemia and hyperkalemia.

Adverse Effects

The most common adverse effects associated with loop diuretics are related to renal effects of the drugs: volume depletion, hypomagnesemia, hypocalcemia, and hypokalemic metabolic alkalosis. Patients who are volume depleted or who are on salt (chloride)-restricted diets are most at risk for loop diuretic–induced metabolic alkalosis. Furosemide and bumetanide are sulfonamide derivatives and may be contraindicated in patients with hypersensitivity to sulfa drugs. Ototoxicity (hearing loss) may occur with loop diuretics, particularly when used intravenously, at high doses, or in combination with aminoglycosides (ethacrynic acid is more ototoxic than furosemide). These ototoxic effects are due to changes in ionic gradients that induce edema of the epithelium of the stria vascularis. Ethacrynic acid also causes gastrointestinal disturbances.

Drug Interactions

Loop diuretics may decrease lithium clearance, resulting in lithium toxicity. Use with angiotensin-converting enzyme inhibitors may result in a precipitous fall in blood pressure, especially in the presence of Na^+ depletion. Diuretic-induced hypokalemia may increase the risk of digoxin toxicity; this occurs because digoxin binds to the K^+-site of the Na^+/K^+-adenosine triphosphatase (ATPase) pump. Under conditions of hypokalemia, there is less K^+ competing with digoxin and digoxin toxicity may occur. Concomitant use with nonsteroidal antiinflammatory drugs reduces the blood pressuring–lowering effects of diuretics owing to the Na^+ reabsorption associated with nonsteroidal antiinflammatory drugs.

●●● THIAZIDES

Hydrochlorothiazide, Indapamide, Metolazone, and Chlorthalidone

Mechanism of Action

Thiazides increase urine output by inhibiting the NaCl cotransporter on the luminal membrane of the earliest portion of the distal convoluted tubule, often called the *cortical diluting segment* (Fig. 9-5). Inhibition of the NaCl cotransporter increases luminal concentrations of Na^+ and Cl^- ions in the late distal tubule; the large Na^+ load downstream promotes K^+ excretion in the late distal tubule and the collecting duct. Thiazides also lead to increased reabsorption of Ca^{++} into the blood and may lead to hypercalcemia. Thus thiazides increase urinary levels of Na^+, K^+, and Cl^- and decrease levels of Ca^{++} in the urine.

Thiazides, as organic acids, are readily filtered and secreted but are less effective at mobilizing fluid than loop diuretics,

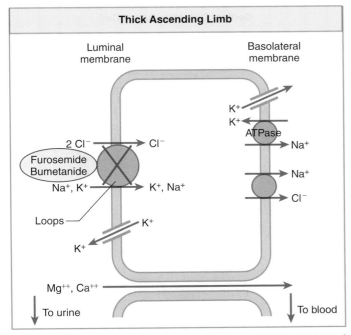

Figure 9-4. The $Na^+/K^+/Cl^-$ symporter is the site of action of loop diuretics.

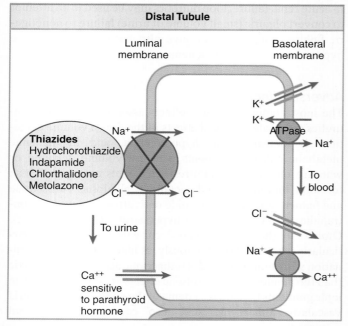

Figure 9-5. Site of action of thiazide diuretics. ATPase, adenosine triphosphatase.

especially at a low (GFR). (Loop diuretics are preferred when creatine clearance is less than 40 to 50 mL/min.) In fact, hydrochlorothiazide decreases GFR without altering renal blood flow.

Clinical Uses

Thiazide diuretics are first-line treatment for hypertension, according to the Seventh Report of the Joint National Committee on Prevention, Detection, Evaluation, and Treatment of High Blood Pressure (JNC-VII). Initially, antihypertensive effects are due to diuresis and volume depletion. Surprisingly, as renal compensation occurs via the renin-angiotensin-aldosterone system, the antihypertensive actions of thiazides continue. It is thought that mobilization of Na^+ makes vessels more pliable and less rigid, producing a decrease in total peripheral resistance. In addition, indapamide has vasodilating properties, which accounts for a portion of its antihypertensive effects. Because thiazides reabsorb calcium, they are a first-line choice for treating idiopathic hypercalciuria to reduce calcium stone formation.

Adverse Effects

Hypokalemia, hyponatremia, hypomagnesemia, and hypercalcemia may occur. Preexisting diabetes mellitus may be aggravated by thiazides. Hyperuricemia that precipitates gout can occur. Triglycerides and low-density lipoprotein cholesterol levels may increase initially but appear to return to pretreatment levels with long-term therapy (indapamide is an exception; it does not appear to increase serum cholesterol). Photosensitivity, decreased libido, and gastrointestinal disturbances may also occur.

Drug Interactions

Drug interactions are the same as for loop diuretics.

PHYSIOLOGY

Parathyroid Hormone

Parathyroid hormone (PTH), synthesized and released by the parathyroid glands, controls the distribution of Ca^{++} and $H_2PO_4^-$ in the body. High levels of PTH cause Ca^{++} transfer from bone to blood. Specifically, PTH enhances Ca^{++} reabsorption within the distal convoluted tubule through G-protein–coupled regulated Ca^{++} channels as well as inhibits tubular reabsorption of phosphate. Finally, PTH also stimulates production of 1,25-dihydroxyvitamin D_3 (calcitriol) within the kidney, which enhances Ca^{++} reabsorption in the gastrointestinal tract.

●●● POTASSIUM-SPARING AGENTS

Spironolactone, Amiloride, and Triamterene

Mechanism of Action

With their effect at the level of the collecting tubules (CTs), these agents are generally considered weak diuretics because most of the filtered Na^+ is reabsorbed upstream (Fig. 9-6). The CTs do, however, determine final urinary Na^+ concentration and are a major site of regulated K^+ and H^+ secretion.

Spironolactone is a steroid analog of the mineralocorticoid aldosterone. As an aldosterone receptor antagonist, spironolactone competes with aldosterone for binding to its cytoplasmic receptor. This antagonism indirectly halts expression of new (spare or silent) Na^+ channels on the luminal membrane, decreases Na^+ conductance, and decreases Na^+/K^+-ATPase pump activity, which is the driving force behind K^+ secretion.

Remember that as Na^+ diffuses through its channels in the CT, it causes an increase in intracellular positive charge,

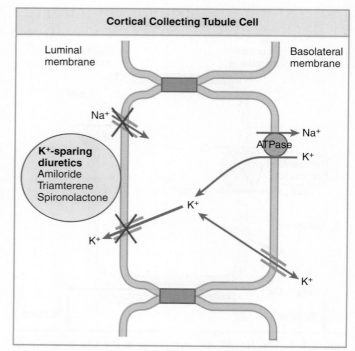

Figure 9-6. Site of action of K^+-sparing diuretics.

which leads to extrusion of K^+ into the lumen. Because Na^+ is usually reabsorbed in exchange for K^+ in the CT, urinary K^+ excretion decreases with the use of spironolactone. Thus inhibition of aldosterone via spironolactone retards K^+ secretion and is thus K^+ sparing. Because aldosterone, through undefined mechanisms, leads to proton extrusion across the luminal membrane of intercalated cells, spironolactone can acidify the urine.

In contrast to spironolactone, amiloride and triamterene have slightly different mechanisms in the CT. These drugs directly block Na^+ channels on the luminal membrane in the CT, resulting in hyperkalemia and acidosis. Again, as these drugs block Na^+ channels at the site of Na^+-dependent K^+ excretion, K^+ is retained in the body (i.e., K^+ is spared). Together, all K^+-sparing diuretics produce small increases in urinary Na^+ and marked decreases in urinary K^+ and H^+.

Clinical Uses

Spironolactone is helpful as an adjunct to other diuretics because of its K^+-retaining properties. As an aldosterone receptor antagonist, spironolactone is also used to treat primary or secondary hyperaldosteronism. Spironolactone has also been shown to increase survival in advanced stages of heart failure and reduce edema and ascites associated with hepatic cirrhosis or nephrotic syndrome.

Triamterene is frequently used in combination with hydrochlorothiazide. This combination enhances the diuretic effect of the thiazide and counteracts the loss of K^+ normally associated with hydrochlorothiazide. As with triamterene, amiloride is used in combination with hydrochlorothiazide. In addition, amiloride has an off-label use for preventing K^+ loss in lithium-induced diabetes insipidus.

Adverse Effects

As a group, K^+-sparing diuretics may cause hyperkalemic metabolic acidosis or azotemia (excessive amounts of urea and other nitrogenous wastes in the blood). Spironolactone is usually not recommended in males because of the drug's antiandrogenic effects, which lead to gynecomastia and lowered libido. Nephrolithiasis (kidney stones) has been reported with triamterene.

PHYSIOLOGY

Role of the Renin-Angiotensin-Aldosterone (RAA) Pathway During Congestive Heart Failure

For patients with congestive heart failure, cardiac output eventually becomes inadequate to provide the necessary O_2 for all the body's tissues. The body attempts to compensate in several ways. One of these compensatory mechanisms involves activation of the RAA pathway, which leads to widespread vasoconstriction and Na^+ reabsorption in an attempt to compensate for the body's perceived "lack of blood flow." Unfortunately, these compensatory mechanisms simply end up placing more stress (i.e., preload and afterload) on an already failing heart. As an antagonist of aldosterone,

spironolactone inhibits one of the end results of RAA activation, that of aldosterone secretion, and thus prevents further sodium and water retention.

CLINICAL MEDICINE

Spironolactone Is More Than Just a Diuretic

Hirsutism and polycystic ovary syndrome occur in females when androgen levels are too high. Having a steroid structure, spironolactone possesses nonspecific antiandrogenic effects. Spironolactone has been used by women to treat excessive hair growth and polycystic ovary syndrome.

●●● HYPONATREMIA

Tolvaptan, Conivaptan

Mechanism of Action and Clinical Uses

The action of the renal system is not just about loss of water via diuretics. Often in pathologies such as congestive heart failure, cirrhosis of the liver with ascites, nephrotic syndrome, renal failure, or syndrome of inappropriate antidiuretic hormone, there is a dilution of serum sodium due to increases in total body water. These diverse pathologies often require active pharmacologic intervention to treat resultant hyponatremia. Orally administered tolvaptan and intravenously administered conivaptan are selective and preferential arginine vasopressin V2 receptor antagonists. As arginine vasopressin antagonists, both drugs lead to aquaresis or excretion of free water and restoration of low sodium concentrations. Other co-administered treatment options can be fluid restriction, hypertonic (3%) saline solution, or diuretics.

Adverse Effects

Because of potential life-threatening adverse effects of overshooting normal sodium levels and inducing hypernatremia-induced osmotic demyelination syndrome, a black box warning has been placed on these drugs, directing their use in hospital settings where plasma sodium concentrations can be monitored frequently. Tolvaptan is metabolized by the cytochrome P450 3A4 isoform. Thus CYP3A4 inhibitors (e.g., ketoconazole, clarithromycin, grapefruit juice) or CYP3A4 inducers (e.g., rifampin, phenytoin, St. John's wort) increase or decrease, respectively, the plasma concentration of this drug that exhibits such a narrow therapeutic window.

●●● COMPLEMENTARY AND ALTERNATIVE MEDICINE

In addition to prescription diuretics, natural diuretics are used by patients to self-treat problems such as menstrual disorders, edema, and hypertension. Although more than 90 natural products are reported to have diuretic activity, only caffeine is routinely included in over-the-counter medications for this purpose because adequate scientific data supporting the safety and efficacy of other products are lacking. However, patients may self-medicate with dandelion, stinging nettle, corn silk, and other natural therapies. A partial listing of the most common natural products with diuretic activity is given in Box 9-2.

●●● TOP FIVE LIST

1. Diuretics that block Na^+ reabsorption at segments proximal to the collecting duct increase Na^+ load in the late proximal tubule and collecting ducts.
2. An increase in Na^+ load leads to urinary excretion of K^+.
3. Urinary loss of K^+ may cause hypokalemia.
4. Blockade of Na^+ reabsorption by loop diuretics and thiazides drives water excretion (diuresis) and is associated with loss of H^+, resulting in alkalosis.
5. Loss of K^+ can be avoided through use of drugs that act primarily at collecting ducts (i.e., K^+-sparing diuretics)—the final site for K^+ secretion.

The major effects of diuretics on urine and blood chemistries are reviewed in Table 9-1. Choosing a diuretic in clinical practice requires a complete patient history (Table 9-2) and will vary according to underlying disease.

Self-assessment questions can be accessed at www. StudentConsult.com.

Box 9-2. NATURAL PRODUCTS HAVING DIURETIC EFFECTS

Caffeine	Foxglove
Chicory	Licorice
Corn silk	Stinging nettle
Dandelion	St. John's wort
Elderberry	

TABLE 9-1. Review of Major Diuretic Classes

DRUG	MECHANISM	URINE LEVELS	BLOOD CHEMISTRY
Carbonic anhydrase inhibitors	Inhibit carbonic anhydrase in the PCT	Elevated Na^+, K^+, Ca^{++}, HCO_3^-, and PO_4	Hypokalemia, acidosis, hyperchloremia
Loop diuretics	Inhibit $Na^+/K^+/2Cl^-$ in the TAL	Elevated Na^+, K^+, Ca^{++}, Mg^{++}, and Cl^- Decreased HCO_3^-	Hypokalemia, alkalosis, hypomagnesemia, hypocalcemia
Thiazides	Inhibit NaCl in the PCT	Elevated Na^+, K^+, and Cl^- Decreased Ca^{++}	Hypokalemia, alkalosis, hypercalcemia, hyperuricemia
K^+-sparing agents	Inhibit Na^+ channels or antagonize aldosterone receptors in the CT	Elevated Na^+ Decreased K^+	Hyperkalemia, acidosis

CT, collecting tubule; *PCT*, proximal convoluted tubule; *TAL*, thick ascending limb of the loop of Henle.

TABLE 9-2. Choice of Diuretics in Clinical Practice

CONDITION	DIURETIC OF CHOICE
Congestive heart failure	Furosemide
Acute pulmonary edema	Furosemide
Hypertension	Hydrochlorothiazide
Hepatic cirrhosis	Spironolactone
Lithium-induced diabetes insipidus	Amiloride
Ca^{++} stones	Hydrochlorothiazide
Idiopathic hypercalciuria	Hydrochlorothiazide
Hirsutism	Spironolactone
Polycystic ovary syndrome	Spironolactone
Idiopathic hypercalcemia	Furosemide
Nephrogenic diabetes insipidus	Hydrochlorothiazide

Inflammatory Disorders 10

CONTENTS

INTRODUCTION TO ANTIINFLAMMATORY DRUGS
ANTIHISTAMINE DRUGS
  H₁ Antagonists
  H₂ Antagonists
NONSTEROIDAL AND STEROIDAL ANTIINFLAMMATORY DRUGS
  NSAIDs
  Steroidal Antiinflammatory Drugs (Glucocorticoids)
INFLAMMATORY DISORDERS OF THE SKIN
  Corticosteroids, T-Cell Immunomodulators (Eczema) and Retinoids (Acne)
ASTHMA
  β₂-Selective Agonists, Mast Cell Stabilizers, Corticosteroids, Leukotriene Receptor Antagonists, and Methylxanthines
GOUT
  Colchicine, Uricosurics, and Xanthine Oxidase Inhibitors
RHEUMATOID ARTHRITIS
  NSAIDs and Disease-Modifying Antirheumatic Drugs
TOP FIVE LIST

●●● INTRODUCTION TO ANTIINFLAMMATORY DRUGS

This chapter is all about a fine line. A little inflammation restores homeostatic balance, fights disease, and drives wound-healing responses. A lot of inflammation results in pathologic conditions such as asthma, rheumatoid arthritis, inflammatory bowel diseases, gout, atherosclerosis, and, quite possibly, cancer. Understanding the mechanisms by which inflammatory mediators regulate tissue damage has identified pharmaceutical targets for the development of drugs that combat unchecked inflammation. Histamine blockers, cyclooxygenase (COX) inhibitors, and glucocorticoids are all examples of drug classes that put the brakes on inflammatory processes.

Tissue damage causes dilation of local blood vessels as well as other characteristic changes, such as increased capillary permeability and accumulation of inflammatory cells at the site of injury. Leukocytes play a central role in initiation of the inflammatory process. Yet, it is the interaction between a wide range of mediators (e.g., histamine, kinins, neuropeptides, cytokines, arachidonic acid derivatives) that is needed to maintain an inflammatory response. Acute and nonspecific inflammation is primarily

mediated by neutrophils and macrophages, whereas lymphocytes, basophils, and eosinophils are generally associated with specific, more chronic types of inflammatory responses. Under normal circumstances, inflammation is localized, is short lived, and resolves spontaneously. However, persistent inflammation indicates an ongoing pathologic state.

Drugs used to treat inflammatory disorders fall into one of the following categories:

1. Antihistamines
2. Broad-spectrum agents, which include nonsteroidal antiinflammatory drugs (NSAIDs) and steroidal antiinflammatory drugs (glucocorticoids)
3. Disease-specific drugs that have uses in conditions such as asthma, gout, and skin disorders

IMMUNOLOGY

Hypersensitivity Reactions

Hypersensitivity reactions result from antigen interactions with humoral antibodies or sensitized lymphocytes. Type I reactions occur when allergens bind to specific immunoglobulin (Ig)E antibodies immobilized on FcεR1 high-affinity IgE receptors, mast cells, or basophils. Activated mast cells release histamine, prostacyclin D₂, and leukotrienes. Type I allergic immediate reactions are associated with allergic rhinitis, bronchial asthma, atopic dermatitis, and systemic anaphylaxis. Type II reactions are cytotoxic and typically involve IgG and IgM antibodies reacting with a tissue antigen and triggering cytotoxicity. An example of a type II reaction is hemolytic anemia, in which certain drugs cause hemolysis of red blood cells. Type III reactions are immunocomplex mediated, in which preformed antigen-antibody complexes are deposited in tissues or blood vessels. This type of hypersensitivity reaction can lead to vasculitis. Finally, type IV hypersensitivity reactions are delayed reactions between sensitized CD4+ or CD8+ T cells and antigens expressed in the proper cellular context. Activation of these CD4+ T cells releases cytokines, which further recruit and activate macrophages, granulocytes, and natural killer cells. Activation of CD8+ T cells can lead to direct cellular cytotoxicity.

●●● ANTIHISTAMINE DRUGS

Histamine is typically found at pathologic levels in the lungs, skin, and the gastrointestinal (GI) tract. It is also released from mast cells and basophils during type I hypersensitivity

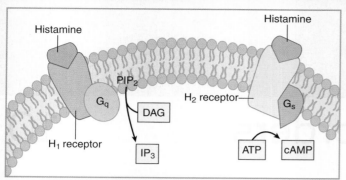

Figure 10-1. Histamine receptor signaling. H_1 receptors are G_q-coupled, whereas H_2 receptors are G_s-coupled. *PIP2*, phosphatidylinositol 4,5-bisphosphate; *DAG*, diacylglycerol; *IP3*, inositol triphosphate *ATP*, adenosine triphosphate; *cAMP*, cyclic adenosine monophosphate.

reactions and in response to certain drugs, venoms, and even trauma.

Histamine receptors belong to the 7-transmembrane G-protein–coupled family of receptors (Fig. 10-1). There are two main histamine receptors—H_1 and H_2—and activation leads to selective effects (Table 10-1). In clinical practice, antagonists of both histamine receptors subtypes are used. Traditionally, H_1-selective antagonists are known as *antihistamines*, whereas H_2 antagonists are known as *H_2 blockers*.

H_1 Antagonists

Sedating Drugs: Diphenhydramine, Promethazine, and Meclizine
Low to Moderately Sedating Drugs: Cetirizine, Chlorpheniramine, Clemastine, and Cyproheptadine
Nonsedating Drugs: Loratadine, Fexofenadine, Desloratadine, and Phenindamine
Topical Nonsedating Drugs: Ketotifen, Levocabastine, Olopatadine, Epinastine, and Azelastine

Mechanism of action

These agents exert their pharmacologic effects through selective competitive antagonism of H_1 receptors and therefore may be ineffective in the presence of high histamine levels.

Clinical use

This class of drugs is most commonly recognized for its effectiveness in relieving allergic symptoms of hay fever, urticaria, and rhinitis. They are also helpful in treating vertigo, motion sickness, and nausea, and many have sedating effects that allow them to be used as sleep aids. The sedating antihistamines impair performance, and in several states in the United States, drivers using these drugs would be considered impaired. It should be noted that drugs such as loratadine and fexofenadine are second-generation H_1 blockers and, unlike first-generation drugs, do not penetrate the central nervous system. As a result, these drugs do not cause drowsiness or provide relief from motion sickness. Several of these nonsedating antihistamines are now available over the counter.

Some antihistamines have been developed specifically for treatment of seasonal allergies (Box 10-1). Moreover, certain antihistamines and/or mast cell stabilizers, including epinastine, azelastine, ketotifen, and olopatadine, are designed as intranasal/ophthalmic preparations for allergic conjunctivitis. Because these formulations often contain benzalkonium chloride, soft contact lenses should be removed before topical administration because this compound is absorbed by the lens material.

Adverse effects

H_1 blockers are associated with muscarinic receptor blockade and accompanying anticholinergic side effects, sedation, and GI distress (less with second-generation drugs). On rare occasions, allergies to H_1 blockers have been reported.

Box 10-1. TOPICAL ANTIHISTAMINE TREATMENTS FOR SEASONAL ALLERGIES

Ocular

Ketotifen
Levocabastine
Olopatadine

Nasal

Azelastine

TABLE 10-1. Characteristics of Histamine Receptor Activation

H_1 ACTIVATION	H_2 ACTIVATION
↑ Capillary dilation → ↓ blood pressure	↑ Gastric acid secretion → ↑ gastrointestinal ulcers
↑ Capillary permeability → ↑ edema	↑ Sinoatrial nodal rate
↑ Bronchiolar smooth muscle contraction	Positive cardiac inotrope
↑ Peripheral nociceptive receptors	↑ Cardiac automaticity
↓ Atrioventricular nodal conduction	

H₂ Antagonists

Cimetidine, Ranitidine, Nizatidine, and Famotidine

Mechanism of action

These drugs are discussed in detail in Chapter 11. H₂ blockers indirectly suppress activity of proton pumps in the gastric mucosa and partially antagonize HCl secretion.

Clinical use

H₂ blockers are used in peptic ulcer disease, gastroesophageal reflux disease, and Zollinger-Ellison syndrome.

Adverse effects

Effects range from GI distress, dizziness, and somnolence to slurred speech and delirium (typically only in the elderly). In particular, cimetidine is a potent inhibitor of cytochrome P450 isoenzymes and interferes with metabolism of common medications (Table 10-2).

●●● NONSTEROIDAL AND STEROIDAL ANTIINFLAMMATORY DRUGS

Nonsteroidal and steroidal antiinflammatory drugs are all about lipids; that is, the bioactive, lipid-derived second messengers that contribute to inflammation. Oxygenated metabolites of arachidonic acid, known as *eicosanoids*, play a central role in the majority of inflammatory reactions; manipulation of their biosynthesis provides the basis of modern antiinflammatory therapy (Table 10-3). Arachidonic acid itself is a

TABLE 10-2. Drug Interactions Caused by H₂ Antagonists That Inhibit Hepatic Microsomal P450

H₂ ANTAGONISTS *INCREASE THE EFFECTS* OF THESE DRUGS BY DECREASING THEIR METABOLISM	H₂ ANTAGONISTS *DECREASE THE EFFECTS* OF THESE PRO-DRUGS BY BLOCKING ACTIVATION BY P450s
Amphetamines	Azole antifungals
Some β-blockers	Codeine
Some benzodiazepines	Hydrocodone
Calcium channel blockers	Oxycodone
Cyclosporine	Tramadol
Mexiletine	
Nateglinide	
Quinidine	
Phenytoin	
Risperidone	
Some selective serotonin reuptake inhibitors	
Sildenafil (and other phosphodiesterase-5 inhibitors)	
Tacrolimus	
Theophylline	
Tricyclic antidepressants	
Warfarin	

TABLE 10-3. Major Actions of Specific Eicosanoids and Therapeutic Uses of Several Eicosanoid Derivatives

EICOSANOIDS	ACTIONS AND USES
Leukotrienes (LTs)	
LTA₄, LTC₄, LTD₄	Increased vascular permeability Anaphylaxis Bronchoconstriction (central role in asthma)
LTB₄	Neutrophil chemoattractant Activation of polymorphonuclear cells Increased free radicals, leading to cell damage
Prostaglandins (PGs)	
PGE₁	Protection of gastric mucosa (**misoprostol**) Maintenance of patency of ductus arteriosus in neonates (**alprostadil**) Vasodilation (used in male impotence to treat erectile dysfunction) (**alprostadil**) Inhibition of platelet aggregation
PGE₂	Uterine smooth muscle contraction (**dinoprostone**) Cervical ripening and abortifacient Vasodilation and increased vascular permeability Sensitization of nociceptive fibers
PGE₂α	Uterine smooth muscle contraction to terminate pregnancy/postpartum uterine bleeding (**carboprost**) Bronchiolar smooth muscle contraction Decreased intraocular pressure (**latanoprost** or **travoprost**) Used primarily as abortifacient and in glaucoma Vasodilation and increased vascular permeability Sensitization of nociceptive fibers
PGI₂	Inhibition of platelet aggregation Vasodilation Used to treat pulmonary arterial hypertension (**epoprostenol**)
Thromboxanes (TXs)	
TXA₂	Platelet aggregation Potent bronchoconstriction Potent vasoconstriction

Therapeutic eicosanoids are in **bold**.
PGE, prostaglandin E; *PGI*, prostacyclin I; *TXA₂*, thromboxane A₂.

20-carbon fatty acid with four double bonds that is released from cell membrane phospholipids by the enzyme phospholipase A₂ (Fig. 10-2). Through further metabolism, arachidonic acid is converted by COX to prostanoid (thromboxane and prostacyclin), by lipoxygenase to leukotriene, or by epoxygenase to hydroxyeicosatraenoic acid. As shown in Figure 10-3, 5-lipoxygenase products can be converted to leukotrienes, which are important mediators of inflammation and chemoattraction.

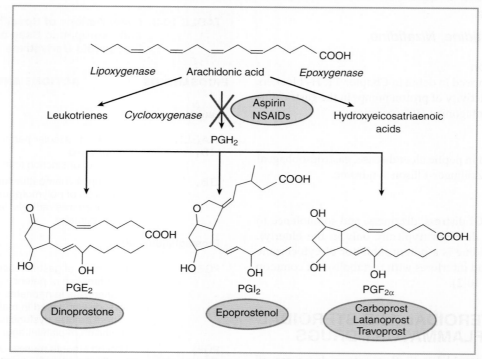

Figure 10-2. Arachidonic acid metabolites. Drugs that inhibit prostaglandin production (in purple) or mimic prostaglandin action (in green). In rare circumstances, inhibition of cyclooxygenase with aspirin and nonsteroidal antiinflammatory drugs (*NSAIDs*) may shunt arachidonic acid to leukotrienes and lead to bronchoconstriction, which is why aspirin and NSAIDs may be contraindicated in asthmatics.

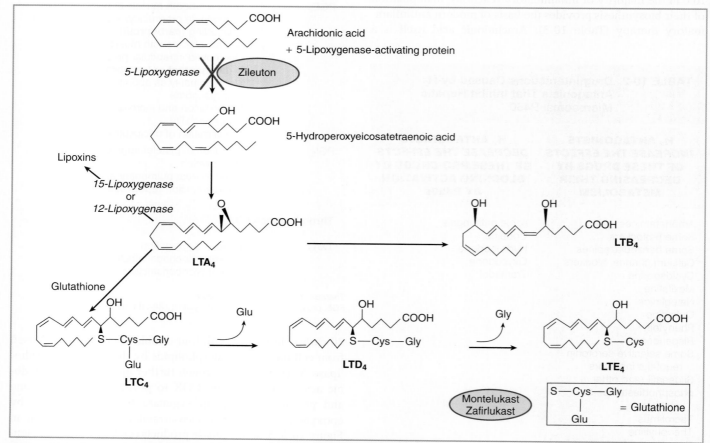

Figure 10-3. Drugs that inhibit leukotriene (*LT*) biosynthesis (zileuton) or antagonize the leukotriene receptors directly (montelukast and zafirlukast). Note how the structure of glutathione (*inset*) is incorporated into *LTA₄*.

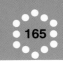

NSAIDs

Nonselective Cyclooxygenase Inhibitors:
Aspirin, Ibuprofen, Indomethacin, Ketorolac,
Ketoprofen, Naproxen, Piroxicam, and
Sulindac
Preferential Cyclooxygenase-2 Inhibitors:
Meloxicam and Etodolac
Selective Cyclooxygenase-2 Inhibitor:
Celecoxib

Mechanism of action

Irreversible inhibition of COX is a unique property of aspirin. Aspirin (acetylsalicylic acid) was the first NSAID to be used in clinical practice (it was initially extracted from the bark of the willow tree). Aspirin covalently and irreversibly acetylates serine-520 of COX to inhibit its activity. All other NSAIDs work through noncovalent mechanisms.

Today, NSAIDs comprise a chemically diverse group of drugs, all of which possess the ability to competitively inhibit the enzyme COX to decrease formation of prostaglandins and thromboxane. COX exists in two isoforms: COX-1, which is expressed in most tissues (especially in platelets, gastric mucosa, and kidneys), and COX-2, which is induced at sites of inflammation. Most NSAIDs work by indiscriminately inhibiting both COX isoforms and thus exhibit analgesic, antipyretic, antiinflammatory, and antiplatelet effects. COX-2–specific inhibitors were developed to, theoretically, capitalize on the antiinflammatory and analgesic properties of NSAIDs while simultaneously bypassing the risk of gastric bleeding associated with COX-1 inhibition. However, recent reports linking COX-2 inhibitors with cardiovascular mortality have lead to removal of rofecoxib (Vioxx) from the market. Some suggest that COX-2–specific inhibitors exert prothrombotic effects via inhibition of endothelial cell function and wound healing. Additional research will elucidate the safety issues surrounding the use of COX-2–specific inhibitors; for now, celecoxib is the only selective COX-2 agent available. In addition, the Food and Drug Administration mandated in February 2005 that all NSAIDs must carry warnings (black box warning) that include the possibility of increased adverse cardiovascular events.

Clinical use

In general, NSAIDs are used as antiinflammatory agents, antipyretics, and analgesics, although not all agents possess these three actions to the same extent. Depending on the desired effect, specific NSAIDs are used to treat rheumatoid arthritis, osteoarthritis, musculoskeletal pain or inflammation, postoperative pain, headaches, dental pain, and dysmenorrhea, and to provide symptomatic febrile relief. For pain, the analgesic strength profile is ketorolac > naproxen > ibuprofen > aspirin. Ketorolac, available as both oral tablets and an intramuscular injection, was developed specifically for postoperative analgesia. Even though high doses of NSAIDs may alleviate symptoms of rheumatoid arthritis, these drugs do not reduce progression of joint disease.

Acetaminophen (e.g., Tylenol), through unknown mechanisms, has antipyretic and analgesic actions similar to aspirin.

However, because it is believed to inhibit a COX-3 isoform, its anti-inflammatory actions are negligible. Acetaminophen is particularly useful in patients with aspirin allergies, peptic ulcer disease, bleeding disorders, and those taking anticoagulant therapies.

Indomethacin is used in neonatal settings to encourage closure of a patent ductus arteriosus. The ductus arteriosus remains patent (open) as a result of enhanced prostanoid production. In fact, one reason NSAIDs should be avoided during pregnancy is that they may cause premature closure of the ductus arteriosus, leading to pulmonary hypertension in the fetus.

Adverse effects

Patients with GI ulcers and/or bleeding should avoid NSAIDs because these conditions might be exacerbated. Taking NSAIDs with food lessens the risk of adverse GI effects. Ketorolac is especially problematic for the GI tract; to avoid GI bleeding, this drug should never be used for more than 5 days in a row. Hypersensitivity to NSAIDs is possible, particularly among patients with a history of nasal polyps or asthma. Cross-reactivity between agents is possible. Caution should be exercised when these drugs are used in patients with asthma because the drugs can lead to unopposed accumulation of leukotrienes, thereby predisposing patients to bronchoconstriction (shunting of arachidonic acid to lipoxygenases; see Fig. 10-2).

NSAIDs are highly protein bound and can displace other drugs from plasma protein binding sites (with the exception of acetaminophen, ibuprofen, and indomethacin). This may increase the toxicity of sulfonylureas, sulfonamides, and phenytoin. Plasma levels of methotrexate and lithium may also be elevated with NSAIDs. Furthermore, long-term use of NSAIDs may lead to nephritis, nephritic syndrome, or acute renal failure, (i.e., via reduction of prostaglandin E_2 and prostacyclin I_2, which normally maintain glomerular filtration rate and renal blood flow). Because of the sodium retention induced by NSAIDs, antihypertensive therapies (e.g., angiotensin-converting enzyme inhibitors, β-blockers, and loop diuretics) are often rendered less effective, and sodium retention may also aggravate symptoms of congestive heart failure. Renal complications are not seen with long-term use of sulindac; however, this drug can lead to pancreatitis. Indomethacin has been associated with thrombocytopenia, agranulocytosis, and central nervous system effects. Long-term diclofenac use is associated with hepatotoxicity. Celecoxib causes hypersensitivity reactions in patients with allergies to sulfonamides. Acetaminophen overdoses can cause hepatotoxicity, a situation that is managed by administering intravenous acetylcysteine (see Chapter 3).

Aspirin's unique mechanism (irreversible inhibition of COX) allows it to be a potent inhibitor of platelet aggregation (through reduction of thromboxane), which has led to its successful use in primary and secondary prevention of cardiovascular and cerebrovascular events (Table 10-4). Recall that the actions of other NSAIDs are not irreversible but are competitive in nature. These disparate properties can be problematic for patients who take aspirin for cardiovascular protection

TABLE 10-4. Unique Properties of Aspirin

PROPERTY	DESCRIPTION
Molecular mechanism	Irreversible covalent bond via acetylation of a serine hydroxyl group near the active site of COX enzymes.
Antiplatelet aggregation	Even a low dose (81-mg baby aspirin vs. 325-mg full dose) exerts irreversible inhibition of TXA_2 synthesis; an elevation in prothrombin time is noted at high doses.
Analgesia	Moderate doses inhibit formation of prostaglandins, which in turn blunts peripheral pain receptor responses to pain mediators such as bradykinin and histamine.
Antipyresis	Pyrogens typically release IL-1, leading to increased PGE_2 in the hypothalamus and increasing the body's set point temperature. At moderate doses, aspirin causes sufficient inhibition of PGE_2 and lowers the set point to normal.
Antiinflammatory	At moderate to high doses, strong inhibition of COX-2 is noted. Aspirin also interferes with cell surface selectins and integrins, thereby inhibiting leukocyte adhesion.
Uric acid excretion	At low to moderate doses, a decrease in renal tubular secretion is noted that leads to hyperuricemia; however, at high doses a reduction of tubular reabsorption is noted, which leads to uricosuria.
Acid-base balance	At high therapeutic doses, a mild uncoupling of the oxidative phosphorylation chain leads to respiratory alkalosis and a compensatory metabolic acidosis. At toxic doses, inhibition of the respiratory center leads to respiratory acidosis, and severe uncoupling of the oxidative phosphorylation chain leads to metabolic acidosis, hyperthermia, and hypokalemia.
Gastrointestinal irritation	Inhibition of PGE_2 leads to gastritis, ulcers, and bleeding.
Salicylism	First signs of toxicity are often tinnitus (ringing in ears), vertigo, and decreased hearing.
Hypersensitivity	Seen most often among those with the triad of asthma, nasal polyps, and rhinitis. Generally manifested as bronchoconstriction, due to leukotriene accumulation.
Reye syndrome	Potentially lethal condition in children that results in hepatotoxicity and/or encephalopathy due to use of aspirin during a viral illness; may be due to shunting of arachidonic acid to leukotrienes and lipoxin metabolites.

COX, cyclooxygenase; *IL*, interleukin; *PGE_2*, prostaglandin E_2; *TXA_2*, thromboxane A_2.

while simultaneously taking chronic NSAID therapy for antiinflammatory effects. If the NSAID reaches the COX active site first, it blocks aspirin's ability to bind, thus preventing the antiplatelet actions of aspirin. In fact, patients taking both ibuprofen and aspirin have a 73% increased risk of death from cardiovascular events compared with patients taking aspirin alone. The bottom line is, if patients need both types of therapies, it is best to administer the "antiplatelet" aspirin first and delay other NSAID therapy for several hours.

Steroidal Antiinflammatory Drugs (Glucocorticoids)

Oral Drugs: Budesonide, Dexamethasone, Methylprednisolone, Prednisolone, and Prednisone

Inhaled (Pulmonary, Nasal) Drugs: Budesonide, Ciclesonide, Beclomethasone, Flunisolide, Fluticasone, Mometasone, and Triamcinolone

Topical Drugs: Betamethasone, Hydrocortisone, Mometasone, and Triamcinolone

Mechanism of action

Unlike NSAIDs, which directly inhibit enzymes that generate pro-inflammatory lipid-derived second messengers, steroids are lipophilic, binding to cytosolic steroid receptors, which translocate into cell nuclei to exert their effects on glucocorticoid-responsive genes. Of particular importance in this chapter on inflammation-mediated lipid-derived second messengers, a major effect of glucocorticoids is the enhanced transcription or translation of a peptide called *lipocortin* that inhibits phospholipase A_2. This enzyme is responsible for mobilizing arachidonic acid from phospholipids in cell membranes. As a result of phospholipase A_2 inhibition, both prostanoids and leukotrienes are inhibited. As discussed in Chapter 5, glucocorticoids also induce immunosuppression by reducing the number and activity of immunocompetent cells in the circulation.

Clinical use

Glucocorticoids cause profound inhibition of inflammatory responses and are used to treat rheumatoid arthritis, inflammatory bowel diseases, asthma, and eczema, to name only a few uses. Various glucocorticoids have been formulated that can be delivered via nasal and oral inhalation for more local, nonsystemic, nontoxic control of asthma or allergic rhinitis.

Adverse effects

Prolonged use of systemic glucocorticoids leads to a "cushingoid state," characterized by central obesity, moon face, hyperglycemia (which may lead to clinically significant diabetes mellitus), osteoporosis, and loss of skin structural integrity (seen as thin skin, easy bruising, and purple striae) as well as muscle weakness and wasting. Growth is often suppressed in children requiring systemic steroids. Adrenal suppression is also a major consideration in long-term corticosteroid users, and therefore a slow, tapered withdrawal must be used. Immunosuppression increases susceptibility to pathogenic and opportunistic infections. Thus, a high index of suspicion for infection must be maintained in patients on long-term corticosteroids because normal indicators of infection (such as inflammation) are suppressed. Other adverse effects include oral or nasal thrush (typically with inhaled corticosteroids), perforation of the nasal septum (with nasally administered corticosteroids), mood changes (euphoria or psychosis), peptic ulceration, and eye disorders (cataracts or glaucoma). With the exception of growth suppression and osteoporosis, inhaled glucocorticoids do not manifest systemic adverse effects, and the inhaled steroids do not have to be tapered. However, they cannot be used as substitutes for systemic formulations.

As unique examples, we will look at four specific inflammatory conditions (acne, asthma, gout, and rheumatoid arthritis) for which additional *disease-specific* antiinflammatory agents are also used.

CLINICAL MEDICINE

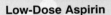

Low-Dose Aspirin

Low-dose aspirin treatment (81 mg) is particularly effective to prevent additional cardiovascular and cerebrovascular accidents in patients who have had myocardial infarctions and strokes. This may be a reflection of the enucleated state of platelets. Platelets do not have nuclei; therefore irreversible inactivation of platelet COX requires synthesis of new platelets (>24 hours) to produce vasoconstrictive and prothrombogenic thromboxanes. This is in contrast to endothelial cells, which can transcriptionally synthesize COX (<8 hours) to primarily generate vasodilatory and antithrombotic prostacyclins.

CLINICAL MEDICINE

Putting It All Together: Anaphylactic Shock

Anaphylactic shock is a life-threatening, type I IgE–mediated systemic reaction in patients who have been previously sensitized to the antigen in question. Typical antigens that can generate anaphylaxis include insect stings, blood products, penicillin, cephalosporins, and food allergens (e.g., eggs, peanuts).

Activated mast cells and basophils release histamine and leukotrienes that induce bronchial constriction, vasodilatation, and vascular permeability. Bronchial constriction induced by leukotrienes lead to airway obstruction, laryngeal edema, bronchospasms and possible asphyxia and hypoxia. Vasodilation and plasma leakage into tissues, mediated by H_1 receptors, leads to hypovolemic shock, hypotension, and angioedema. First-line treatment for anaphylactic shock is intramuscular administration of epinephrine to increase total peripheral resistance (raising blood pressure and reducing edema). In addition, antihistamines and glucocorticoids may be administered.

●●● INFLAMMATORY DISORDERS OF THE SKIN

Corticosteroids, T-Cell Immunomodulators (Eczema), and Retinoids (Acne)

Three common skin disorders, eczema, acne, and psoriasis, also have inflammatory components. In the case of eczema, topical steroids are usually the first line of therapy. Another option is topical T-cell immunomodulators, such as tacrolimus or pimecrolimus. These drugs block T-cell activation and prevent release of inflammatory cytokines. However, these products carry warnings regarding the possible increased risk of cancer associated with their use. These are the same drugs discussed in Chapter 5 as immunosuppressants to prevent organ rejection after transplantation.

Inflammatory acne may be treated with retinoic acid (vitamin A) derivatives, such as oral isotretinoin and topical tretinoin. These drugs reduce sebaceous gland size, reduce sebum production, and regulate cell proliferation and differentiation. Because of teratogenicity, numerous stipulations have been placed on isotretinoin before a prescription for this product can be dispensed. In addition to its teratogenicity, concerns over depression and suicidal ideation, elevated triglycerides, hepatitis, back pain, and visual disturbances have been raised with isotretinoin. The retinoic acid derivatives may cause excessive skin dryness, cheilitis, pruritus, and photosensitivity. Additional drugs used to treat acne are described in Table 10-5.

Psoriasis is commonly treated by topically administered keratolytics (salicylic acid, the active metabolite of aspirin), corticosteroids (halobetasol, clobetasol, betamethasone), vitamin D analogues (calcitriol, calcipotriene), and retinoids (tazarotene) and systemically delivered retinoids (acitretin). Remember that retinoids are vitamin A analogues. Second-line treatments for more virulent psoriatic lesions include coal tar, methotrexate, cyclosporine derivitives, and now new biologic recombinant fusion proteins. As examples, alefacept and efalizumab are dimeric fusion proteins that reduce T-cell activation and leukocyte adhesion, respectively. Alafacept is a fusion protein of human leukocyte function antigen (LFA-3) with IgG1 that binds to CD-2 to prevent LFA/CD activation of T cells. Efalizumab is a monoclonal antibody to CD11a, which as a subunit of LFA prevents LFA binding to intracellular adhesion molecule and leads to reduced leukocyte adhesion, bind to lymphocyte antigen CD2 and CD11a, respectively. These recombinant therapies reduce multiple inflammatory mediators, including interleukins (IL) and tumor necrosis factor (TNF) through down-regulation of circulating immune and inflammatory cells.

●●● ASTHMA

β_2-Selective Agonists, Mast Cell Stabilizers, Corticosteroids, Leukotriene Receptor Antagonists, and Methylxanthines

According to the National Institutes of Health, asthma is primarily a disease of inflammation, with secondary bronchoconstriction. In addition to inhaled (or oral, if necessary)

TABLE 10-5. Pharmacotherapy in Acne

DRUG	MODE OF APPLICATION	MECHANISM COMMENTS	COMMENTS
Benzoyl peroxide	Topical	Releases free radical oxygen to oxidize bacterial proteins in sebaceous follicles, decreasing the number of anaerobic bacteria and decreasing the irritating free fatty acids produced by those bacteria	Bleaches fabrics
Sulfur, resorcinol, and salicylic acid	Topical	Keratolytic and mildly antibacterial	
Antibacterials	Topical, oral	Examples: erythromycin, tetracyclines, clindamycin, metronidazole	
Azelaic acid	Topical	Antimicrobial activities	May cause erythema, burning, pruritus
Adapalene	Topical	Modulates cellular differentiation, keratinization, and inflammatory processes	Retinoid-like compound Less irritating than tretinoin
Tazarotene	Topical	Modulates differentiation and proliferation of epithelial tissue Antiinflammatory activities	Retinoid
Tretinoin	Topical	Causes keratinocytes in follicle to be less adherent, for easier removal Irritating to skin	A "flare" is seen after initial treatment
Isotretinoin	Oral	Decreases sebum production; inhibits *Propionibacterium acnes* Inhibits inflammation Increased differentiation of keratinization	Cheilitis, skin desquamation, muscle stiffness, arthralgias, hypertriglyceridemia, aggressive/violent behavior, teratogenicity

corticosteroids, mast cell stabilizers, such as cromolyn, are antiinflammatory options for patients with mild disease (Box 10-2). With these drugs, mast cells are no longer able to release inflammatory leukotrienes, cytokines, or histamine. Mast cell stabilizers are extremely safe agents; their antiinflammatory effects are less than those of glucocorticoids, but they may be used in conjunction with corticosteroids in an effort to reduce corticosteroid dosages. Cough, dry throat, and headache may be associated with their use. Keep in mind that, although a therapeutic response may be observed in 2 weeks, it will likely take 4 to 6 weeks until maximal benefits are seen. Not all patients respond to mast cell stabilizers, and children are more likely than adults to respond favorably.

Another strategy for asthmatics is to antagonize leukotriene C_4 and leukotriene D_4 receptors (as reviewed in Fig. 10-3). Orally active leukotriene receptor antagonists, such as montelukast and zafirlukast, may be used. In addition, inhibition of 5-lipoxygenase, the rate-limiting step in leukotriene synthesis, with the orally active drug zileuton, can also be used to treat asthma. However, not all patients respond to these classes of drugs, with elderly patients responding least well.

When used to treat asthma, inhaled corticosteroids alter gene transcription such that the number of β_2-receptors expressed in the lungs increases, mucus production decreases, inflammation is inhibited by decreased synthesis of proinflammatory cytokines, vascular permeability decreases, and cellular recruitment also decreases (fewer mast cells, macrophages, lymphocytes, and eosinophils). Corticosteroids are used in asthma to control and reverse inflammation as well as for long-term suppression of inflammation. Although corticosteroids are the most effective antiinflammatory agents used to treat asthma, it may take as long as 8 weeks until maximal effects are observed. Oral corticosteroids may also be used for short-term control of acute exacerbations. Finally, intranasally administered corticosteroids (including ciclesonide, flunisolide, fluticasone propionate) are used to prophylactically manage allergic rhinitis (seasonal allergies), which often exacerbates asthma symptoms.

In addition to chronic airway inflammation, bronchoconstriction occurs in asthma. Thus bronchodilators are first-line treatments for asthmatics. Specifically, β_2-selective agonists, such as albuterol or pirbuterol, are used to treat acute bronchoconstriction. These drugs relax activated bronchial smooth muscle cells by inducing a G_s-mediated increase in cyclic adenosine monophosphate (cAMP). Subsequent activation of protein kinase A results in phosphorylation (and surprisingly inactivation) of myosin light chain kinase, which prevents formation of myosin/actin-mediated smooth muscle contraction (see Chapter 6). Side effects include tremors and tachycardia, but the consequences of severe bronchoconstriction can be life-threatening. In addition to the short-acting

Box 10-2. ADDITIONAL MAST CELL STABILIZERS USED IN TREATMENT OF SEASONAL ALLERGIES AND ASTHMA

Ocular

Lodoxamide
Pemirolast

Nasal

Cromolyn

Pulmonary

Cromolyn

β2-agonists mentioned above that are used for acute situations, longer acting agents such as levalbuterol, formoterol, and salmeterol are used prophylactically. Paradoxically, these long-acting β2 agonists carry warnings that when asthma exacerbations do occur, they can be very severe. This is believed to be due to down regulation and desensitization of β2 receptors when agonists are used long term. Some Food and Drug Administration–approved drugs combine a long-acting bronchodilator with an antiinflammatory corticosteroid in a single formulation. These formulations are approved for management of asthma as well as chronic obstructive pulmonary disease. These combination therapies negate the risks associated with the long-lasting β2-agonists alone with regard to exacerbating asthma symptoms because corticosteroids upregulate β2 receptor expression. However, patients should still be advised that these combinations thepaies could put them at risk for increased asthma-related mortality.

For some asthmatics, methylxanthines such as theophylline may be effective bronchodilators. Theophylline inhibits cAMP phosphodiesterase, indirectly elevating cAMP, analogously to the β2-agonists. Theophylline has a narrow therapeutic index, and serum concentrations must be monitored periodically. Adverse effects include nausea and vomiting, headache, hyperglycemia, hyperkalemia, tachycardia, arrhythmias, tremors, severe neurologic toxicities (which can include seizures), and death. Theophylline is metabolized by hepatic microsomal P450 isoenzymes, and concomitant use with P450 inhibitors increases the risk of theophylline toxicity. Finally, anticholinesterases such as tiotropium or ipratropium may have limited success as bronchodilators in some asthmatic or chronic obstructive pulmonary disease (chronic bronchitis or emphysema) patients. Mechanistically, these drugs antagonize muscarinic receptors, diminishing inositol triphosphate (IP_3)-regulated sarcoplasmic reticulum–released calcium and subsequently reduce calcium/calmodulin-mediated bronchoconstriction (see Chapter 2 or Chapter 6 regarding the phospholipase C/IP_3 signaling cascade).

A final strategy makes use of a new biologic reserved for patients whose symptoms are inadequately controlled with inhaled corticosteroids. Omalizumab is a recombinant humanized monoclonal antibody that selectively blocks IgE receptors and thus reduces histamine release. Malignant neoplasms, injection site reactions, and the possibility of anaphylactic reactions are possible with this drug.

The National Institutes of Health has established guidelines for treating asthma based on symptom severity. Step therapy guidelines are listed in Table 10-6.

PATHOLOGY

Acne

The etiology of acne involves several pathophysiologic changes. (1) Androgen production increases sebaceous gland activity. (2) Sebum (glycerides, wax esters, and cholesterol) is produced in sebaceous glands. (3) These triglycerides and diglycerides are metabolized by *Propionibacterium acnes* to fatty acids, which cause inflammation. (4) Plugging of the follicle and abnormal desquamation of follicular epithelial cells may further exacerbate inflammation.

●●● GOUT

Colchicine, Uricosurics, and Xanthine Oxidase Inhibitors

Gout, which is the most common inflammatory disorder in men older than 40 years, occurs when urate crystals are deposited within joints, often because of underexcretion or overproduction of uric acid. In addition, gout may occur as a secondary complication of myeloproliferative diseases or kidney disorders or as a result of enzymatic defects.

Antiinflammatory NSAIDs such as ibuprofen, ketorolac, and indomethacin are effective in reducing gout joint pain. In addition to NSAIDs to manage joint pain, colchicine is often used. Even though colchicine relieves pain of acute gout attacks, it is not an analgesic. Instead, colchicine decreases motility of leukocytes and other inflammatory cells within joints by interfering with microtubule assembly. Ultimately, this reduces the deposition of urate crystals that perpetuate inflammatory responses. When properly administered, colchicine provides pain relief within 12 hours. However, colchicine treatment is limited by severe GI distress, bone marrow toxicity, and myopathy or peripheral neuritis.

Two strategies to diminish uric acid load are also effective treatments for gout. Uricosuric drugs (probenecid and sulfinpyrazone) are particularly effective for patients who are "underexcretors" of uric acid because these drugs work by inhibiting uric acid transporters in renal proximal tubules that normally reabsorb uric acid. The net result of these drugs is that uric acid excretion is enhanced. These drugs are best used prophylactically and should not be used during acute attacks because kidney stones may form. Temporary urinary alkalization and good hydration for the first few days of therapy minimize the risk of kidney stones. Recall that salicylates inhibit the uricosuric effects of these drugs.

The second pharmacologic strategy to diminish uric acid load is to inhibit uric acid synthesis. Xanthine oxidase (Fig. 10-4) is the enzyme that converts soluble xanthine and hypoxanthine into insoluble uric acid. Allopurinol and febuxostat are xanthine oxidase inhibitors that are particularly useful in patients who are "overproducers" of uric acid. These drugs are also administered prophylactically to cancer patients who are receiving cytotoxic purine mimetics. Allopurinol is associated with an unusually high incidence of nonallergic skin rash when administered concomitantly with ampicillin. In addition, xanthine oxidase inhibitors are contraindicated in patients taking drugs that are xanthine oxidase substrates, including azathioprine, mercaptopurine, or theophylline.

In management of pediatric patients with nonsolid or solid tumors, antineoplastic chemotherapy may be associated with tumor lysis syndrome, which results in toxic levels of plasma uric acid. In these cases, therapies to reduce existing uric acid stores may be preferred to reducing uric acid synthesis. Rasburicase is a recombinant uric acid oxidase enzyme that catalyzes oxidation and subsequent degradation of endogenous uric acid stores. Significant adverse effects of this intravenously administered biologic include vomiting, fever, and methemoglobinemia (increased levels of methemoglobin in blood).

TABLE 10-6. Stepwise Approach to Managing Asthma in Adults and Children Older Than 5 Years

CLASSIFY SEVERITY: CLINICAL FEATURES BEFORE TREATMENT OR ADEQUATE CONTROL			MEDICATIONS REQUIRED TO MAINTAIN LONG-TERM CONTROL	
Step	**Day Symptoms/Night Symptoms**	**PEF or FEV$_1$/PEF Variability**	**Daily Medication**	
Severe persistent (step 4)	Continual/frequent	$\leq$60%/>30%	*Preferred treatment:* High-dose inhaled corticosteroids *plus* Long-acting inhaled β$_2$-agonists *plus* corticosteroid tablets or syrup (if needed) long term (make repeated attempts to reduce systemic corticosteroids and maintain control with high-dose inhaled corticosteroids)	
Moderate persistent (step 3)	Daily/>1 night/wk	>60% to <80%/>30%	*Preferred treatment:* Low- to medium-dose inhaled corticosteroids and long-acting inhaled β$_2$-agonists *Alternative treatment:* Increase inhaled corticosteroids within medium-dose range *or* Low- to medium-dose inhaled corticosteroids and either leukotriene modifier or theophylline	
Mild persistent (step 2)	>2/wk but <1/day/>2 nights/mo	$\geq$80%/20% to 30%	*Preferred treatment:* Low-dose inhaled corticosteroids *Alternative treatment:* Cromolyn, leukotriene modifier *or* Sustained-release theophylline to serum concentration of 5–15 μg/mL	
Mild intermittent (step 1)	$\leq$ 2 days/wk/$\leq$2 nights/mo	$\geq$80%/<20%	No daily medication needed Severe exacerbations may occur, separated by long periods of normal lung function and symptoms	

FEV, forced expiratory volume in 1 second; *PEF*, peak expiratory flow.
From Busse W, et al: National Asthma Education & Prevention Program: Expert Panel Report: Guidelines for the Diagnosis and Management of Asthma—Update Selected Topics 2002, p 116. National Heart, Lung, & Blood Institute, U.S. Department of Health & Human Services, Bethesda, MD, NIH Pub. 02-5074, June 2003.

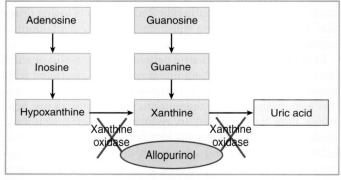

Figure 10-4. Mechanism of action for allopurinol, which leads to reduction in uric acid load.

●●● RHEUMATOID ARTHRITIS

NSAIDs and Disease-Modifying Antirheumatic Drugs

Rheumatoid arthritis is a chronic inflammation of the synovium of peripheral joints. It is primarily a disease mediated by proinflammatory cytokines. Activated CD4+ T cells invade and infiltrate the joint. These cells release IL-2, IL-6, and interferon-γ, which chemoattract B cells and macrophages. Activated B cells (plasma cells) release rheumatoid factor, which initiates cartilage and bone damage. Activated macrophages within the synovium release IL-1 and TNF-α, which further degrade the joint by causing synovial

TABLE 10-7. Disease-Modifying Antirheumatic Drugs (DMARDs)

DRUG	MECHANISM	ADVERSE EFFECTS
Infliximab	Monoclonal antibody that neutralizes TNF-α, thus suppressing TNF-induced proliferation of immune cells and macrophages	Hypersensitivity reaction Serious infection Heart failure Increased risk of cancer
Certolizumab pegol	A PEGylated Fab′ fragment of a humanized TNF inhibitor monoclonal antibody	Infection, malignancies
Golimumab	Monoclonal antibody to TNF-α, golimumab in combination with methotrexate is more effective than methotrexate alone	Infection, malignancies
Adalimumab	Monoclonal antibody for TNF-α	Serious infections Increased risk of cancer Lupus-like syndrome
Etanercept	Recombinant form of TNF receptor that binds circulating TNF	Hypersensitivity reaction Serious infections Increased risk of cancer
Anakinra	IL-1 receptor antagonist	Infection Headache Gastrointestinal distress
Tocilizumab	Monoclonal antibody for IL-6 receptor	Respiratory tract infection Nasopharyngitis Increased liver enzymes and BP Increased tumor risk
Abatacept	Inhibits T-cell activation and subsequent production of multiple inflammatory cytokines including interferon-γ, IL-2, and TNF	Malignancies Infections
Gold salts (e.g., auranofin)	Reduce migration of macrophage phagocytosis and cause stabilization of lysosomes	Rash Leukocytopenia Proteinuria Pruritus Persistent diarrhea
D-Penicillamine	Hypothesized to inhibit T helper cell function Decreases circulating IgM rheumatoid factor	Gastrointestinal distress, intolerance Autoantibodies Vasculitis Neurologic symptoms
Hydroxychloroquine	Inhibits locomotion of neutrophils and chemotaxis of eosinophils	Dermatitis Cardiomyopathy Hematologic abnormalities Visual disturbances
Sulfasalazine	Unknown	Allergic myocarditis Hemolytic anemia Exfoliative dermatitis
Methotrexate	Interferes with folic acid synthesis and inhibits proliferating inflammatory cells	Gastrointestinal distress Hepatotoxicity Bone marrow depression
Azathioprine	Inhibits purine synthesis	Bone marrow depression
Leflunomide	Inhibits pyrimidine synthesis	Diarrhea Hypertension Respiratory tract infection Alopecia Gastrointestinal upset
Cyclosporine	Inhibits IL-2 production and inhibits T-cell activation	Hypertension Hirsutism Renal dysfunction

BP, blood pressure; *Ig*, immunoglobulin; *IL*, interleukin; *PEG*, polyethylene glycol; *TNF*, tumor necrosis factor.

endothelial cells and fibroblasts to proliferate, neovascularize, and remodel the joint. These cytokines also activate osteoclasts to proteolyze bone surrounding the joint. Thus it is no surprise that NSAIDs, which inhibit COX-induced proinflammatory prostanoids and thromboxanes, are effective treatments for rheumatoid arthritis. Similarly, orally active glucocorticoids can be used to diminish chronic inflammation in patients with rheumatoid arthritis.

Disease-modifying antirheumatic drugs (DMARDs) are also used (Table 10-7). DMARDs are the only drugs capable of halting the underlying disease processes. Recent additions to DMARDs include monoclonal antibodies or receptor antagonists for circulating pro-inflammatory cytokines. A few of the most effective biologic DMARDs are listed below.

- Infliximab, adalimumab, certolizumab pegol, and golimumab neutralize antibodies that target TNF-α. These humanized monoclonal antibodies prevent binding of TNF-α to its receptor. Infliximab is admistered intravenously, in contrast to the other antibodies, which are administered subcutaneously.
- Etanercept, a recombinant form of the TNF receptor that binds to circulating TNF, prevents interaction with endogenous receptors. (It is of interest that both approaches, TNF-directed antibodies and recombinant TNF receptors, share a common effect [reduction of circulating TNF] through distinct mechanisms.)
- Adalimumab, a monoclonal antibody that targets TNF-α.
- Anakinra, an IL-1 receptor antagonist, is a recombinant, nonglycosylated version of a human IL-1 receptor antagonist bioengineered from cultures of genetically modified *Escherichia coli* using recombinant DNA technology.
- Tocilizumab, a recombinant monoclonal antibody targeting IL-6, is administered once per month intravenously for patients who do not respond to anti-TNF therapies.
- Abatacept is a soluble recombinant fusion protein of the extracellular domain of the human cytokine T lymphocyte–associated antigen 4 linked to IgG1. Abatacept is a costimulation modulator that inhibits T-cell activation by binding to cell surface markers (CD80 and CD86) on leukocytes. Without this costimulation, full T-cell activation is prevented and subsequent production of multiple inflammatory cytokines, including interferon-γ, IL-2, and TNF is significantly diminished.

There is, however, a warning that all TNF inhibitors can cause serious infections and sepsis, especially when combined with IL-1 antagonists. These drugs may also increase the risk of cancer. Finally, some of these TNF/IL-1 blockers/inhibitors are also indicated for Crohn disease, ankylosing spondylitis, or psoriatric arthritis.

CLINICAL MEDICINE

Orphan Diseases and Biologics

Biologics are now being developed for chronic inflammatory orphan diseases such as cryopyrin-associated periodic syndrome. These rare inherited chronic inflammatory disease syndromes are often induced by cold temperatures and are the result of mutations in a gene that encodes cryopyrin, which produces IL-1β. New therapies for this disease include anakinra, the recombinant IL-1 receptor antagonist as well as rilonacept, a dimeric fusion protein of the ligand binding domain of human IL-1 receptor in sequence with an IL-1 receptor accessory protein coupled to IgG1. Both recombinant therapeutic approaches reduce cryoporin-dependent, IL-1–induced chronic inflammation.

●●● TOP FIVE LIST

1. Inflammation is a physiologic process that fights disease and promotes wound healing responses. Unchecked inflammation is a pathologic crisis that is often an underlying cause of atherosclerosis, inflammatory bowel disease, asthma, and rheumatoid arthritis.
2. Inflammatory mediators are often lipid second messengers. Oxygenated derivatives of arachidonic acid include prostaglandins, thromboxanes, and leukotrienes. NSAIDs inhibit COX activity, the enzyme that forms prostaglandins and thromboxanes. Inhibitors of leukotriene synthesis (Zileuton) and antagonists of leukotriene receptors (Montelukast, Zafirlukast) can be effective in asthmatics.
3. H_1 (histamine)-receptor blockers are effective for allergies and can be obtained over the counter or in prescription strengths.
4. Inflammatory acne is often treated with retinoic acid derivatives.
5. Monoclonal antibodies that target the cytokine TNF-α are effective for patients with rheumatoid arthritis.

Self-assessment questions can be accessed at www. StudentConsult.com.

Gastrointestinal Pharmacology

11

CONTENTS

GASTROESOPHAGEAL REFLUX DISEASE
   Antacids
   Alginic Acid
   H_2 Blockers
   Proton Pump Inhibitors
   Prokinetic Drugs
PEPTIC ULCER DISEASE
INFLAMMATORY BOWEL DISEASE
NAUSEA AND VOMITING
DIARRHEA
CONSTIPATION
IRRITABLE BOWEL SYNDROME
COMPLEMENTARY AND ALTERNATIVE MEDICINE
TOP FIVE LIST

This chapter is all about the pump: the H^+/K^+ pump that regulates stomach acidity (Fig. 11-1). Drugs that inhibit the pump are effective agents for both gastroesophageal reflux disease (GERD) and peptic ulcer disease. These agents can either directly inhibit the pump or inhibit the second messengers (cyclic adenosine monophosphate [cAMP] and calcium) that activate the pump.

●●● GASTROESOPHAGEAL REFLUX DISEASE

GERD, or "heartburn," affects nearly 60 million Americans on an intermittent basis, with 25 million people having daily symptoms. The typical cause of GERD is decreased lower esophageal sphincter tone, resulting in acid reflux. Substances including chocolate, caffeine, cholesterol, alcohol, and nicotine can all decrease esophageal sphincter pressure and exacerbate GERD. Drugs can also be culprits. Pharmacologic agents known to aggravate GERD are listed in Box 11-1.

Pharmacologic treatments for GERD include reducing stomach acidity by antacids, H_2 blockers, or proton pump inhibitors (PPIs) as well as prokinetic drugs that increase lower esophageal sphincter smooth muscle tone. Mild and transient GERD can be treated with over-the-counter medications, whereas chronic, recalcitrant cases require prescription-strength medications.

Antacids

Antacids, including aluminum hydroxide, magnesium hydroxide, and calcium carbonate, can be quite effective against occasional GERD. Antacids increase gastrointestinal (GI) pH. However, as with any over-the-counter medication, adverse effects (Table 11-1) and drug interactions may occur (e.g., aluminum, magnesium, and calcium may form insoluble complexes with tetracyclines or fluoroquinolones, reducing bioavailability of the antibiotics). Because GI pH is elevated by antacids, absorption of numerous other drugs may be limited. It is recommended that antacid administration be separated from other drugs by at least 2 hours.

Alginic Acid

Alginic acid reduces the adverse effects of reflux by forming a viscous foam on the top of the gastric contents—a mechanical barrier—that protects the esophagus.

Unfortunately, the effects of antacids and alginic acid are short lived, so the drugs have to be administered four times daily (usually with meals and at bedtime).

ANATOMY

Regulation of Stomach Acid Release

Neural release of acetylcholine and gastrin stimulates release of acid from the parietal cells of the gastric mucosa by activating the H^+/K^+-adenosine triphosphatase (ATPase) pump via a Ca^{++}-dependent protein kinase. In addition, acetylcholine and gastrin induce histamine release from enterochromaffin-like cells, which then stimulate the H^+/K^+-ATPase pump (through paracrine stimulation of H_2 receptors on parietal cells). In contrast to acetylcholine and gastrin, H_2 receptors stimulate the H^+/K^+-ATPase pump via activation of adenylate cyclase to form cAMP and stimulate protein kinase A. Protein kinase A induces fusion of tubulovesicles within the canicular membrane of the parietal cell to release protons into the gastric lumen. Inhibition of muscarinic, gastrin, or histamine receptors leads to inhibition of acid secretion by the pump. In addition, activated prostaglandin E_2 receptors on parietal cells reduce pump activity via G_i inhibition of adenylate cyclase.

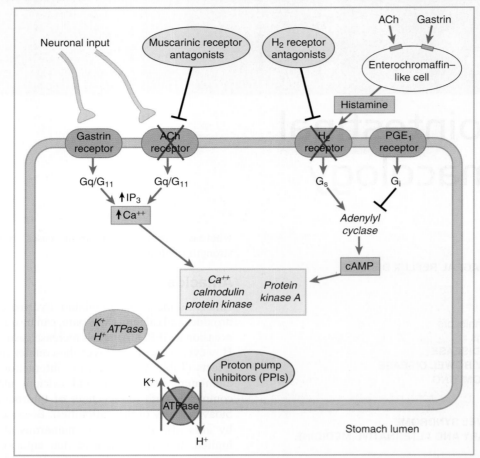

Figure 11-1. Sites of action of drugs that inhibit H^+/K^+ pump activity. This pump is responsible for transporting hydrogen ions (acid) into the stomach lumen. *ACh*, acetylcholine; *PGE2*, prostaglandin E_1; *cAMP*, cyclic adenosine monophosphate; *ATP*, adenosine triphosphate.

Box 11-1. DRUGS THAT DECREASE LOWER ESOPHAGEAL SPHINCTER TONE AND CONTRIBUTE TO GASTROESOPHAGEAL REFLUX DISEASE

Anticholinergics	Nitrates
Benzodiazepines	Opioids
Ca^{++} channel blockers	Progesterone
Dopaminergic agents	Theophylline
Estrogens	

TABLE 11-1. Adverse Effects Associated with Antacids

DRUG	EFFECT
Aluminum hydroxide	Constipation Binds to phosphate in gastrointestinal tract; may lead to bone damage
Magnesium hydroxide	Diarrhea
Calcium carbonate	Stimulates gastrin; acid rebound Hypercalcemia, milk alkali syndrome (hypercalcemia, alkalosis, kidney stones)

H_2 Blockers

Cimetidine, Famotidine, Nizatidine, and Ranitidine

Note that H_2 blockers all end in "-tidine" and are not the H_1 receptor antagonists that alleviate allergic symptoms (see Chapter 10).

Mechanism of action

Histamine H_2 receptor antagonists are now available both over the counter and with a prescription. These drugs antagonize parietal cell H_2 receptors, diminishing cAMP and resultant H^+/K^+ pump activity. H_2 receptor antagonists block basal levels of gastric acid secretion *and may partially block* meal-stimulated secretion (which is gastrin mediated). Over-the-counter doses are effective for intermittent heartburn if there is no evidence of esophagitis. Pharmacokinetic differences among common H_2 receptor antagonists are listed in Table 11-2.

Adverse effects

H_2 receptor antagonists are usually well tolerated. Adverse effects on the central nervous system are more common in the elderly (anxiety, confusion, dizziness, headache). Cimetidine may cause some adverse endocrine effects,

TABLE 11-2. Typical H₂ Receptor Antagonists

DRUG	COMMENT
Cimetidine	Significant P450 inhibitor Can lead to toxic drug interactions as a result of inhibition of benzodiazepines, warfarin, and phenytoin
Famotidine	Does not interfere with P450
Nizatidine	Does not interfere with P450
Ranitidine	Weaker P450 inhibition than cimetidine

TABLE 11-3. Typical Proton Pump Inhibitors

DRUG	COMMENT
Omeprazole	Available over the counter as well as in prescription strengths for healing esophageal lesions
Lansoprazole	High bioavailability
Rabeprazole	Does not interfere with P450
Pantoprazole	Also available as an intravenous formulation
Esomeprazole	S isomer (and active form) of omeprazole
Dexlansoprazole	Dual release formulation

particularly in men (decreased libido, impotence, gynecomastia). Cimetidine may also possess immunomodulatory activities such that it is sometimes administered (off label) to eliminate warts that have been refractory to other treatments. Because of the superior acid inhibition and safety profile of PPIs (see the following section), the use of prescription H₂ antagonists has markedly declined.

Proton Pump Inhibitors

Dexlansoprazole, Esomeprazole, Lansoprazole, Omeprazole, Pantoprazole, and Rabeprazole

Note that these drug names all end in "-prazole."

Mechanism of action

In cases of chronic GERD with evidence of esophagitis, PPIs, which directly inhibit the gastric mucosal cell H^+/K^+ pump, may be prescribed. After absorption, these drugs bind irreversibly and covalently, via sulfhydryl groups, to the H^+/K^+ pump to inhibit both basal- and meal-stimulated gastric acid production. As a result, the pH in the stomach is elevated and remains above pH 4, even postprandially (after meals).

Adverse effects

Overall, these drugs are well tolerated; GI disturbances are the most commonly reported adverse effects. Keep in mind, however, that hypochlorhydria (inadequate production of HCl by parietal cells) causes gastrin to be released and that resultant hypergastrinemia causes gastric tumors in rodents via a trophic effect on enterochromaffin-like cells. Long-term use of PPIs in humans has been associated with atrophic gastritis, which also may predispose patients to gastric tumors. Patients carrying *Helicobacter pylori* appear to be at greatest risk. Because acid is needed to absorb many vitamins and minerals, long-term use of PPIs leads to deficiencies and complications associated with low absorption of calcium, iron, magnesium, and vitamin B_{12}.

All currently used PPIs are pro-drugs and are converted to the active drug in the parietal cell canaliculus (tubular "canals" in which HCl is secreted). PPIs are listed in Table 11-3.

Prokinetic Drugs

Metoclopramide and Bethanechol

Mechanism of action

In addition to PPIs, severe GERD can be treated with prokinetic agents that increase lower esophageal sphincter tone, including dopamine antagonists (e.g., metoclopramide) or muscarinic cholinergic receptor agonists (e.g., bethanechol). Metoclopramide has antidopaminergic and cholinomimetic effects. The drug acts as a dopamine receptor antagonist, with highest affinity for D_1, D_4, and D_5 receptors. As a result of its actions, metoclopramide inhibits smooth muscle relaxation normally produced by dopamine, which in turn enhances cholinergic responses in the myenteric plexus of the enteric nervous system. In addition, metoclopramide increases lower esophageal sphincter tone and the force of peristaltic contractions. All together, gastric emptying is accelerated, which provides some symptomatic improvements.

Adverse effects

Unfortunately, metoclopramide is associated with a high incidence of adverse effects, many stemming from the drug's anti-dopaminergic actions (extrapyramidal movements, gynecomastia, menstrual irregularities, galactorrhea). Its use is not recommended for more than 12 weeks because of the risk of tardive dyskinesia.

CLINICAL MEDICINE

Patients May Self-Medicate

Physicians should be aware that overuse of H₂ antagonists or PPIs can mask underlying disease, including Barrett esophagus (a premalignancy leading to esophageal adenocarcinoma), peptic ulcer disease, or Zollinger-Ellison syndrome (an oversecretion of acid and pepsin). Furthermore, acid suppression by H₂ antagonists or PPIs can lead to overgrowth of *Candida* or bacteria (including *Clostridium difficile*) within the GI tract. H₂ antagonists are also recognized as independent risk factors for pneumonia.

PEPTIC ULCER DISEASE

Peptic ulcers of the duodenum and the stomach are the result of multiple inflammatory stresses that damage the GI mucosa, including *Helicobacter pylori* infection, nonsteroidal antiinflammatory drugs (NSAIDs, which diminish prostaglandin E_2 synthesis), and long-term use of glucocorticoids.

For patients with a history of peptic ulcer disease who take NSAIDs, several alternative treatment options are available:
- Synthetic prostaglandin E_1 analogs (misoprostol) with NSAIDs
- PPIs with NSAIDs
- Celecoxib, the cyclooxygenase-2 selective inhibitor

Celecoxib should be used preferentially to NSAIDs. Celecoxib may preferentially exert fewer effects on cyclooxygenase-1–dependent antiinflammatory prostaglandins in the GI tract.

Misoprostol enhances mucosal defenses by stimulating mucus and bicarbonate production. In addition, misoprostol increases local blood flow by promoting vasodilation. Misoprostol is classified as pregnancy category X (absolutely contraindicated) because it induces uterine contractions and can cause miscarriage.

The primary therapeutic approaches to ulcer healing involve concomitant use of PPIs and H_2 receptor blockers to alleviate symptoms plus two or more antimicrobials to eradicate *H. pylori*. The antiinfectives most often used in these multidrug regiments include the following:
- Tetracycline
- Amoxicillin
- Clarithromycin
- Metronidazole

Bismuth subsalicylate (e.g., Pepto-Bismol) is also frequently added. Bismuth subsalicylate protects the gastric tract by stimulating endogenous production of prostaglandins. In addition, bismuth subsalicylate has antimicrobial actions against some strains of enteric bacteria. Adverse effects from bismuth subsalicylate include dark-colored stools and tongue. Bismuth may interfere with absorption of tetracyclines. Because of the salicylate component of bismuth subsalicylate, tinnitus (ear ringing) may occur. Patients with a history of asthma or sensitivity to salicylates should avoid using products containing this active ingredient. Bismuth subsalicylate may increase bleeding in patients taking anticoagulants. Use of bismuth subsalicylate is contraindicated in children because of the risk of Reye syndrome. Recently, a combined formulation of bismuth subcitrate potassium (a bismuth salt of citric acid), metronidazole, tetracycline, and omeprazole has been approved to treat duodenal ulcer disease.

Another option for managing peptic ulcer disease is sucralfate (ammonium salt of sulfated disaccharides), which forms a protective barrier at the ulcer lesion. Fortunately, the drug is not absorbed systemically, so adverse effects other than GI disturbances are uncommon. However, the drug must be administered four times per day—1 hour before meals and at bedtime. Numerous drug interactions are likely because sucralfate binds nonspecifically to positively charged molecules, so administration should be separated from all other drugs by giving other agents at least 2 hours before sucralfate.

MICROBIOLOGY

Peptic Ulcer Disease

Even though individuals can be tested for *H. pylori*, a positive test may not correlate with peptic ulcer disease.

These tests include:
- Release of $^{14}CO_2$ in breath from ^{14}C urea
- Immunoglobulin G antibodies to *H. pylori*
- Endoscopy followed by culture

INFLAMMATORY BOWEL DISEASE

Ulcerative colitis (limited to the colon and rectum) and Crohn disease (may occur anywhere from mouth to rectum) are inflammatory bowel diseases (IBDs) that can be treated but not cured at present. One line of treatment focuses on controlling inflammation; another line of treatment involves immunosuppression. Some pharmacologic agents may induce remission, whereas others may also help maintain remission. Patients with severe gastric disease may have altered absorption of drugs, and doses may require adjustment. First-line treatment options for ulcerative colitis are described in Table 11-4. Note that these drugs are based on mesalamine.

Initial therapeutic options for ulcerative colitis include sulfasalazine or mesalamine (5-aminosalicylic acid). Sulfasalazine is hydrolyzed by GI flora to both sulfapyridine (a sulfa antibiotic) and mesalamine. Therapeutic effects may be related to antibacterial properties of sulfapyridine and antiinflammatory properties of mesalamine. Mesalamine inhibits cyclooxygenase and prostaglandin production and can be obtained in several formulations that deliver it to different regions of the small or large bowel.

Corticosteroids may be used when sulfasalazine or mesalamine derivatives are ineffective. Although sulfasalazine and corticosteroids are equally effective, antiinflammatory effects occur more rapidly with corticosteroids. Corticosteroids may

TABLE 11-4. Drugs Used to Manage Ulcerative Colitis

DRUG	COMMENT
Sulfasalazine	Adverse effects are numerous and are related to those normally found with sulfonamides.
Mesalamine	Has fewer side effects than sulfasalazine because there is no sulfa moiety. This drug is most efficacious in proximal regions of the gastrointestinal tract.
Olsalazine	Two molecules of mesalamine are linked by a disulfide bond, which is cleaved by intestinal bacteria. Associated with severe diarrhea.
Balsalazide	Bacteria hydrolyze release of mesalamine in distal portions of the gastrointestinal tract.

be administered intravenously, orally, or rectally to induce remission. Budesonide, approved for treating exacerbations of Crohn disease, is extensively metabolized by first-pass metabolism in the liver, thereby limiting the adverse side effects generally associated with corticosteroid use. The pharmacology of corticosteroids is discussed in Chapter 10. Immunosuppressants, such as azathioprine, cyclosporine, and 6-mercaptopurine, are used when corticosteroids fail to induce remission of IBD. The pharmacology of these drugs is discussed in Chapters 5 and 10.

As a last resort, infliximab, a monoclonal antibody that targets tumor necrosis factor (TNF)-α may be used to manage severe Crohn disease. This drug is administered parentally to suppress inflammation mediated by TNF. Infliximab use is limited by the occurrence of serious infections and malignancies, including tuberculosis and lymphoma. Patients should avoid vaccinations with live virus vaccines while receiving this therapy. Owing to the biologic origin of this drug, hypersensitivities may occur. This medication may cause dizziness; caution is warranted while driving or performing activities that require alertness, coordination, or physical dexterity. Additional adverse effects include heart failure and lupuslike syndromes. Infliximab is usually given in combination with other immunosuppressants to reduce the likelihood that neutralizing antibodies will form to the anti-TNF monoclonal antibody. For patients intolerant to infliximab, new Food and Drug Administration–approved biologics have been added to the treatment options for patients with Crohn disease. These biologics include subcutaneously administered monoclonal antibodies to human TNF (adalimumab and certolizumab pegol). In addition, a last resort treatment, natalizumab, which is used in the treatment of multiple sclerosis, can also be used for the treatment of Crohn disease. Natalizumab is an antibody inhibitor of α₄ integrin, which mediates adhesion and activation of leukocytes. Natalizumab is a last resort treatment because it has been associated with progressive multifocal leukoencephalopathy, a viral infection of the brain. The Food and Drug Administration had withdrawn this biologic from the marketplace after it was linked to progressive multifocal leukoencephalopathy, but it has recently returned to the market under a special restricted-access program.

●●● NAUSEA AND VOMITING

Nausea and vomiting, which can be triggered by GI, infectious, neurologic, metabolic, or psychogenic diseases, can be treated with a multitude of drug classes (Table 11-5). They include mixed-function antimuscarinics/antihistamines, antidopaminergics, serotonin receptor (5HT3) antagonists, substance P/neurokinin receptor antagonists and cannabinoids (drabinol). Drabinol contains Δ^9tetrahydrocannabinol, the active ingredient in marijuana. Some states in the United States have recently legalized the use of medical marijuana to treat nausea/vomiting complications of antineoplastic chemotherapeutics. It is easier to prevent nausea than to stop vomiting. Patients receiving chemotherapeutic agents require efficient treatment of nausea and vomiting. Often, severe emesis (vomiting) associated with chemotherapy requires use of drug combinations. Specific combination therapies include

- Metoclopramide + diphenhydramine + dexamethasone
- Prochlorperazine + lorazepam
- 5HT3 antagonists + dexamethasone + lorazepam

●●● DIARRHEA

The first line of defense in managing diarrhea is rehydration. Diarrhea is a complication of either increased intestinal secretions or decreased intestinal absorption of carbohydrates and resultant water. Increased chloride and water secretions frequently occur from bacterial or parasitic toxin-induced opening of cAMP-induced chloride channels. In fact, cholera toxin adenosine diphosphate ribosylates the α-subunit of G_s, which inhibits the guanosine triphosphatase function of the stimulatory G-protein, thus constitutively activating G_s to generate cAMP and open chloride channels.

Severe bacterial diarrhea induced by *Shigella, Salmonella, Campylobacter, Cholera,* or *Staphylococcus* can be treated with antibiotics, including tetracycline, ampicillin, and erythromycin. Noninvasive strains of *Escherichia coli* can be treated with rifaximin, a GI-selective oral antibiotic. However, most diarrhea is self-limiting and often viral in nature (rotavirus is a frequent cause of acute gastroenteritis in children) and may well be a mechanism by which the body rids itself of harmful bacterial or viral toxins. Additional therapies used to manage diarrhea are listed in Table 11-6 and include opiate derivatives and anticholinergic agents.

MICROBIOLOGY

Traveler's Diarrhea

It is conservatively estimated that one in five travelers worldwide will experience an acute episode of diarrhea. Pathogens responsible for traveler's diarrhea are often noninvasive *Escherichia coli, Shigella, Campylobacter jejuni*, protozoa, or viruses. Treatment is focused on rehydration and not reduction of loose stool.

●●● CONSTIPATION

Constipation is not a disease; rather, it represents another underlying pathologic condition. It may be associated with metabolic or endocrine disorders (diabetic neuropathies, hypothyroidism); pregnancy (decreased gut motility); and neurogenic, psychogenic, or drug-induced events. Drugs used to speed GI motility are listed in Table 11-7. Remember that obstructions (impaction) should be removed before laxatives are used and that long-term use of laxatives may result in electrolyte imbalances and reduced peristaltic motility.

●●● IRRITABLE BOWEL SYNDROME

Another potentially debilitating GI condition, irritable bowel syndrome (IBS), may be associated with either constipation or diarrhea. In fact, symptoms often fluctuate between the two extremes. Note that IBS and IBD (Crohn and ulcerative colitis) are different conditions. The etiology of IBS is still undefined, and

TABLE 11-5. Drugs Used to Treat Nausea and Vomiting

DRUG	COMMENT
Antimuscarinics/Antihistamines (Mixed Function)	
Scopolamine	Patch applied behind ear for motion sickness Predominantly blocks muscarinic cholinergic receptors in dorsal vagal complex
Dimenhydrinate	Drug of choice for children Metabolized to diphenhydramine (an antihistamine) moiety
Meclizine	Antihistaminic and anticholinergic actions
Diphenhydramine	Central blockade of H_1 receptors
Hydroxyzine	Antihistamine
Doxylamine	Antihistamine; often used to manage nausea and vomiting in pregnant women
Antidopaminergics	
Prochlorperazine	Phenothiazine that blocks dopamine receptors in chemoreceptor trigger zone Can cause sedation, liver dysfunction, and dystonias, especially in children with viral illnesses
Metoclopramide	Dopaminergic antagonist action raises the threshold of activity in the chemoreceptor trigger zone
Serotonin Receptor (5HT3) Antagonists	
Ondansetron, granisetron, dolasetron, alosetron*	Block afferent vagal fibers in upper gastrointestinal tract as well as central vomiting center to prevent emesis Generally well tolerated, do not induce sedation; minimal autonomic side effects Often used postoperatively or for chemotherapy-induced nausea Safe for children
Palonosetron*	Only drug in this class that is approved for delayed nausea and vomiting associated with chemotherapy because of its long $t_{1/2}$ Use with caution in those at risk for QT prolongation
Phosphated carbohydrate solutions	Used for mild symptoms May elevate blood sugar (like drinking a cola)
Cannabinoids	Used for chemotherapy-induced nausea when all other regimens have failed Act on receptors in the vomiting center of brain May cause numerous central nervous system adverse effects (mood changes, anxiety, memory loss, fear, confusion, motor incoordination, hallucinations, euphoria, sedation, paranoia) Can cause hypotension and tachycardia Tolerance may develop to side effects but not to antiemetic effects

Dronabinol	Δ^9 tetrahydrocannabinol the active ingredient in marijuana
	    Binds to cannabinoid receptors
	The endogenous cannabinoid receptor agonist in humans is arachidonylethanolamide, a
	    derivative of the same arachidonic acid that is metabolized into prostaglandins and leukotrienes

Nabilone	Fewer euphoric effects than dronabinol
Substance P/Neurokinin-1 Receptor Antagonists	
Aprepitant	May be combined with 5HT3 antagonists and dexamethasone for treatment of severe chemotherapy-induced nausea and vomiting While effective, inhibits CYP3A4 and induces CYP2C9, causing drug interactions
Corticosteroids	Inhibit production of prostaglandins, which can be highly emetogenic Effective, but adverse effects limit utility

*Note that drug names end in "-setron."

patients often experience symptoms of depression and anxiety (treated with selective serotonin receptor inhibitors or tricyclic agents). Antispasmodic muscarinic receptor antagonists (dicyclomine or hyoscyamine) are often used to manage abdominal cramping.

For constipation, patients can be treated with multiple regimens, including increased dietary fiber, exercise, increased fluid intake, and stool softeners. For constipation-predominant IBS in women, an aggressive treatment involves tegaserod, a 5HT4 receptor partial agonist, which speeds GI mobility. However, the use of tegaserod was recently discontinued because of increased incidence of cardiovascular events (myocardial infarction, stroke, unstable angina). Patients with constipation-predominant IBS may now be treated with lubiprostone, a

TABLE 11-6. Pharmacologic Therapies Used in Management of Diarrhea

AGENT	COMMENT
Rehydrating solutions	Provide rehydration and electrolyte replacement to reduce mortality World Health Organization suggests rehydration is critical for preventing complications associated with diarrhea
Opiate derivatives	Do not use opiates if bacterial enteritis is suspected
Loperamide	Acts only on peripheral opioid receptors May also have antisecretory properties
Diphenoxylate	Combined with atropine (to discourage opioid abuse) in a product called Lomotil
Paregoric	Rarely used owing to abuse potential
Anticholinergics	
Atropine	Blocks vagal tone and prolongs gut transit time Used with diphenoxylate
Bismuth subsalicylate	Possesses antisecretory, antibacterial, and anti-inflammatory properties
Somatostatin Analogs	
Octreotide	A somatostatin analog that blocks release of serotonin and other vasoactive peptides Used in symptomatic treatment of carcinoid tumors that secrete histamine, bradykinin, serotonin Can cause gallbladder and biliary tract complications Administered via injection
Adsorbents	Examples include kaolin, pectin, attapulgite, polycarbophil, and bile acid resins
Lactase enzymes	Used for osmotic diarrhea resulting from lactose intolerance
Proton pump inhibitors or H$_2$ blockers	May be used to manage chronic diarrhea that occurs after meals, which may be caused by increased acid secretion after eating Prescription doses should be tried and, if effective, relief will be noticed in 3 days

prostaglandin E$_1$ derivative, which selectively activates pH- and voltage-dependent CIC-2 Cl$^-$ channels expressed on apical GI epithelial cells. Activation of these chloride channels leads to a chloride-rich intestinal fluid that augments GI motility. Opioid/anticholinergic regimens (loperamide and diphenoxylate/atropine) are often recommended for diarrhea-predominant IBS. In addition, alosetron, a 5HT3 antagonist is approved for use in women with diarrhea-predominant IBS. For unknown reasons, bioavailability in men is 50% lower than in women. This drug is a last resort and is appropriate for only a small percentage of patients with the most severe disease because of the serious constipation and ischemic colitis that sometimes result. In fact, because of these serious adverse effects, alosetron was temporarily removed from the marketplace but was later reintroduced in a lower dose with stricter guidelines.

●●● COMPLEMENTARY AND ALTERNATIVE MEDICINE

Increasingly greater evidence illustrates the utility of probiotics—healthy bacterial microorganisms—for managing diarrhea, IBD, and IBS. *Lactobacillus* and *Bifidobacterium* are the two most commonly studied genera.

Level 1 evidence supports the use of probiotics for preventing and treating diarrhea, including antibiotic-associated diarrhea, *Clostridium difficile* pseudomembranous colitis, and rotaviral gastroenteritis. The mechanisms of action for probiotics may include the following:

- Competing with harmful bacterial species for space and nutrients in the colon
- Secreting bacteriocins that act as antimicrobial agents to eliminate harmful pathogens
- Producing short-chain fatty acids that lower colonic pH
- Stimulating the immune system to secrete immunoglobulin A antibodies and protective cytokines
- Stimulating peristalsis

New lines of evidence suggest that inflammatory bowel diseases are caused by abnormalities within normal gut flora. Such alterations may be caused by the following:

- Persistent infection (at the moment *Mycobacterium paratuberculosis* is a leading candidate)
- Slight imbalances among "normal" GI flora
- Defective mucosa that is continuously stimulated by gut bacteria
- A lack of oral tolerance to one's own normal GI flora (essentially, an allergy develops to one's own normal flora)

Numerous clinical trials have found probiotics effective at maintaining remission in patients with ulcerative colitis, Crohn disease, and pouchitis (inflamed surgical pouch after IBD bowel resection). Anecdotal evidence suggests that probiotics may be effective in inducing remission in these IBDs as well.

Clinical evidence also finds probiotics effective for restoring appropriate gut function in patients with both constipation-predominant and diarrhea-predominant IBS. Some investigators have found increased GI colonization by clostridia in patients with IBS, a situation that probiotics may help resolve.

TABLE 11-7. Drugs That Speed Gastrointestinal Motility

AGENT	COMMENT
Bulk-forming agents	Soften stool by retaining water Bowel obstruction can result if not consumed with adequate fluids Flatulence common
Psyllium hydrophilic colloids	Often administered to children
Methylcellulose	
Polycarbophil	
Malt soup extract	
Emollients	
Docusate	Facilitate mixing of aqueous and fatty materials within gastrointestinal tract Used to prevent constipation or to reduce straining when stooling (e.g., after hemorrhoid surgery, childbirth)
Mineral oil	Oil coating on stools promotes easier passage Inhibits colonic reabsorption of water Oil may leak from anal sphincter Should not be used for more than 2 weeks or in debilitated patients (risk of aspiration)
Opioid Receptor Antagonists	
Methyl naltrexone	A μ-opioid antagonist for treatment of opioid-induced constipation (palliative care) Selective for peripheral and not central opioid receptors; does not cross blood-brain barrier
Alvimopan	Selective antagonist of peripheral μ-opioid receptors; used short term to accelerate gastrointestinal recovery after bowel resection surgery with primary anastomosis
Osmotic agents	Exert osmotic effects to pull water into intestines May cause flatulence, cramps, diarrhea, and electrolyte imbalances
Lactulose	Oral syrup formulation
PEG	Often used for bowel evacuation before gastrointestinal procedures Also used for intermittent constipation Formulations that contain PEG plus electrolytes prevent salt imbalances and are preferred in patients with congestive heart disease, angina, and renal or liver disease
Glycerin	Suppositories often used for osmotic actions in children
Stimulants	Increase activity of gut by acting as irritants Should only be used intermittently May cause severe cramping and fluid and electrolyte disturbances
Bisacodyl	Oral and rectal formulations
Senna	Proposed laxative of choice for opioid-induced constipation May be associated with melanosis coli, a black pigment that infiltrates the colon wall
Casanthranol, castor oil	Stimulates secretions, decreases glucose absorption, promotes gastrointestinal motility
Saline cathartics	Magnesium and sodium salts Often used for bowel evacuation before gastrointestinal procedures May cause electrolyte disturbances Magnesium may accumulate in patients with renal dysfunction Sodium may worsen congestive heart failure

Some of these agents are not routinely recommended by health care professionals (e.g., castor oil). However, patients may use them as "old-time remedies" because many are available over the counter.
PEG, polyethylene glycol.

●●● TOP FIVE LIST

1. Histamine H₂ blockers and PPIs limit GERD.
2. Antibiotics that eradicate *H. pylori* are given concomitantly with H₂ blockers and PPIs to treat peptic ulcer disease.
3. Ulcerative colitis and Crohn disease are two severe forms of IBD treated with antiinflammatory and immunosuppressive drugs.
4. Combinatorial drug therapy (antidopaminergic, antihistaminic, antimuscarinic, 5HT3 antagonistic, corticosteroid) often is used to treat severe nausea and vomiting.
5. The first line of defense for diarrhea is rehydration.

Self-assessment questions can be accessed at www. StudentConsult.com.

Endocrine Pharmacology 12

CONTENTS

ANTERIOR PITUITARY HORMONES
Adrenal Disorders
Thyroid Disorders
Growth-Related Disorders
Prolactin Disorders
POSTERIOR PITUITARY HORMONES
Vasopressin Analogs (Desmopressin)
WOMEN'S REPRODUCTIVE HEALTH AND DISORDERS
Pregnancy
Contraception
Menstrual Disorders, Endometriosis, and Uterine Fibroids
Osteoporosis
MEN'S REPRODUCTIVE DISORDERS
Erectile Dysfunction
Hypogonadism/Andropause
Benign Prostatic Hyperplasia
PANCREATIC DISORDERS
Diabetes Mellitus
Oral Agents for Type 2 Diabetes
New Drugs for Diabetes
COMPLEMENTARY AND ALTERNATIVE MEDICINE
TOP FIVE LIST

This chapter is all about the axis—the hypothalamus/pituitary axis. The keys to understanding endocrine pharmacology are the feed-forward and feed-back mechanisms that govern how "releasing" factors in the hypothalamus control the release of hormones in the pituitary that then target multiple organs within the body. This interplay of hormonally regulated signals is summarized in Table 12-1. Pharmacologically, pathologic alterations in these hormones can be corrected by recombinant or synthetic analogs of these hormones.

●●● ANTERIOR PITUITARY HORMONES

Adrenal Disorders

Stress triggers the hypothalamus to release corticotropin-releasing hormone, which is a positive stimulus for the secretion of adrenocorticotropin hormone (ACTH) from the anterior pituitary (Fig. 12-1). Circulating ACTH stimulates the adrenal gland to release glucocorticoids that control basic body functions and metabolic activities (Table 12-2).

The released glucocorticoids feed back to negatively regulate the hypothalamus and the anterior pituitary to diminish release of corticotropin-releasing hormone and ACTH and complete the feedback loop.

PHYSIOLOGY

The Hypothalamus Is Connected to the Pituitary

Neurosecretory neurons originating within the hypothalamus release oxytocin and vasopressin from the posterior pituitary. In contrast, nerve fibers converge on the median eminence within the hypothalamus, releasing hypothalamic hormones that travel via portal vessels to the anterior pituitary. Once there, these hypothalamic hormones trigger the release of pituitary hormones. These anterior pituitary hormones include growth hormone, adrenocorticotropic hormone, thyroid-stimulating hormone, prolactin, dopamine, follicle-stimulating hormone, and luteinizing hormone. These anatomic connections are depicted in Figure 12-1.

ANATOMY

The Adrenal "Zone"

The adrenal cortex is composed of three histologic zones with separate functions. The outer zone is the zona glomerulosa, which produces mineralocorticoids such as aldosterone. The middle zone, the zona fasciculata, produces glucocorticoids such as cortisol. The inner zone, the zona reticularis, primarily produces precursors of estrogens and androgens. Remember that the adrenal *medulla* releases epinephrine and norepinephrine.

Cushing Syndrome (Hypercortisolism)
Aminoglutethimide, Metyrapone, High-dose Ketoconazole, and Mitotane

Cortisol serves as the primary glucocorticoid in humans. Increased levels of cortisol from the adrenal gland can lead to hypertension, hyperglycemia, impotence, hirsutism, osteoporosis, and mood changes. Patients may also exhibit moon facies (an abnormally swollen face). Increased cortisol concentrations can be a result of overproduction of ACTH from an overactive hypothalamus (Cushing disease) or from an adrenal or ectopic tumor that secretes ACTH. First-line treatment, where warranted, is surgical resection of the tumor. For patients who are not surgical candidates or during the interim until surgery can be performed,

TABLE 12-1. Signals on the Hypothalamic-Pituitary Axis

HYPOTHALAMUS	PITUITARY	TARGET ORGAN	HORMONES/CELL SIGNAL
Corticotropin-releasing hormone	Adrenocorticotropic hormone	Adrenal cortex	Glucocorticoids, mineralocorticoids, androgens
Thyrotropin-releasing factor	Thyroid-stimulating hormone	Thyroid	Thyroid hormones (T_3, T_4)
Growth hormone–releasing factor and growth hormone inhibitory hormone (somatostatin)*	Growth hormone	Liver Adipose	Insulinlike growth factor (mediates most growth effects of growth hormone)
Dopamine*	Prolactin	Mammary glands	Breast milk production
Gonadotropin-releasing hormone	Follicle-stimulating hormone and luteinizing hormone	Ovary Testes	Estrogen, progesterone, testosterone
Oxytocin[†]	Oxytocin	Uterus Mammary tissue	Induction of labor, lactation
Vasopressin[†]	Vasopressin	Renal tubules Smooth muscle	Water reabsorption via aquaporin channels ↑ cAMP

*Although nearly all the hypothalamic hormones listed stimulate release of pituitary hormones, dopamine and somatostatin are exceptions. In this context, dopamine acts as an inhibitory factor, preventing release of prolactin and somatostatin prevents release of growth hormone.
[†]Oxytocin and vasopressin are synthesized within cell bodies located in the hypothalamus, but long axons transport the hormones for release by the posterior pituitary.
T3, triiodothyronine; T4, thyroxine; cAMP, cyclic adenosine monophosphate.

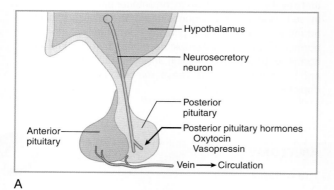

A

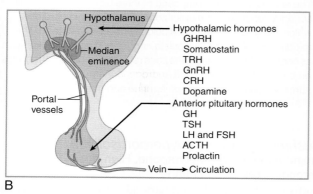

B

Figure 12-1. A, The posterior pituitary releases hormones directly from the hypothalamus. **B,** Hormones secreted by the anterior pituitary gland are released from resident cells in response to signals from the hypothalamus. *GHRH*, growth hormone–releasing hormone; *TRH*, thyrotropin releasing hormone; *GnRH*, gonadotropin-releasing hormone; *CRH*, corticotropin-releasing hormone; *GH*, growth hormone; *TSH*, thyroid-stimulating hormone; *LH*, luteinizing hormone; *FSH*, follicte stimulatin hormone; *ACTH*, adrenocorticotropic hormone.

TABLE 12-2. Actions of Glucocorticoids

GLUCOCORTICOID EFFECT	TARGET TISSUE
Increases blood glucose	Liver
Increases hepatic glycogen	Liver
Protein catabolism	Muscle
Reduces inflammation and suppresses immune responses	Macrophages and lymphocytes
Stimulates gastric acid secretions	Stomach
Stimulates gluconeogenesis	Liver
Stimulates lipolysis	Adipose

pharmacologic intervention with drugs that inhibit cholesterol metabolism is the course of therapy.

Steroid-modifying drugs such as aminoglutethimide and metyrapone and high doses of ketoconazole can be used to treat Cushing syndrome. Each of these drugs inhibits one or more enzymes involved in cortisol synthesis (Fig. 12-3).

Aminoglutethimide inhibits cholesterol desmolase, the first and rate-limiting step responsible for converting cholesterol to pregnenolone. Metyrapone inhibits 11-hydroxylase activity, the last step in cortisol synthesis. Ketoconazole, at much higher doses than normally used for antifungal activity, inhibits both 11- and 17-hydroxylases.

Adverse effects of aminoglutethimide include extreme sedation, gastrointestinal (GI) disturbances (nausea), and severe skin rashes. Adverse effects occurring with metyrapone include nausea, vomiting, hirsutism, acne (enhanced production of androgens resulting from cortisol blockage), and hypertension (because of accumulation of 11-deoxycortisol). Therefore the two drugs are often used together for maximal efficacy and to allow dose reductions of each. Ketoconazole can also be used at high doses. Notice that antagonism of 17-hydroxylase with ketoconazole can lower testosterone levels, causing gynecomastia and reduced libido in men. Ketoconazole also elevates hepatic enzymes.

PHYSIOLOGY

Aldosterone and the Adrenal Gland

In contrast to glucocorticoids, which are stimulated via adrenocorticotropic hormone from the anterior pituitary, the mineralocorticoids are regulated by means of ion sensors within the adrenal gland itself. A decrease in plasma Na^+ concentration or a decrease in extracellular fluid volume induces the adrenal gland to secrete aldosterone, which causes the kidney to retain sodium and excrete potassium and protons. The retention of Na^+ leads to an antidiuretic effect, which restores extracellular fluid volume.

The adrenal gland can also be stimulated to secrete aldosterone via circulating angiotensin II (see Fig. 12-2). Production of angiotensin II is itself a consequence of ion sensors within the juxtaglomerular apparatus of the afferent arteriole, which releases renin, the rate-limiting enzyme that degrades angiotensinogen to angiotensin I. Angiotensin I is hydrolyzed by angiotensin-converting enzyme to angiotensin II. Angiotensin II is both a potent vasoconstrictor and a stimulus for release of aldosterone.

When necessary, mineralocorticoid replacement therapy can be accomplished with aldosterone mimetics such as fludrocortisone. In contrast, spironolactone and eplerenone are pharmacologic agents that act as aldosterone receptor antagonists.

Other drug strategies for managing Cushing disease include adrenolytics (drugs that cause atrophy of the adrenal gland) such as mitotane. Mitotane therapy typically requires hospitalization so that plasma and urinary cortisol levels can be closely monitored. Steroid replacement therapy may be required in these patients. Lethargy, somnolence, and other adverse central nervous system effects are experienced by most patients. Also used to manage hypercortisolism are neuromodulators (e.g., cyproheptadine, bromocriptine, valproate, and octreotide—although none of these agents has been consistently effective) and glucocorticoid blockers (e.g., spironolactone, mifepristone). Remember that neither glucocorticoid blocker is specific for antagonizing only the glucocorticoid receptors. Spironolactone also blocks aldosterone receptors, and mifepristone (better known as RU-486 or the "morning after pill") is an antagonist of progesterone receptors.

Addison Disease (Adrenal Insufficiency)
Hydrocortisone and Fludrocortisone

Symptoms of adrenal insufficiency are observed only after more than 90% of the adrenal gland is nonfunctional. The most common cause of adrenal insufficiency is long-term glucocorticoid use (hypothalamic-pituitary axis suppression because of feedback inhibition). Specifically, pharmacologic levels of glucocorticoids can negatively regulate the hypothalamus and diminish ACTH levels. This is particularly important in patients who abruptly stop taking high-dose

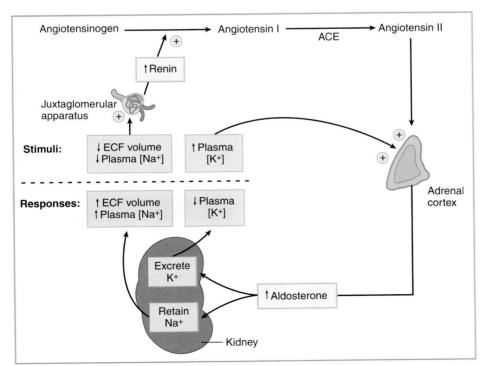

Figure 12-2. Role of renin and angiotensin in regulating aldosterone secretion by the adrenal cortex. Renin is an enzyme that converts angiotensinogen to angiotensin. *ACE*, angiotensin-converting enzyme; *ECF*, extracellular fluid.

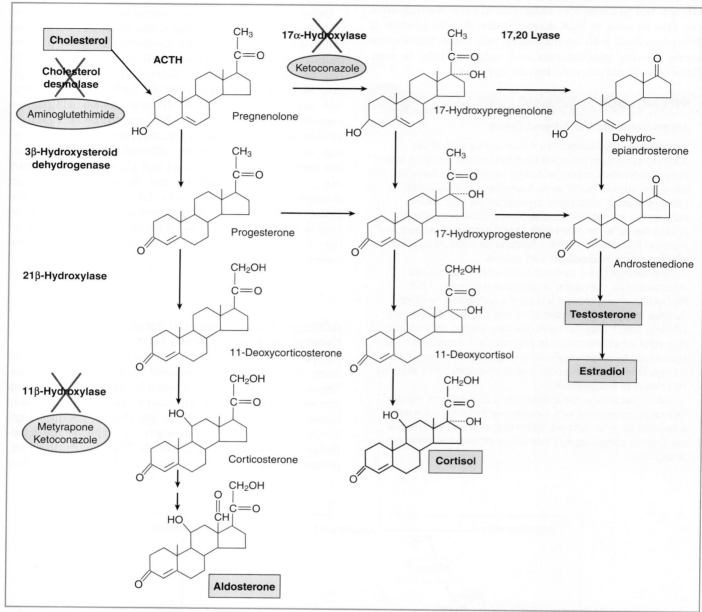

Figure 12-3. Biosynthetic pathway of adrenal steroids. Drugs that inhibit cholesterol biosynthesis will, by definition, lower production of cortisol and thus are first-line treatments for Cushing disease. However, note that these drugs affect testosterone production. *ACTH*, adrenocorticotropic hormone.

glucocorticoids (immunosuppressive treatment) because their adrenal glands are no longer capable of producing adrenal steroids. Another condition of adrenal insufficiency is Addison disease, in which diminished ACTH leads to diminished adrenal gland function.

The major uses of corticosteroids with glucocorticoid activity are as immunosuppressives and as adjuvants to combinatorial cancer chemotherapeutic regimens (see Chapter 5). In cases of adrenal insufficiency, hydrocortisone is usually given for its combined glucocorticoid and mineralocorticoid effects. Major side effects of long-term corticosteroid therapy are listed in Box 12-1, and the mechanisms of action of the corticosteroids are described in Figure 12-4. If mineralocorticoid replacement is also needed for adrenal insufficiency, fludrocortisone is

Box 12-1.   SIDE EFFECTS OF LONG-TERM CORTICOSTEROID TREATMENT

Sodium retention
Edema
Muscle wasting
Growth suppression
Cataracts
Peptic ulcer disease
Osteoporosis
Hypokalemia
Increased risk of infections
Iatrogenic (treatment-induced) Cushing syndrome

administered. Side effects associated with fludrocortisone typically are those associated with Na$^+$ retention and fluid overload.

Hirsutism

Finasteride and Flutamide

The zona reticularis of the adrenal gland is a site of steroid dysregulation that leads to hirsutism. Overproduction of adrenal androgens in females can lead to husky voice, menstrual irregularities, and male pattern baldness. Treatments include finasteride, which inhibits 5α-reductase to prevent conversion of testosterone to dihydrotestosterone. Flutamide, which inhibits tissue uptake of androgens, decreases binding of androgen to cytosolic receptors. (These drugs are discussed further under Men's Reproductive Disorders.)

BIOCHEMISTRY

Cholesterol as the Master Steroid

To appreciate the drugs that regulate adrenal dysfunction, an understanding of cholesterol metabolism is required. As depicted in Figure 12-3, cholesterol is the precursor of all adrenal steroids. Cholesterol and its metabolites are the substrates for multiple enzymes. Thus inhibition of specific enzymes in these interrelated metabolic pathways can decrease specific metabolic and reproductive steroids at the expense of others. Cholesterol desmolase and the 17α- and 11β-hydroxylases are critical pharmacologic targets. Cholesterol is also the precursor of vitamin D and bile acids (not depicted in Fig. 12-3).

PHYSIOLOGY

Steroid-Mediated Signal Transduction

The mechanism of action of cell-permeable (lipophilic) glucocorticoids is mediated by cytosolic steroid-binding receptors, as depicted in Figure 12-4. When bound to glucocorticoids, the steroid-binding receptor translocates to the nucleus. Binding the glucocorticoid also changes the confirmation of the steroid receptor, exposing a selective DNA binding domain. This transactivating complex binds to specific glucocorticoid regulatory elements on the 5′ untranslated region of DNA to repress or enhance transcription of immunosuppressive or anti-inflammatory cytokines, respectively. Hence, steroid receptors act as transcription factors.

Thyroid Disorder

Thyroid-stimulating hormone (thyrotropin) from the anterior pituitary stimulates follicular cells of the thyroid to produce the thyroid hormones (triiodothyronine and thyroxine; Fig. 12-5). The activated thyrotropin receptor is coupled via G_s to produce cyclic adenosine monophosphate (cAMP), which regulates expression of precursors to T_4. Specifically, iodide (I$^-$) is removed from the circulation by the thyroid gland and oxidized to iodine via actions of the enzyme thyroperoxidase. Iodine then crosses into the colloid, a secretory matrix comprising a large glycoprotein, thyroglobulin. Iodine molecules bind

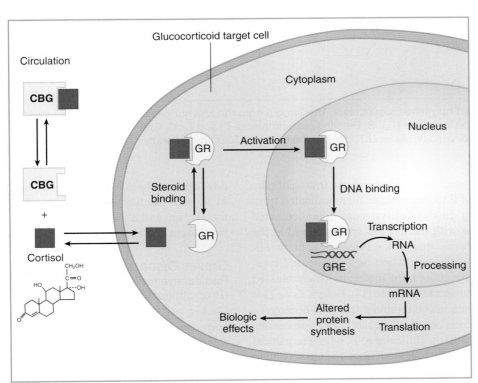

Figure 12-4. Cell and molecular biologic features of cytosolic glucocorticoid receptors. Only free cortisol (*purple boxes*) crosses the plasma membrane. After cortisol binds to the intracellular glucocorticoid receptor (*GR*), the steroid-receptor comlplex enters the nucleus and assumes a shape that permits DNA binding. *CBG*, cortisol-binding globulin; *GRE*, glucocorticoid response element.

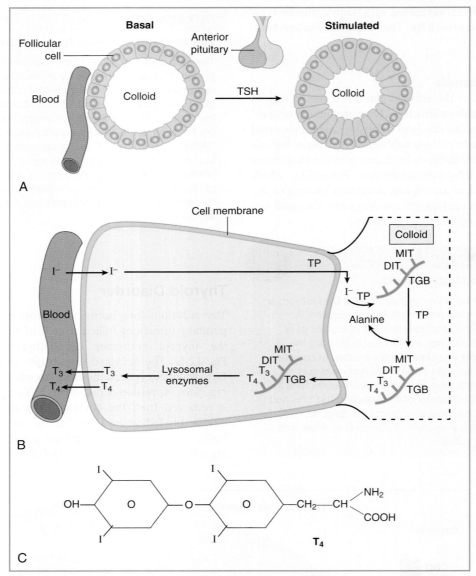

Figure 12-5. A, Thyroid hormone biosynthesis. Thyrotropin from the anterior pituitary stimulates thyroid follicular cells to produce triiodothyronine (T_3) and thyroxine (T_4). **B,** Detailed biosynthesis of T_3 and T_4. **C,** Chemical structure of T_4 (T_3 simply lacks one of the iodines). *MIT*, monoiodinated tyrosine; *DIT*, diiodinated tyrosine; *TGB*, thyroglobulin; *TP*, thyroperoxidase; *TSH*, thyroid-stimulating hormone.

to the numerous tyrosine residues found on thyroglobulin. Through the activity of thyroperoxidase, monoiodinated tyrosines combine to form diiodinated tyrosines. Monoiodinated tyrosines can combine with diiodinated tyrosines within the colloid to form a molecule that, when released, is known as *triiodothyronine* (T_3). Likewise, when two diiodinated tyrosines combine within the colloid, the molecule, when released from the thyroid, is known as *thyroxine* (T_4). Before T_3 or T_4 is released, thyroglobulin must be removed from the hormones. This occurs in the follicular cells because the T_3 or T_4 precursors are endocytosed back into the follicular cells, where functional T_3 and T_4 are subsequently released from the glycoprotein through actions of lysosomal enzymes. Finally, newly synthesized thyroid hormones are released into the circulation.

T_3 and T_4 can be thought of as master regulators of metabolism, oxygen consumption, energy, and growth and development. Both hyperdysregulation and hypodysregulation of thyroid function leads to major, but opposite, changes in metabolism and heart function. Signs and symptoms of hyperthyroidism and hypothyroidism are reviewed in Table 12-3.

Graves Disease (Hyperthyroidism)
Radioactive Iodide and Thionamides (Propylthiouracil and Methimazole)

Causes of hyperthyroidism include thyroid-stimulating hormone–secreting pituitary tumors, pituitary resistance to T_4, and thyroid goiters. Graves disease, an autoimmune syndrome in which antibodies to the thyrotropin receptor stimulate T_4 production and release, is another cause of hyperthyroidism. Note that patients with hyperthyroidism often have weight loss despite an increased appetite. When patients come to the emergency department with severe

TABLE 12-3. Symptoms of Hyperthyroidism and Hypothyroidism

HYPERTHYROIDISM SYMPTOMS	HYPOTHYROIDISM SYMPTOMS
Nervousness	Lethargy, slow cerebration
Weight loss	Weight gain
Diarrhea	Constipation
Tachycardia	Bradycardia
Insomnia	Sleepiness
Increased appetite	Anorexia
Heat intolerance	Cold intolerance
Oligomenorrhea (sparse and infrequent menstrual cycles)	Menorrhagia (heavy menstrual cycles)
Muscle wasting	Weakness
Goiter	Dry, coarse skin
Exophthalmos (bulging eyes)	Facial edema

hyperthyroidism—thyrotoxicosis, or thyroid storm—the first step is to stabilize the patient. Symptoms are controlled with β-blockers, aspirin, and corticosteroids. Then, the underlying clinical problem is addressed as discussed in the following section.

Treatments for hyperthyroidism include surgery and radioactive iodide isotopes (^{131}I), which destroy overactive thyroid tissue. However, a consequence of thyroid removal or destruction is hypothyroidism.

Pharmacologic treatments that may be used until surgical removal of thyroid tissue or as management during a thyrotoxic crisis include drugs that are substrates for thyroid peroxidase, which block oxidation of iodide in the thyroid gland and prevent subsequent synthesis of T_3 and T_4. These drugs are known as *thionamides* (propylthiouracil and methimazole). Patients using these drugs are at risk for maculopapular and pruritic rashes, arthralgia, and fever. Hypersensitivity reactions can be severe and may include thrombocytopenia, pancytopenia, aplastic anemia, and agranulocytosis. Hypersensitivity reactions occur suddenly, often within the first 3 months of therapy. Therefore white blood cell counts should be closely monitored. Patients should be counseled to see their physicians if they experience any flulike symptoms.

Another pharmacologic treatment of hyperthyroidism is potassium iodide. Sudden exposure to excess serum iodide inhibits oxidation or organification of iodide, thus diminishing thyroid hormone biosynthesis. The exact mechanism of this action is unknown. For a short period, T_3 and T_4 release is inhibited. However, within 2 weeks of continued exposure to large amounts of iodide, the thyroid gland escapes this blockade and hormone biosynthesis continues.

Hypothyroidism
T_3 and/or T_4 Replacement (Levothyroxine, Liothyronine)
Hypothyroidism during pregnancy can result in miscarriage or mental retardation (cretinism). The cause of the hypothyroidism usually is inadequate iodine levels during the first trimester of pregnancy, which is preventable. Pregnant women should ingest approximately 220 μg of iodine, a little higher than the typical average daily intake of 160 μg. As many as 6 of 100 miscarriages may be due to thyroid insufficiency. Also of importance, 10% of all women older than age 65 years develop hypothyroidism. Women are five times more likely to develop thyroid insufficiency than are men.

Treatments for hypothyroidism include natural thyroid extracts or synthetic T_4. Natural thyroid extracts contain a mixture of T_3 and T_4 from animal sources (hog, sheep, cow). Absorption and bioavailability are unpredictable, and hypersensitivity reactions can occur. On the other hand, synthetic T_4 (levothyroxine) contains T_4 only; this drug is chemically stable, relatively nonantigenic, and easily converted to the more active T_3 form with defined kinetics. Levothyroxine is highly protein bound and has a relatively long half-life ($t_{1/2}$) of 9 days in hypothyroid patients. It may take up to 30 days to reach a steady-state level of replacement. Drugs such as rifampin, carbamazepine, and phenytoin can increase metabolism and removal of synthetic T_4 via P450 induction.

There are also synthetic T3 replacement therapies. Liothyronine contains T_3. This drug has a shorter $t_{1/2}$, leading to faster dose titration. This drug is also quickly eliminated in cases of overdose. However, liothyronine also has a slightly higher incidence of cardiac adverse effects compared with T_4 synthetic drugs. Liothyronine may be preferred in patients who are unable to convert T_4 to T_3. The many drug interactions for thyroid hormones are listed in Box 12-2.

Growth-Related Disorders
Sermorelin, Somatropin, and Mecasermin Lanreotide, Octreotide and Pegvisomant
Sermorelin, somatropin, and mecasermin are given for growth hormone deficiency syndromes, and lanreotide, octreotide, and pegvisomant are used to treat growth hormone excess.

Box 12-2. THYROID HORMONE–DRUG INTERACTIONS

- Drugs that induce cytochrome P450 enzymes, such as phenytoin, carbamazepine, and rifampin, may increase metabolism and biliary excretion of thyroid hormone.
- Calcium and iron products chelate oral thyroid hormone preparations in the gastrointestinal tract, diminishing their effectiveness. Raloxifene may also decrease absorption of thyroid hormones.
- Soy flour, soy isoflavones, high-fiber diets, and some legumes inhibit absorption of thyroid hormones.
- Warfarin doses should be decreased because thyroid hormones may increase degradation of vitamin K clotting factors.
- Effects of β-agonists, stimulants, and decongestants should be monitored because thyroid hormones potentiate sympathetic effects on the heart.
- Thyroid hormones may increase the dose requirement for insulin and oral hypoglycemic drugs.

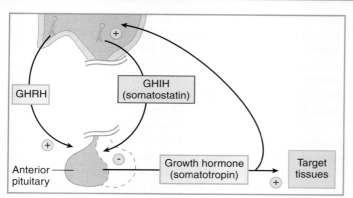

Figure 12-6. Growth hormone feedback inhibition. *GHIH,* growth hormone inhibitory hormone (somatostatin); *GHRH,* growth hormone–releasing hormone.

Growth hormone–releasing hormone induces the anterior pituitary to secrete growth hormone (somato**tropin**). Growth hormone induces its own feedback inhibition by stimulating growth hormone inhibitory hormone (somato**statin**) release from the hypothalamus (Fig. 12-6). Recombinant DNA versions of growth hormone (somatotropin) can be used to treat growth hormone deficiency (dwarfism). Several different recombinant products are available and differ from in terms of route of administration (intramuscular or subcutaneous) and frequency of injection (three to seven times per week). A growth hormone–releasing hormone biologic, sermorelin (consisting of the first 29 amino acids of growth hormone–releasing hormone), is available for patients who have a hypothalamic deficiency. In addition, an insulinlike growth factor therapy, mecasermin, has been approved for children who may not necessarily have a growth factor deficiency but may be resistant to the effects of growth hormone due to the production of neutralizing antibodies to growth hormone. Mecasermin is also used for children with severe insulinlike growth factor-1 deficiency. Mecasermin is administered subcutaneously before meals to avoid a hypoglycemic response. This is yet another example of how targeting a signal transduction cascade (insulinlike growth factor-1 tyrosine kinase receptors) yields a novel therapeutic strategy.

In contrast, synthetic forms of growth hormone inhibitory hormone (somastatin), such as lanreotide and octreotide, are effective for managing growth hormone excess (acromegaly or gigantism). Acromegaly is often the result of a benign pituitary tumor; pharmacologic treatment is often initiated because of inadequate responses to surgery and radiation. These biologics are 40 times more potent at inhibiting growth hormone secretion than is endogenous somatostatin. However, subcutaneously administered lanreotide and intramuscularly administered octreotide are associated with abdominal cramps, reduced gallbladder contractility, gallstones, reduced serum levels of vitamin B_{12}, and altered absorption of dietary fats. A newer, more specific therapy uses a growth factor receptor antagonist such as pegvisomant to treat acromegaly. Injection site reactions, flulike symptoms, diarrhea, and elevated liver enzyme levels can occur. Hepatoxicity must therefore be closely monitored.

Prolaction Disorders

Dopamine Receptor Agonists and Antagonists

Dopamine receptor agonists include bromocriptine, pergolide, and the newer agents cabergoline, pramipexole, and ropinirole. A more detailed discussion of dopamine agonists can be found in Chapter 13.

Hyperprolactinemia (increased prolactin secretion) in women presents as menstrual dysfunction, lack of ovulation, and inappropriate lactation. Hyperprolactinemia can also induce lactation in men. The most common cause of hyperprolactinemia is drug induced. Drugs that have been implicated most often are those with dopamine receptor antagonist properties (e.g., haloperidol, metoclopramide). In addition, even selective serotonin reuptake inhibitors and oral contraceptives can induce hyperprolactinemia. Pharmacologic treatment of hyperprolactinemia uses dopamine receptor agonists such as bromocriptine, pergolide, and the newer agents cabergoline, pramipexole, and ropinirole. Dopamine receptor agonists reduce prolactin secretion by the anterior pituitary. Adverse effects include GI distress (abdominal pain, diarrhea), dizziness, headache, and fatigue. Patients should be warned that all dopamine receptor agonists can cause sudden sleep attacks. Newer drugs seem to target the D_2-like receptor subtypes preferentially over the D_1-like receptors and seem to have a lower incidence of side effects.

Sometimes it is desirable to facilitate breast milk production in lactating women. Metoclopramide, a dopamine receptor antagonist that leads to prolactin release from the anterior pituitary, has been used on a short-term basis for this purpose.

●●● POSTERIOR PITUITARY HORMONES

Vasopressin Analogs (Desmopressin)

As depicted in Figure 12-7, vasopressin (also known as *antidiuretic hormone*) controls fluid balance in response to osmoreceptor stimulation. Desmopressin is a long-acting synthetic analog of vasopressin. Oral and nasal spray formulations are available and are used to treat both centrally mediated diabetes insipidus and enuresis. In both situations, it is desirable to form less urine. Desmopressin accomplishes this by enhancing water reabsorption from renal tubules. The adverse effect is hyponatremia, or "water intoxication." Patients should be cautioned to ingest only enough fluid to satisfy their thirst.

Vasopressin antagonists, such as conivaptan, are reviewed in Chapter 9 as agents to treat hypernatremia.

Oxytocin

Oxytocin is the other hormone released from the posterior pituitary. Its primary role is to induce labor and stimulate contraction of smooth muscles in the breast during lactation to facilitate milk ejection. Clinically, oxytocin is used to facilitate labor. Unborn infants must be monitored closely for signs of fetal distress during oxytocin infusions because of severe contractions. Because of structural similarities with vasopressin, oxytocin causes fluid retention in the mother.

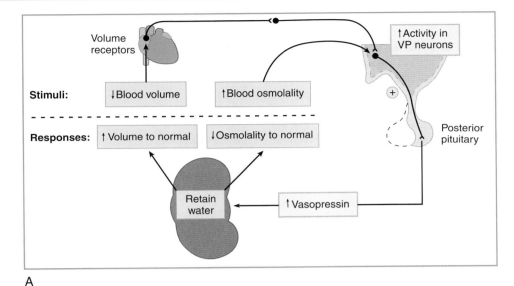

A

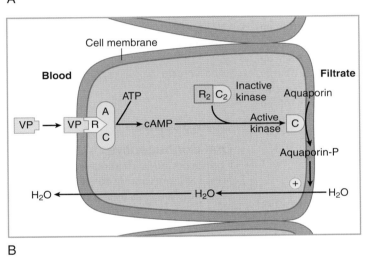

B

Figure 12-7. Feedback control mechanisms (**A**) and signaling cascades (**B**) regulated by vasopressin. *VP*, vasopressin; *AC*, adenylyl cyclase; *R₂C₂*, inactive protein kinase A holoenzyme (*R*, regulatory subunit; *C*, catalytic); *ATP*, adenosine triphosphate; *cAMP*, cyclic adenosine monophosphate.

PHYSIOLOGY

Vasopressin

Increased blood osmolarity, sensed by osmoreceptors within the hypothalamus, activates release of vasopressin (also called *antidiuretic hormone* [ADH]) from the posterior pituitary. As depicted in Figure 12-7, circulating vasopressin activates G_s-coupled V_2 vasopressin receptors within the tubules of the nephron to produce cAMP. Activation of cAMP-regulated protein kinase A leads to insertion of additional aquaporin water channels in the luminal membrane of renal tubules that reabsorb water and limit diuresis, thereby reducing blood osmolarity. Desmopressin is a long-acting, synthetic, nasally administered ADH analog that is used to treat central diabetes insipidus, a medical condition characterized by decreased ADH levels, resulting in large volumes of dilute urine.

●●● WOMEN'S REPRODUCTIVE HEALTH AND DISORDERS

Pregnancy

Oxytocin, Dinoprostone, Misoprostol, β₂-Agonists, Gonadotropic Hormones, and Clomifene

As previously mentioned, oxytocin, synthesized in the hypothalamus and released from the posterior pituitary, induces or augments labor. Prostaglandin E analogs, such as dinoprostone and misoprostol, can also be given vaginally to "ripen" the cervix and augment labor.

In contrast, β₂-agonists, such as ritodrine and terbutaline, can be used to mitigate uterine contractions and manage preterm labor. However, tachycardia, palpitations, and hyperglycemia can result. Magnesium sulfate, which antagonizes Ca^{++} to prevent actin-myosin interactions, and Ca^{++} channel blockers (e.g., nifedipine) can also be used to suppress uterine contractions. In cases of premature birth, glucocorticoids such as betamethasone are given to mothers during labor to hasten fetal lung development and decrease the incidence of respiratory distress syndrome.

As previously discussed, to facilitate lactation, metoclopramide, a drug with dopamine receptor antagonist actions, can be administered to stimulate prolactin release. In contrast, methylergonovine or methysergide, ergot alkaloids, can be used to suppress lactation. As expected, ergot alkaloids should never be given to nursing mothers. Ergot alkaloids can cause chest pain and vasoconstriction.

Multiple hormonal strategies are used to manage in vitro fertilization and in vivo ovulation and implantation as well as hypothalamic hypogonadism. As examples, urinary and synthetic forms of follicle-stimulating hormone (FSH) and human chorionic gonadotropin (which is similar to luteinizing hormone [LH]) are used to manage ovulation in women with hypogonadism and aid in vitro fertilization programs. The use of gonadotropic hormones can, in rare circumstances, lead to "a hyperstimulation syndrome," characterized by ovarian enlargement, ascites, and shock. These treatment strategies can result in multiple births or spontaneous abortions. Other approaches to manage female infertility by hormonal ovarian stimulation include clomifene, a selective estrogen receptor modulator (SERM). Clomifene increases production of gonadotropins by inhibiting the negative feedback on the hypothalamus by estrogens.

Pregnancy and the Food and Drug Administration

For more than 20 years, the Food and Drug Administration has required that all new drugs be assigned a pregnancy category that illustrates the safety for use during pregnancy. This rating scale is shown in Box 12-3; specific drugs to avoid are listed in Table 12-4. The Food and Drug Administration has announced that this system is being phased out; manufacturers are now required to describe the adverse effects in both humans and animals as well as the risks associated with not using the drug to treat a given medical condition.

Box 12-3. DRUG SAFETY DURING PREGNANCY

- Category A: Controlled studies in women fail to demonstrate a risk to the fetus in the first trimester; the possibility of fetal harm appears remote.
- Category B: Either animal studies do not indicate a risk to the fetus and there are no controlled studies in pregnant women *or* animal studies indicate a fetal risk but controlled studies in pregnant women fail to demonstrate a risk.r
- Category C: Either animal studies indicate fetal risk and there are no controlled studies in women *or* there are no available studies in animals or women.
- Category D: There is positive evidence of fetal risk but there may be situations where benefits might outweigh the risks.
- Category X: Definite fetal risk based on animal or human studies or human experience; the risk clearly outweighs any benefit in pregnant women.

TABLE 12-4. Some Drugs to Avoid During Pregnancy

DRUG	CONSEQUENCE
Androgens	Ambiguous genitalia
Antineoplastics	Teratogenic
Benzodiazepines	Cleft palate (first trimester; especially diazepam); central nervous system depression, withdrawal symptoms
Fluoroquinolones	Cartilage damage
Isotretinoin	Craniofacial, central nervous system, and cardiac abnormalities
Lithium	Cardiac defects (first trimester)
Salicylates	Delay onset of labor, increase bleeding during delivery, premature closure of patent ductus arteriosus
Tetracyclines	Stained teeth, skeletal system abnormalities
Thalidomide	Teratogenic

Contraception

Oral Contraceptives

Contraception is all about negative feedback. Estrogens suppress FSH, preventing development of a dominant follicle that ultimately leads to ovulation. Progestins suppress LH, blocking ovulation. In addition, progestins thicken the cervical mucus, reduce ovum movement, and thin the endometrium, thereby reducing the likelihood of implantation. Most oral contraceptives are composed of combinations of synthetic estrogens and progestins. It is now suggested that the progestin component of oral contraceptives primarily prevents conception, whereas the estrogen component augments the actions of progestins. For the most part, the estrogen is ethinyl estradiol (EE, the major estrogen produced by the ovaries) or mestranol, which is metabolized by the liver into EE. On the other hand, there are substantial differences in pharmacologic effect among various progestins used in oral contraceptives. Progestins may differ in their relative estrogenic and androgenic effects (Table 12-5).

Various formulations achieve monophasic, biphasic, or triphasic dosing levels throughout the female cycle. The "phasic" formulations were designed to reduce progestin exposure in the earlier stages of the menstrual cycle to lower the incidence of adverse effects.

Oral contraceptives can also be administered to achieve hormonal balance, regulate menstrual cycling, and control endometriosis. The major effects of both too much and too little estrogenic and progestin activities are listed in Table 12-6. These are the types of common side effects observed when patients begin taking oral contraceptives.

It is not uncommon for users of oral contraceptives to experience the following adverse effects: migraine, breast

TABLE 12-5. Differing Pharmacologic Effects of Progestins Used in Oral Contraceptives

Progestins	RELATIVE EFFECTS		
	Progestinic	Estrogenic	Androgenic
Desogestrel and levonorgestrel	++++	—	+++
Ethynodiol diacetate and norethindrone acetate	++	+++	++
Norgestrel and norgestimate	++	—	++

++++, Pronounced effect; +++, moderate effect; ++, low effect; —, no effect.

TABLE 12-6. Symptoms of Estrogen and Progestin Excess and Deficiency

ESTROGEN		PROGESTIN	
Excess	Deficiency	Excess	Deficiency
Nausea, bloating Cervical mucorrhea Polyposis Chloasma (age spots) Hypertension Migraine Breast fullness or tenderness Edema	Early or mid-cycle breakthrough bleeding Spotting Hypomenorrhea	Increased appetite Weight gain Tiredness, fatigue Hypomenorrhea or hypermenorrhea Acne, oily scalp Hair loss, hirsutism Breast regression Depression Vaginal yeast infection	Late breakthrough bleeding Amenorrhea

tenderness, elevated blood pressure, adverse effects on lipids, nausea and vomiting, intolerance to contact lenses, weight gain, hirsutism, and chloasma (brown patches of irregular size and shape on the face). Estrogen-containing oral contraceptives decrease breast milk production and should be avoided in breastfeeding women.

Oral contraceptives are contraindicated in patients with thrombotic disorders, cardiovascular disease, impaired liver function, breast cancer, or pregnancy and in heavy tobacco smokers. Adverse drug reactions include thrombotic disease, pulmonary emboli, myocardial infarction, cerebral hemorrhage, gallbladder disease, and hepatic tumors. The risk of deep vein thrombosis and pulmonary emboli dramatically increases with smokers who use high-dose estrogen formulations. Symptoms of severe adverse events are listed in Table 12-7.

Drugs that induce cytochrome P450 metabolism, such as rifampin, griseofulvin, and older generation antiepileptic drugs, speed estrogen metabolism and thus significantly diminish the efficacy of oral contraceptives. Patients should be counseled to use additional alternative contraceptives or switch to high-dose estrogen contraceptives.

For patients in whom estrogen is contraindicated (those who smoke or who are breastfeeding), progestin-only (mini-pills) contraceptives are available (e.g., norethindrone, norgestrel). However, for maximal effects, progestin-only pills must be started on the first day of menses and taken at the same time each day. This type of contraception has a

TABLE 12-7. Symptoms Experienced by Oral Contraceptive Users That Could Indicate Serious Adverse Effects (Mnemonic: ACHES)

SYMPTOM	CONDITION
Abdominal pain	Gallstones, blood clot, pancreatitis
Chest pain, shortness of breath, coughing blood	Blood clot in lung, myocardial infarction
Headaches	Stroke, hypertension, migraine
Eye problems	Stroke, hypertension, vascular occlusion
Severe leg pain	Blood clot

higher incidence of irregular bleeding and ectopic pregnancy compared with combination oral contraceptives. Keep in mind that with progestin-only pills, ovulation may not be suppressed.

In addition to oral contraceptives, progestins can be deposited intramuscularly for long-lasting contraception. Drugs such as medroxyprogesterone can be administered every 3 months via intramuscular injection. Depot medroxyprogesterone has been associated with significant, sometimes irreversible, loss of bone density. Similarly, levonorgestrel-containing intrauterine devices and subcutaneous implants can be inserted for long-lasting contraception (3 to 5 years).

Other combinatorial estrogen plus progestin formulations have been developed, including the vaginal ring, which releases EE and etonogestrel; the transdermal patch, which releases EE and norelgestromin; and a combination oral contraceptive that contains EE plus drospirenone. Drospirenone is a progestin whose mechanism resembles that of spironolactone. As a result, there is less water retention and associated weight gain. Patients should not take drospirenone with other medications that retain potassium because the drug has mineralocorticoid activity that influences water and electrolyte balance. Oral contraceptives have now been formulated for 3- to 12-month continuous hormonal therapy (EE plus levonorgestrel). High doses of progestins formulated with or without EE can be used as emergency postcoital contraceptive approaches.

It should not be surprising that besides the various progesterone analogues/agonists described above, progesterone-receptor antagonists have also been developed. Mifepristone is a progesterone receptor antagonist that can be used as an abortifacient.

Menstrual Disorders, Endometriosis, and Uterine Fibroids

Premenstrual syndrome is a group of symptoms related to the menstrual cycle. Women who experience severe dysmenorrhea (painful menstrual cramps) are often treated with EE-containing hormonal contraceptives. Table 12-8 lists treatment options for managing symptoms of severe premenstrual syndrome.

Gonadotropin-releasing hormone (GnRH, alluded to in Table 12-1 and Figure 12-1 and often referred to as *LH-releasing hormone*) regulates LH and FSH production in the antituitary pituitary gland. Paradoxically, long-term treatment with GnRH analogs/agonists, such as subcutaneously or intravenously administered leuprolide, nasal-administered

TABLE 12-8. Premenstrual Syndrome

SYMPTOM	TREATMENT
Anxiety	Benzodiazepines
Breast tenderness	Vitamin E, bromocriptine (dopamine agonist), leuprolide (gonadotropin-releasing hormone agonist), danazol (mastodynia)
Depression/irritability	Selective serotonin reuptake inhibitors
Dysmenorrhea and cramps	Oral contraceptives, nonsteroidal antiinflammatory drugs
Insomnia	Antihistamines, tricyclic antidepressants
Migraines	Low-dose estrogen, nonsteroidal antiinflammatory drugs
Mood swings	Lithium, carbamazepine, valproate
Weight gain, bloating	Spironolactone, drospirenone

nafarelin, and subcutaneously implantable goserelin, can actually induce hypogonadism by down-regulating GnRH receptor expression. These GnRH peptide analogues are used to treat endometriosis, uterine fibroids, and central precocious puberty (very early secondary sex characteristics). As described in Chapter 5, GnRH agonists are also used as an endocrine therapy for androgen-dependent prostate cancers. See Table 5-3 to review other hormonal agonists and antagonists used for endocrine therapy of cancer.

Other therapeutic approaches to manage endometriosis are danazol and cetrorelix. Danazol is a modified testosterone structure (ethisterone) that inhibits ovarian steroidogenesis. Other uses for danazol include menorrhagia, fibrocystic breast disease, and breast pain. Adverse effects include hirsutism, weight gain, and edema. Danazol should be discontinued during pregnancy and breastfeeding and in patients with hepatic dysfunction. Cetrorelix is a GnRH antagonist administered subcutaneously.

Menopause
Hormonal Replacement Therapy

Permanent amenorrhea occurs when ovarian follicles no longer respond to FSH. This loss in ovarian function leads to a decline in ovarian estrogen secretion. Menopausal women still make some adrenal-derived estrogens (estrone, E_1) from androstenedione; however, these forms of estrogen are only one third the potency of EE, and there are no cyclic variations throughout the monthly cycle as there formerly were with EE.

Women entering menopause often experience vasomotor instability (hot flashes) when the lack of estrogen leads to surges in LH and FSH, which affect thermoregulation of the hypothalamus. In addition, menopausal women are frequently bothered by urinary and vaginal irritation (dryness, atrophy, dyspareunia).

Hormone replacement therapies composed of estrogens (conjugated, synthetic, natural) and progestins are used to manage symptoms. Topical vaginal formulations are treatments of choice for women with symptoms of urogenital irritation. For those with hot flashes, systemic hormone replacement therapies may be prescribed. Formulations most often include either oral tablets or transdermal patches, although depot oil injections, lotions, and gels are also available. Women with an intact uterus also receive progestins with their estrogen replacement therapy—either in a continuous fashion or in a cyclic manner during the second half of the month. The continuous progestin formulations prevent bleeding, whereas the cyclic formulations cause bleeding reminiscent of menstrual cycles. The reason progestins are added to estrogen replacement therapies is that, without progestins, estrogen therapy is associated with a higher risk of endometrial cancer.

Medroxyprogesterone is the most commonly used progestin during menopause, but norethindrone acetate and progesterone also are used. Progesterone causes sedation in some women because it is metabolized to allopregnanolone, a compound that acts at γ-aminobutyric acid$_A$ (GABA$_A$) receptors (see Chapter 13). Capsule formulations of progesterone may contain peanut oil and therefore are contraindicated in women who are allergic to peanuts.

CLINICAL MEDICINE

Risks Associated with Hormone Replacement Therapy

Outcomes from the Women's Health Initiative (WHI) trial found that hormone replacement therapy increased the risk of heart disease, breast cancer, and stroke (although the risk of colon cancer was reduced).

Specifically, during the WHI, an oral combination product containing conjugated estrogens with medroxyprogesterone, was used. Additional studies have suggested that hormone replacement therapy increases the risk of breast cancer and makes the cancer more difficult to detect by increasing breast tissue density.

Currently, it is recommended that hormone replacement therapy (1) be used at the lowest possible dose, for the shortest possible time, in women with vasomotor symptoms and (2) be avoided in women with a significant risk of breast cancer or heart disease. Moreover, continuous use of progesterone may increase the risk of breast cancer compared with intermittent use. When discontinuing hormone replacement therapy, it is recommended that the drugs be gradually tapered for 6 to 8 weeks to reduce the likelihood of vasomotor adverse effects.

Adverse effects of hormone replacement therapy include nausea, vomiting, breakthrough vaginal bleeding, edema, breast tenderness or enlargement, gallbladder disease, elevated blood pressure, thromboembolic disease, hyperkalemia, and glucose intolerance. Patients should notify their health care professionals if they have pain in the groin or calves, sharp chest pain, shortness of breath, abnormal vaginal bleeding, sudden or severe headache, dizziness or fainting, visual or speech disturbance, yellowing of skin or eyes, breast lumps, or severe depression; these symptoms can be signs of serious adverse effects.

PHYSIOLOGY

Clasts Versus Blasts

Bone tissue is continually in a state of dynamic flux. This is due in part to the fact that osteoclasts signal osteoblasts and osteoblasts signal osteoclasts.

Osteoclasts release proteases that dissolve bone mineral and collagen matrix, a process known as *bone resorption.* The process clears away damaged bone. Simultaneously, osteoclasts secrete growth factors that act as chemoattractants for osteoblasts.

Osteoblasts fill in bone cavities with new bone matrix. Osteoblasts release cytokines to attract osteoclasts and continue the dynamic remodeling of bone. The entire process can be hormonally regulated to modulate release or absorption of calcium into bone matrix and thus indirectly regulate serum calcium levels.

Osteoporosis

Calcium Supplements, Hormone Replacement Therapy, Selective Estrogen Receptor Modulators (Raloxifene), Bisphosphonates, and Calcitonin

Osteoporosis affects nearly 45 million Americans, of whom nearly 70% are women. Osteoporosis is a gradual loss of bone mass, leading to "trauma-less" fractures, the most common of which occur in vertebrae and the most serious in the hip. The main physiologic regulators of bone density are listed in Table 12-9.

BIOCHEMISTRY

Organ-Specific Modification of Vitamin D(s)

Ergosterol (provitamin D_2)	Ultraviolet light $\longrightarrow$	Ergocalciferol (vitamin D_2)	Liver $\longrightarrow$	25-Hydroxyergocalciferol (25-[OH]-D_2)	Kidney $\longrightarrow$	1,25-Dihydroxyergocalciferol (1,25-[OH]$_2$-D_2)
7-Dehydrocholesterol (provitamin D_3)	Skin via $\longrightarrow$ Ultraviolet light	Cholecalciferol (vitamin D_3)	Liver $\longrightarrow$	Calcifediol (25-[OH]-D_3)	Kidney $\longrightarrow$	Calcitriol (1,25-[OH$_2$]-D_3)

Treatment of osteoporosis usually begins with prevention. Calcium and vitamin D supplements should be encouraged as well as weight-bearing exercise. Caffeine and nicotine should be discouraged. Each calcium salt contains different amounts of elemental calcium (Table 12-10). This is important because most adult women require between 1000 and 1200 mg elemental calcium daily. Therefore intake of supplements must be adjusted to ensure the optimal dose of calcium.

Calcium carbonate is relatively insoluble and requires an acidic environment to be absorbed. On the other hand, calcium citrate is readily soluble and does not require a low pH for absorption, so calcium citrate is a preferred calcium supplement in patients with low gastric acid production (e.g., patients with achlorhydria or who take antacids, H₂-blockers, or proton pump inhibitors or who are post-bariatric surgery). High doses of calcium may cause constipation and kidney stones (the latter usually occur only in the presence

TABLE 12-9. Hormonal Regulators of Bone

HORMONE	MECHANISM	PREDOMINANT EFFECT
Calcitonin	Secreted from thyroid to inhibit osteoclast bone resorption	Prevents bone loss
Estrogen	Blocks the interleukin-6 receptor, a potent cytokine associated with bone resorption; inhibits parathyroid hormone activity; increases apoptosis of osteoclasts	Prevents bone loss
Parathyroid hormone	Secreted from parathyroid gland in response to low serum calcium concentrations; increases osteoclast activity	Stimulates bone resorption with chronic exposure (hyperparathyroidism)
Vitamin D	Increases calcium absorption (gastrointestinal tract) and increases calcium reabsorption (kidney)	Prevents bone loss

TABLE 12-10. Variations Among Calcium Salts

CALCIUM SALT	ELEMENTAL CALCIUM (%)
Calcium carbonate	40
Calcium citrate	24
Calcium lactate	18

of large amounts of oxalate). Calcium can interfere with absorption of a variety of drugs, such as the following:

- Iron
- Tetracyclines
- Fluoroquinolones
- Bisphosphonates
- Phenytoin
- Fluoride

Inadequate levels of vitamin D or inadequate sun exposure causes abnormal bone mineralization (rickets in children, osteomalacia in adults). Vitamin D_2 and vitamin D_3 are metabolized via actions of the liver and kidneys to their active forms, 1,25-dihydroxyergocalciferol and calcitriol, respectively. Calcitriol is the most potent form of vitamin D. Vitamin D_3 is the form found in many multivitamins, but it must be metabolized by the liver and kidneys to its more active form, calcitriol. Calcitriol is used especially by patients with renal or hepatic dysfunction. Adverse effects associated with vitamin D excess begin with weakness, headache, and bone pain and progress to polyuria, polydipsia, weight loss, and symptoms associated with hypercalcemia (cardiac arrhythmias). The number of persons with very low vitamin D levels is increasing (possibly from reduced sun exposure with high use of sunscreen) and has been associated with chronic fatigue syndrome, cancer, depression, heightened pain sensitivity, and colds or flu. Nearly 70% of all Americans have insufficient levels of vitamin D. Indeed, the U.S. government has recently released new vitamin D guidelines (2011). Previous guidelines were based only on the amount of vitamin D necessary to prevent rickets, not on the amount necessary for adequate health.

Raloxifene is a SERM that can be used to promote bone mineralization. This drug acts as an agonist at some tissues and as an antagonist at other tissues. Specifically, raloxifene functions as an estrogen agonist in bone and liver but acts as an estrogen receptor antagonist in breast and uterine tissues. Thus raloxifene diminishes endometrial and breast cancer development while stimulating bone mineralization. As a bonus, raloxifene improves high-density lipoprotein/low-density lipoprotein ratios. Tamoxifen, described in Chapter 5, is a SERM that is antagonistic for breast tissue but agonistic for uterine tissue as well as bone. Compared with hormone replacement therapy, raloxifene does not stimulate uterine or endometrial tissues, does not require coadministration of progestins, and does not cause breast swelling or tenderness.

Despite its low risk of causing reproductive cancers, raloxifene still can increase the risk of deep vein thrombosis and thromboemboli. Raloxifene also can decrease the absorption of T_4; therefore, for the large subset of women who have hypothyroidism and osteoporosis, raloxifene and thyroid hormone administration should be separated by 12 hours. Raloxifene may cause hot flashes and leg cramps.

Another therapeutic approach for osteoporosis are the bisphosphonates. These drugs actively adsorb to the hydroxyapatite of bone to become part of the bone matrix. These "reinforced" bones are more resistant to the proteolytic actions of osteoclasts. Alendronate or risedronate are available in once-per-week formulations. Ibandronate is a monthly orally administered bisphosphonate therapy, and zoledronic acid is a once-yearly intravenous infusion bisphosphonate therapy. Notice that most of the bisphosphonates end in "-dronate." The bioavailability of orally administered bisphosphonates is poor; food and antacids further diminish absorption through the GI tract. Therefore the drugs should be taken with water, first thing in the morning, on an empty stomach, at least 30 minutes before breakfast. Patients must also be instructed to maintain an upright position for at least 30 minutes after taking the drugs to minimize esophageal irritation. The major adverse side effects are esophageal erosion and peptic ulcer disease. Rare but serious eye problems have also been reported. In addition, serious jaw necrosis has been reported by cancer patients using some intravenous bisphosphonate therapies. Other bisphosphonates are used to treat Paget disease or hypercalcemia of malignancy, including etidronate, pamidronate, tiludronate, and zoledronic acid. Overall, bisphosphonates reduce the risk of vertebral fractures

TABLE 12-11. Pharmacologic Treatments for Erectile Dysfunction

	SILDENAFIL	TADALAFIL	VARDENAFIL
Duration of activity	Up to 5 h	Up to 36 h	Up to 5 h
Time to onset	60 min	30 min	16 min
Common side effects	Headache Flushing Bluish vision	Headache Dyspepsia Back pain	Headache Flushing

significantly; however, concern is increasingly mounting about the way the drugs may hinder healing of bone fractures when they do occur.

Synthetic salmon calcitonin also can be administered to limit bone loss. Calcitonin inhibits osteoclast-induced bone resorption via activation of G_s-meditated cAMP. Calcitonin helps maintain homeostasis by opposing the actions of parathyroid hormone. Calcitonin also has antinociceptive properties, with analgesia occurring in as little as 5 days. Hypersensitivity reactions (anaphylactic shock, laryngeal edema, angioedema, bronchospasm) may occur from an immune response to the foreign antigen.

Another new therapy for osteoporosis is a recombinant truncated form of parathyroid hormone (teriparatide), administered subcutaneously. Although somewhat of a paradox, continuous administration of parathyroid hormone causes bone resorption, whereas intermittent dosing preferentially stimulates new bone formation. Teriparatide is administered subcutaneously daily and thus stimulates bone formation. However, this parathyroid analog has been associated with osteosarcoma, and long-term safety is a concern. Patients should discontinue use after 2 years. Patients often experience dizziness or tachycardia after injections, although these effects typically subside after the first few doses. Teriparatide is the only drug that stimulates new bone formation; other drugs simply slow bone loss.

●●● MEN'S REPRODUCTIVE DISORDERS

Erectile Dysfunction

Phosphodiesterase-5 Inhibitors

Phosphodiesterase-5 (PDE5) inhibitors include sildenafil, tadalafil, and vardenafil. Note that the names all end in "-afil."

Erectile dysfunction can be caused by numerous abnormalities: endocrine, neurologic, vascular, psychologic, and structural. Medications can also contribute. The most common drugs used to treat erectile dysfunction are the PDE5 inhibitors, which facilitate vasodilation. These drugs prevent catabolism of cyclic guanosine monophosphate (cGMP). Remember that nitric oxide–induced smooth muscle relaxation and resultant vasodilation is cGMP dependent. For the most part, differences between agents are pharmacokinetic in nature (Table 12-11).

Keep in mind that because tadalafil has a long duration of activity, any side effects that occur may last for extended periods.

Dosage must be lowered for all three PDE5 inhibitors in patients who take potent P450 CYP3A4 inhibitors, and these drugs are contraindicated in patients who use nitrates. In addition, the PDE5 inhibitors must be used cautiously, if at all, in patients who take α-blockers for hypertension or benign prostatic hyperplasia because of the risk of hypotension and dizziness. Men should seek medical attention if priapism (continuous erection of the penis) develops because permanent damage could ensue. There are increasing concerns about visual disturbances, including optic neuritis. PDE5 inhibitors may inhibit PDE6, which is the phosphodiesterase found in photoreceptors.

Alprostadil, a PGE_1 analog, enhances cavernous arterial blood flow and is another option for treating erectile dysfunction. This drug comes in various injectable formulations as well as urethrally inserted pellets. Penile fibrosis and pain can occur with regular use. Priapism also may occur.

Hypogonadism/Andropause

Testosterone replacement therapy has long been used as a treatment for male hypogonadism. Testosterone replacement therapy in aging, but otherwise healthy, men is receiving new attention in the management of andropause (weakness, fatigue, reduced muscle mass, osteoporosis, sexual dysfunction, depression, insomnia, and memory impairment associated with aging in men).

Testosterone replacement therapies come in numerous forms: transdermal patches, gels, subcutaneous pellets, injectables, and transbuccal delivery systems. The oral dose form is noticeably absent from this list. Oral testosterone formulations are avoided because of hepatic injury. Adverse effects associated with testosterone replacement therapy include acne, cardiovascular disease, gynecomastia, testicular atrophy, and advancement of benign prostatic hypertrophy or prostate cancer.

It should not be surprising that the same hormones (FSH, human chorionic gonadotropin) used to manage ovulation in women can also be used in men to stimulate the Leydig gland to synthesize testosterone and enhance spermatogenesis and increase fertility.

Benign Prostatic Hyperplasia

α₁-Adrenergic Receptor Blockers and 5α-Reductase Inhibitors

α₁-Adrenergic Receptor Blockers: Doxazosin, Prazosin, Terazosin, Alfuzosin, Silodosin, and Tamsulosin

5α-Reductase Inhibitors: Dutasteride and Finasteride

α₁-Adrenergic receptor blockers and 5α-reductase inhibitors are the drugs of choice for managing symptomatic benign prostatic hyperplasia. Benign prostatic hyperplasia is experienced by most men older than 50 years and can manifest as increased urinary urgency, incomplete bladder emptying, incontinence, and nocturia. Of course, all patients with benign prostatic hyperplasia symptoms should be evaluated for prostate cancer. First-generation α₁-receptor blockers (doxazosin, prazosin, terazosin) relax prostatic smooth muscle as well as vascular smooth muscle, thereby accounting for some of their side effects (hypotension, dizziness). On the other hand, newer α₁-receptor blockers (alfuzosin, silodosin, tamsulosin) are more selective for prostatic smooth muscle but may be associated with decreased amount and release of ejaculate fluid. Alfuzosin prolongs the cardiac QT interval, and CYP3A4 P450 inhibitors (including clarithromycin, ketoconazole, itraconazole, ritonavir) increase alfuzosin and silodosin concentrations.

5α-Reductase inhibitors, drugs that inhibit conversion of testosterone to more active dihydrotestosterone, such as dutasteride and finasteride, are also used to manage benign prostatic hypertrophy. In fact, because it takes 6 to 9 months for 5α-reductase inhibitors to reach their maximal effects, they are often combined with α-receptor blockers, at least for a few months, because the α-receptor blockers alleviate troublesome voiding symptoms almost immediately. Adverse effects associated with decreased production of dihydrotestosterone are sexual in nature (impotence, decreased libido, gynecomastia). These drugs are contraindicated in pregnant women—meaning that men should not give blood for 6 months after taking these medications and pregnant health care workers should avoid handling the tablets because of the risk of fetal anomalies in male fetuses.

Numerous drugs and natural products may be responsible for worsening urinary symptoms in men, such as the following:
- Opiates
- Anticholinergics (tricyclic antidepressants, sedating antihistamines, muscle relaxants)
- Sympathomimetics (pseudoephedrine, ma huang, ephedrine)

PHYSIOLOGY

Dysfunctional Signaling Leads to Type 2 Diabetes

Insulin resistance is attributable to unknown genetic or environmental changes and is often associated with obesity, aging, and a sedentary lifestyle. The molecular mechanisms underlying type 2 insulin resistance are unknown but are speculated to include inappropriate phosphorylation of insulin receptor substrates that uncouple insulin receptors from downstream targets. Impaired insulin receptor signaling results in diminished transcription of critical gene products (GLUT4 protein) essential for proper plasma membrane internalization and processing of glucose. Dysfunctional lipid or glucose metabolism (free fatty acids, glycosphingolipids) may ultimately be responsible for impaired insulin receptor signaling. Notably, there has been a rise in type 2 diabetic symptoms in adolescents worldwide, correlating with a change in diet as Western fast-food culture becomes more prevalent.

BIOCHEMISTRY

Sites of Insulin Action

Insulin facilitates glucose utilization by the following mechanisms:
- Increasing glucose uptake by peripheral tissues
- Increasing glycogen synthesis, thereby decreasing gluconeogenesis in the liver
- Increasing lipogenesis, decreasing lipolysis in adipose tissue
- Increasing protein synthesis in muscle

●●● PANCREATIC DISORDERS

Diabetes Mellitus

Insulin, Sulfonylureas and Meglitinides, Biguanides and Thiazolidinediones, and α-Glucosidase Inhibitors

Diabetes mellitus is the inability to properly manage glucose metabolism (glucose intolerance) because of either the inability to produce and secrete insulin as a result of autoimmune destruction of pancreatic β-cells (type 1) or the inability of peripheral tissues to respond to circulating insulin as a result of diminished or impaired insulin receptor signaling (type 2).

For the most part, patients with type 1 diabetes are managed by insulin replacement therapy and diet, whereas patients with type 2 diabetes are initially managed by diet and oral agents that improve insulin secretion or insulin sensitivity. Because elevated glucose levels progressively damage pancreatic β-cells, patients with type 2 diabetes often are subsequently managed with insulin therapy.

A multiplicity of interconnected metabolic disorders is ultimately responsible for the high morbidity and mortality rates of uncontrolled diabetes. Insulin deficiency and insulin resistance both lead to hyperglycemia. Hyperlipidemia and hypertension are often accompanying problems that must be addressed. Tight glucose control is known to reduce both microvascular and macrovascular diabetic complications (e.g., neuropathies, gastroparesis, paresthesias). However, tight glucose control also increases the risk of hypoglycemic events.

Patients with type 1 diabetes have polyuria, nocturia, polydipsia, unexplained weight loss, weakness, and dry skin. In contrast, patients with type 2 diabetes are often obese and have increased appetite, blurred vision, frequent urinary tract infections, and numbness or tingling in extremities (peripheral neuropathy).

CLINICAL MEDICINE

Monitoring of Patients with Diabetes

A fasting glucose plasma concentration greater than 126 mg/dL is diagnostic of diabetes. A postprandial glucose level greater than 200 mg/dL after a glucose tolerance test (ingestion of 75 g of glucose) is also consistent with diabetes. Glucose levels greater than 180 mg/dL can result in urinary glucose excretion.

In addition to plasma or urinary glucose determination, glycosylated hemoglobin can be used for long-term monitoring of diabetic patients. Intermittent diabetic screenings should be initiated in patients older than 30 years who are at risk for diabetes (e.g., those who are obese, have a family history of diabetes, belong to a high-risk population, or are hypertensive or hyperlipidemic).

Many devices are being developed for noninvasive blood glucose testing to minimize the pain and inconvenience of routinely checking plasma glucose concentrations. In addition to insulin and proper control of blood sugar, tight blood pressure management and cholesterol control are important. Aggressive blood pressure control reduces adverse cardiovascular events and decreases the risk of macrovascular diabetic complications. Many patients with type 2 diabetes are also given angiotensin-converting enzyme inhibitors for renal protection and β-blockers and statins for cardiovascular protection.

Insulin

Insulin is administered subcutaneously via multiple formulations in patients with type 1 diabetes and in approximately 30% of patients with type 2 diabetes who are insulin dependent because of progressive dysfunction of pancreatic β-cells.

Differences between insulin formulations are largely pharmacokinetic. There are synthetic insulin formulations that cover ranges of action from 3 to 24 hours. Rapid or short-acting formulations are taken with meals (lispro, aspart, glulisine), in contrast to intermediate- and long-acting preparations (detimer, glargine) that are used to manage glucose throughout the day. These synthetic insulins have one or two amino acid changes that keep insulin in a monomeric state (lispro), increase absorption (aspart), diminish degradation (detemir, glargine), or lead to faster onset of action (lispro, aspart, glulisine) compared with regular (natural or unadulterated) insulin. Some formulations of insulin contain protamine and zinc or acetate to prolong duration of action. Allergic reactions may develop to protamine. In contrast to the subcutaneous formulations previously mentioned, regular insulin can be administered intravenously as well. The major adverse reaction to all insulin formulations is hypoglycemia, which is associated with sweating, tachycardia, palpitations, tremors, confusion, and seizures. Immediate ingestion of sugar (glucose tablets) can resolve symptoms within 15 minutes. Weight gain is a long-term adverse effect associated with increased insulin levels because insulin is lipogenic (promotes fat storage).

Oral Agents for Type 2 Diabetes

Patients with type 2 diabetes are managed pharmacologically by the following actions:

- Increasing pancreatic insulin secretion with sulfonylureas or meglitinides
- Decreasing hepatic gluconeogenesis with biguanides
- Improving insulin sensitivity in peripheral tissues with thiazolidinediones
- Preventing breakdown of complex carbohydrates into simple sugars with α-glucosidase inhibitors

Sulfonylureas and Meglitinides

Examples of sulfonylureas include glyburide, glipizide, and glimepiride. Meglitinides include repaglinide and nateglinide.

The mechanism of action of both sulfonylureas and meglitinides is to inhibit adenosine triphosphate–dependent K^+ channels in pancreatic β-cells, which results in membrane depolarization and subsequent calcium influx. This calcium influx leads to augmented insulin release in functional β-cells (Fig. 12-8A). These drugs are known as *insulin secretogogues*.

Glyburide, glipizide, and glimepiride are second-generation sulfonylureas. Initially, 60% to 70% of patients respond to sulfonylureas, but many patients develop secondary pancreatic β-cell failure. As with insulin therapy, the major adverse side effect of sulfonylureas is hypoglycemia. Other common adverse effects include nausea, vomiting, dyspepsia, pruritus, erythema, urticaria, and skin rash.

Meglitinides prescribed for patients with type 2 diabetes include repaglinide and nateglinide. The main difference between sulfonylureas and meglitinides is that meglitinides have a rapid onset of action as well as a short duration of activity. This makes meglitinides ideal for patients with postprandial hyperglycemia. Thus these drugs are taken just before meals to reduce postprandial hyperglycemia. Note that if a meal is skipped, the drugs should be skipped as well. Hypoglycemia is the most common adverse effect but occurs less often than with sulfonylureas. Because meglitinides do not contain a sulfa chemical moiety, they can be taken by patients with sulfa allergies.

Because repaglinide is extensively metabolized by the cytochrome P450 3A4 isotype, drugs that induce or inhibit this P450 should be avoided or closely monitored. Specifically, drugs that inhibit P450 3A4 (e.g., azoles, erythromycin, fluoxetine, paroxetine, cimetidine, protease inhibitors, gemfibrozil) can increase the risk of repaglinide-induced hypoglycemia. In contrast, drugs that induce P450 3A4 transcription (e.g., rifampin, barbiturates, carbamazepine, phenytoin, St. John's wort) can reduce the therapeutic efficacy of repaglinide.

Biguanides

Metformin. The major mechanism of action for biguanides is inhibition of hepatic glucose production. These drugs may also decrease intestinal glucose absorption and increase peripheral insulin sensitivity. They are first-line agents in obese patients with type 2 diabetes. Unlike sulfonylureas, which promote weight gain (by increasing insulin levels), biguanides

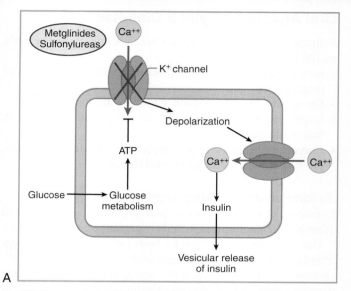

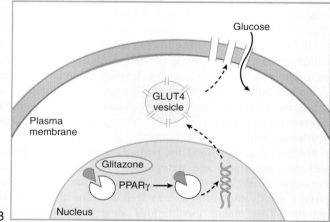

Figure 12-8. A, Mechanism of action for sulfonylureas and metglinides. These insulin secretagogues increase β-cell insulin secretion by inactivating adenosine triphosphate (*ATP*)-dependent potassium channels, which leads to depolarization, influx of Ca⁺⁺, and resultant enhanced insulin secretion. **B,** Mechanism of action for thiazolidinediones. These glitazone drugs (pioglitazone and rosiglitazone) activate the peroxisome proliferator-activated receptor-γ (*PPARγ*), a nuclear receptor found in adipose, skeletal muscle, and liver. PPARγ activates transcription of insulin-response genes that control glucose and lipid metabolism as well as synthesis of the glucose transporter, GLUT4. Newly transcribed and translated GLUT4 is packaged within vesicles for insertion into the plasma membrane. Functional GLUT4 reduces insulin resistance in muscle by increasing glucose uptake, thereby removing glucose from the circulation.

may promote weight loss. Metformin is a biguanide and is often used in combination with sulfonylureas for maximal effectiveness. The major adverse effect associated with metformin is diarrhea and other GI distress. Lactic acidosis also is a concern, and the drug should be avoided by those at risk (those with acutely decompensated congestive heart failure, renal or liver disease, or alcoholism; those who are older than 80 years of age; those who have been given radiologic contrast media).

Thiazolidinediones
Pioglitazone and Rosiglitazone

Thiazolidinediones are a great example of how target identification has led to a group of useful drugs. Peroxisome proliferator-activated receptor-γ (PPARγ) is a nuclear receptor and transcriptional regulator for insulin-responsive genes that control glucose and lipid metabolism (see Fig. 12-8B). Thus therapeutics that selectively activate PPARγ can be used to bypass dysfunctional insulin receptors by transcribing more GLUT-4 receptors. Specifically, pioglitazone and rosiglitazone reduce blood glucose levels by decreasing insulin resistance in skeletal muscle and adipose tissues. Drugs that activate PPARγ increase expression of GLUT4, the transporter that moves glucose into cells. Thiazolidinediones can be used as a monotherapy along with diet and exercise for patients with type 2 diabetes. In addition, thiazolidinediones are often combined with sulfonylureas and biguanides but must be used cautiously with insulin; this combination may cause fluid retention and congestive heart failure. As a bonus, pioglitazone reduces triglyceride levels while elevating high-density lipoprotein.

α-Glucosidase Inhibitors
Acarbose and Miglitol

The α-glucosidase inhibitors, such as acarbose and miglitol, delay the breakdown of ingested complex carbohydrates into glucose by inhibiting α-glucosidase, an enzyme found within the brush border epithelium of the small intestine. These drugs are particularly useful to diminish postprandial hyperglycemia.

The major side effects of these drugs are GI because of their mechanism of action: diarrhea occurs from unabsorbed carbohydrates, abdominal pain, flatulence, and intestinal obstruction. Patients with concomitant inflammatory bowel disease should not use these drugs.

New Drugs for Diabetes

Pramlintide, Exenatide, Liraglutide, Sitagliptin, and Saxagliptin

As new targets (hormones and receptors) are discovered, new opportunities for drug therapies are created. Three new injectable biologics and new oral drugs have been approved for treating diabetes. Pramlintide can be used adjunctively for type 1 and type 2 diabetic patients. Pramlintide is a synthetic analog of amylin, a neuroendocrine hormone that boosts insulin secretion. Physiologically, amylin slows gastric emptying, suppresses glucagon secretion and postprandial hyperglycemia, and enhances satiety. Pramlintide allows insulin doses to be reduced. However, the risk of severe hypoglycemia is increased.

Exenatide and liraglutide are now approved for patients with type 2 diabetes. These biologics were developed after studying glucagon-like peptide-1 from the Gila monster. Exenatide and liraglutide are similar in function to the GI hormone glucagon-like peptide-1 and are referred to as an *incretin mimetics*. Incretin mimetics are hormones that increase insulin secretion. Exenatide and liraglutide stimulate release of insulin, slow gastric emptying, suppress glucagon secretion to reduce postprandial hyperglycemica, and may help restore satiety responses that are impaired in type 2 diabetics.

Adverse effects include nausea and bloating as a result of slowed gastroparesis. Pancreatitis has been reported with exenatide. Possible induction of thyroid C-cell tumors has been noted with liraglutide. Importantly, no other diabetic medications stimulate insulin secretion and induce weight loss. The recent discovery that incretins can be degraded by dipeptidylpeptidases has led to the development of orally administered dipeptidylpeptidase-4 antagonists (sitagliptin, saxagliptin) that slow the inactivation of natural incretins. Taken together, these are excellent examples of how biologic strategies (exenatide, liraglutide) as well as more traditional pharmaceutical development strategies (sitagliptin, saxagliptin) are being used for the same target (incretins).

CLINICAL MEDICINE

Diabetic Ketoacidosis

Patients with diabetes do not respond well to cortisol- or catecholamine-induced stress. When an insulin deficit is coupled with increased levels of a stress hormone and a precipitating factor (acute illness, surgery), the vicious cycle of diabetic ketoacidosis may begin.

Exacerbated hyperglycemia induces osmotic diuresis and dehydration. Insulin deficiency induces fat mobilization and release of fatty acids, which are oxidized to acidic ketones. Diminished glomerular filtration rate because of dehydration further worsens glucose and ketone elimination, worsening hyperosmolality. Osmotic diuresis also causes loss of potassium, sodium, phosphate, and bicarbonate. This hypovolemia decreases tissue perfusion, leading to lactic acid accumulation, which further worsens the ketoacidosis. Vomiting may result, which further exacerbates dehydration. This metabolic ketoacidosis leads to hyperventilation, known as *Kussmaul respirations* (shallow and fast breaths) as well as "acetone breath." Over time, Kussmaul breathing may reduce P_{CO_2} levels, leading to a compensatory respiratory alkalosis.

Diabetic ketoacidosis presents with lethargy, hyperventilation, tachycardia, fruity breath, altered mental status, nausea, thirst, decreased urine output (secondary to a decrease in glomerular filtration rate), and dry mucous membranes. Patients have elevated ketone levels as well as a significant anion gap. Patients require immediate treatment, including rehydration, rapid-onset forms of insulin, and careful management of electrolyte and acid-base balance. Typically, patients with type 1 diabetes mellitus are at risk of diabetic ketoacidosis.

COMPLEMENTARY AND ALTERNATIVE MEDICINE

Fenugreek is a cooking spice that is sometimes used therapeutically to enhance breast milk production. Hypoglycemic actions are possible, and the herbal product should be used cautiously by diabetics. In addition, the herb may have anticoagulation properties, which could be problematic in patients taking anticoagulants or those with bleeding disorders. Because fenugreek is a member of the legume family, there also is a theoretical risk of cross-hypersensitivity in patients who are allergic to peanuts.

St. John's wort is used by some women who experience mild depression at various times throughout their monthly cycles. However, drug interactions occur between this natural supplement and selective serotonin reuptake inhibitors, tricyclic antidepressants, monoamine oxidase inhibitors, L-tryptophan, and dopaminergic agonists, potentially leading to serotonin syndrome (confusion, agitation, fever, tremor, spasm).

Other alternative therapies used by some women include dong quai for controlling hot flashes and black cohosh for alleviating cramps, hot flashes, and vaginal dryness. These alternative therapies have adverse side effects. Dong quai has a laxative effect, may cause photosensitivity, and increases bleeding tendencies, whereas black cohosh may upset the stomach, and its long-term effects are unknown. Black cohosh should not be confused with blue cohosh, which is relatively toxic and induces uterine contractions or menstruation. Phytoestrogens from soy products (isoflavones) may also help hot flashes. Accepted therapies for treating premenstrual syndrome include aerobic exercise and calcium, magnesium, and vitamin E supplementation.

Many men treat benign prostatic hypertrophy with saw palmetto. The natural product seems to aid some in management of nocturia, weak urinary stream, and difficulty postponing the urge to urinate. However, despite its efficacy, prescription medications usually work better. Saw palmetto may increase the risk of bleeding in patients taking anticoagulants or antiplatelet agents.

TOP FIVE LIST

1. The anterior pituitary releases multiple factors that control growth (growth hormone), adrenal function (adrenocorticotropic hormone), thyroid function (thyroid-stimulating hormone), and reproductive organs (LH, FSH, prolactin). The posterior pituitary produces vasopressin (antidiuretic hormone) and oxytocin, which control fluid balance and labor, respectively.

2. Thyroid storm (thyrotoxicosis) can be managed with a combination of thionamides, β-blockers, aspirin, and corticosteroids.

3. For osteoporosis in women, SERMs, bisphosphonates, and calcium supplements may be safer treatments than traditional hormone replacement therapy, which can have significant cardiovascular side effects.

4. Preventing breakdown of cGMP with phosphodiesterase inhibitors is an effective therapy for erectile dysfunction.

5. Type 1 diabetes may be controlled by diet and insulin, whereas type 2 diabetes may be managed by a combination approach with sulfonylureas, meglitinides, biguanides, thiazolidinediones, α-glucosidase inhibitors, and incretin mimetics.

Self-assessment questions can be accessed at www. StudentConsult.com.

Central Nervous System 13

CONTENTS

CENTRAL NERVOUS SYSTEM PHARMACOLOGIC MOLECULAR TARGETS
ANESTHETICS
　Mechanisms of Anesthetic Action
　Inhalation Anesthetics
　Intravenous Anesthetics
　Local (Regional) Anesthesia
MUSCLE RELAXANTS
　Neuromuscular Blockers
　Spasmolytics
ANTICONVULSANTS
　Underlying Pathophysiology of Epilepsy
　Treatment of Seizure Disorders
ANTIDEPRESSANTS AND TREATMENT OF BIPOLAR DISORDER
　Biogenic Amine Theory of Affective Disorder
　Tricyclic Antidepressants
　Selective Serotonin Reuptake Inhibitors and Serotonin and Norepinephrine Reuptake Inhibitors
　Monoamine Oxidase Inhibitors
　Treatment of Mania and Bipolar Disorder
ANTIPSYCHOTICS
　Dopamine Hypothesis of Schizophrenia
　Antipsychotic Therapeutics
NEURODEGENERATION AND MOVEMENT DISORDERS
　Parkinson Disease
　Alzheimer Disease
　Multiple Sclerosis
　Huntington Chorea
OPIOIDS
　Endogenous Opioid System and Pain Management
　Opioid Analgesics
　Management of Migraine Headache Pain
SEDATIVE-HYPNOTIC AND ANXIOLYTIC AGENTS
　GABA Receptor Modulators
　Benzodiazepines
　Nonbenzodiazepine GABA$_A$ Receptor Modulators
　Barbiturates
　Other Anxiolytics
ABUSED RECREATIONAL DRUGS
　Abused Drugs as False Messengers
COMPLEMENTARY AND ALTERNATIVE MEDICINE
TOP FIVE LIST

This chapter is all about managing chemical imbalances in the brain. In most cases, neurologic and psychiatric disorders are the manifestation of perturbed neurochemical homeostasis. Unlike the autonomic nervous system, the CNS is not a simple organization. The autonomic nervous system is a simple opposition system in which the parasympathetic objective is "rest and digest," and the sympathetic is "fight or flight" (see Chapter 6). The central nervous system (CNS) in contrast, is complex and characterized by neurochemical nuances. The CNS, beyond its complex organization of billions of cells with a seemingly infinite number of connections, is noteworthy for its diverse number of neurotransmitter systems. There are more than 20 neurotransmitter systems and multiple receptors for each neurotransmitter. There is tremendous diversity in organization, structure, and function of the brain. When any one of the systems goes awry, it can be manifested as a distinct clinical entity—whether neurologic (epilepsy, Parkinson disease) or psychiatric (depression, Alzheimer disease). In many cases, the etiology (e.g., loss of nigrostriatal dopamine neurons in Parkinson disease) or underlying pathology is not known or understood (e.g., schizophrenia). However, years of clinical trial and error, as well as rational drug design, have brought us to the point of effective drug therapies. Although simplified, Table 13-1 provides an overview of key neurotransmitters in the CNS and clinical manifestations believed to occur as a result of chemical imbalances.

●●● CENTRAL NERVOUS SYSTEM PHARMACOLOGIC MOLECULAR TARGETS

As discussed in Chapters 2 and 6, a variety of molecular drug targets are composed of selective protein subtypes: ion channels, 7-transmembrane, G-protein–coupled receptors, neurotransmitter channels and signal transduction, and biosynthetic enzymes (Fig. 13-1). Because so many different types of molecular targets and diseases are of unknown etiology, CNS therapies generally treat the symptoms rather than the cause. In addition, selective receptor agonists have been developed to treat patients with one disorder, whereas selective receptor antagonists are used to treat patients with another disorder. For example, dopamine agonists are used for Parkinson disease, whereas dopamine antagonists are a central component of antipsychotic neuroleptic therapies.

TABLE 13-1. Simplified View of Chemical Imbalances in the Brain

NEUROTRANSMITTER	TOO MUCH	TOO LITTLE
Acetylcholine	Delirium/confusion, psychoses	Alzheimer disease
Dopamine	Psychoses, Tourette syndrome/tics, chorea	Parkinson disease, ADD/ADHD, depression
GABA	CNS depression, respiratory depression, sedation	Seizures, movement disorders
Glutamate	Seizures, neuronal degeneration	Schizophrenia, depression, cognitive impairment
Norepinephrine	Anxiety, panic, anorexia, excitability, insomnia	Depression, ADD/ADHD
Serotonin	Sleep, hallucinations, decreased appetite, anxiety	Depression, OCD, pain sensitivity, anxiety

ADD, attention deficit disorder; *ADHD*, attention deficit–hyperactivity disorder; *CNS*, central nervous system; *GABA*, γ-aminobutyric acid; *OCD*, obsessive-compulsive disorder.

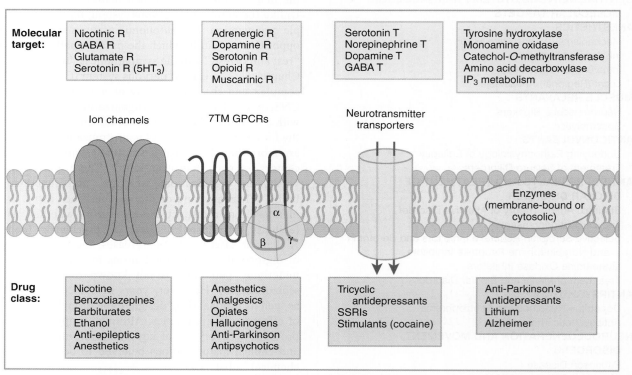

Figure 13-1. Drugs and molecular targets in the central nervous system. This figure summarizes the receptors, channels, transporters, and enzymes that are subject to regulation in central nervous system disorders. Specific pharmacologic classes are listed at the bottom. Note that in the case of ion channels, the channel itself is the receptor and binding of the ligand modulates the channel. *R,* receptor; *T,* transporter. *GABA,* γ-aminobutyric acid; *IP₃,* inositol triphosphate; *SSRIs,* selective serotonin reuptake inhibitors.

Alternatively, it also is common to tackle a given CNS disorder with drugs having widely disparate mechanisms of action. As an example, both barbiturates and inhalant anesthetics are used as general anesthetics despite the fact that these are two distinct and seemingly independent classes of compounds. Finally, it will come as no surprise that many of these compounds produce untoward side effects. Adverse effects occur because receptors are widely distributed and serve not only different functions but also are differentially localized. Therefore patient compliance becomes an important factor in delivering pharmacologic therapies for CNS disorders.

Another important aspect of CNS pharmacotherapy is the balance between stimulation versus inhibition. This occurs at two levels—agonists versus antagonists—at any given receptor system. Indeed, this is a common theme throughout this text. However, opposing neuronal systems must be carefully balanced. This concept was first visited when considering the autonomic nervous system and the opposing sympathetic and parasympathetic pathways (see Chapter 6). The same concept applies in the CNS. For example, γ-aminobutyric acid (GABA) is the major inhibitory neurotransmitter in the brain. This is opposed, in large measure, by excitatory glutamatergic systems (where glutamate is the neurotransmitter). Therefore pharmacotherapeutic approaches must balance the therapeutic and toxicologic aspects of disrupting this delicate relationship.

●●● ANESTHETICS

Mechanisms of Anesthetic Action

Anesthesia is all about excitable membranes. Given that nerve activity, pain, the autonomic nervous system, voluntary muscle control, involuntary muscle reaction (twitching, spinal reflex), and conscious thought all depend on membrane depolarization, they can all be regulated by common drugs. Therefore if membrane biophysics are interfered with, an altered state will be created—figuratively and literally. As a result, the field of anesthesia is designed around decreasing membrane reactivity in such a way as to decrease pain or reduce consciousness, all without decreasing bodily processes to the point at which the patient no longer breathes.

The central intent of general anesthesia is to create a reversible surgical state characterized by loss of consciousness and pain sensation (or involuntary response). In practice, this is accomplished in two general ways—through inhalation agents (anesthetic gases) and intravenous agents (predominantly GABA modulators). The mechanisms of action of the general anesthetics have been a point of contention since the first public demonstration of ether anesthesia in 1846. Until recently, it was assumed that these agents nonspecifically modulated membrane fluidity characteristics and so stabilized membrane activity—inhibiting action potentials. Of course, molecular biology and signal transduction pathways provide more satisfying and physiologic mechanisms. There is growing evidence that whatever their mechanism of action, anesthetics work by modulating ligand-gated ion channels (see Fig. 13-1) either by activating GABA channels (hyperpolarizing cells) or by blocking excitatory receptors (such as N-methyl-D-aspartate [NMDA]-glutamate receptors).

Inhalation Anesthetics

Desflurane, Isoflurane, Nitrous Oxide, and Sevoflurane

Note that most of these drug names end in "-ane."

Inhalation anesthetics are represented by the prototypical halogenated hydrocarbons halothane, desflurane, sevoflurane, and isoflurane (Table 13-2). (Early general anesthetics such as ether [which is highly flammable] and chloroform [which has toxic properties] are no longer used as general anesthetics. The same is true of halothane—the prototype of this class of agents.) The use of general anesthetics is driven by two important concepts—minimum alveolar concentration (MAC) and the blood/gas partition coefficient. MAC is the concentration of anesthetic agent that renders 50% of patients immobile during surgery. As noted in Table 13-2, this is measured as the percentage of the agent in inspired air. MAC is a direct measure of the potency of a drug. This is therefore the value considered in choosing the dose for administration. MAC is influenced by the age and physiologic state of the patient and by the presence of other pharmacologic agents. In fact, although nitrous oxide produces only weak anesthetic effects, it is widely used adjunctively for its "second gas" effect to enhance coadministered anesthetic agents.

The blood/gas partition coefficient is a function of solubility of the agent in blood and is a measure of how quickly the inhalation anesthetic equilibrates between the lungs and blood and ultimately the target site in the brain. Therefore an agent with a low blood/gas coefficient (e.g., desflurane) equilibrates quickly because it prefers to be in the gas phase. The blood/gas coefficient is *inversely* related to the rate of induction of anesthesia and recovery from anesthesia. In other words, the lower the blood/gas coefficient, the faster the induction and the faster the recovery. Keep in mind that there are other important partitioning coefficients (such as the blood/fat ratio) that determine the long-term fate of an agent (volume of distribution). Similarly, the rate of metabolism is an important factor. All inhalational general anesthetics decrease blood pressure, depress ventilatory responses to CO_2, increase intracranial pressure, and relax skeletal muscles.

Nitrous oxide is a weak anesthetic agent. To induce general anesthesia as a single agent would require high concentrations (essentially >100%) of nitrous oxide, which are possible only under hyperbaric conditions. It is used frequently in outpatient dentistry because it provides analgesia and sedation at concentrations that can be reached under normal atmospheric pressure.

TABLE 13-2. Inhalation Anesthetic Agents

DRUG	MOA	MAC	BLOOD/GAS COEFFICIENT	SIDE EFFECT	COMMENT
Desflurane	Ion channels	6.0	0.45	↓ BP	Rapid onset and recovery
Enflurane	Ion channels	1.6	1.8	↓ BP	Reduced use in recent years
Halothane	Ion channels	0.75	2.3	↓ BP	Malignant hyperthermia; tolerated by children; bronchodilator; metabolized by cytochrome P450; hepatitis
Isoflurane	Ion channels	1.2	1.4	↓ BP	Widely used
Sevoflurane	Ion channels	2.0	0.65	↓ BP	Rapid onset and recovery; tolerated by children; bronchodilator

MOA, mechanism of action; *MAC*, minimum alveolar concentration; *BP*, blood pressure.

ANATOMY

Effects of Anesthesia on Nerve Fibers

Recall that nerve fibers come in a variety of types based on size and function (A, B, and C fibers). Local anesthetics are particularly safe and efficacious because they target the smaller fibers (Aδ, B, and C fibers) that are responsible for sensory (pain, temperature) and autonomic functions without affecting motor functions and proprioception (Aα, Aβ, and Aγ). This is why people can chew after dental procedures but cannot feel anything.

Intravenous Anesthetics

Ketamine, Methohexital, Propofol, and Thiopental

Parenteral anesthetics (Table 13-3) are noteworthy in that they are administered intravenously and act quickly. In addition, in nearly all cases, their mechanisms of action are more precisely characterized because they have known binding sites on ligand-gated ion channels (Fig. 13-2). The predominant class is the barbiturates (thiopental, methohexital). These agents work by enhancing GABA-stimulated Cl⁻ channel activity. These Cl⁻ channels (GABA ligand-gated Cl⁻ channel; see Fig. 13-2) open and lead to an influx of Cl⁻ that inhibits neuronal firing.

Although the precise mechanism of action of propofol is unknown, this agent is also believed to work through GABA receptors. Propofol has a fast onset of action and a fast recovery time with less of a "hangover" effect than that of barbiturates. This property is useful for outpatient surgery because it allows patients to be discharged rapidly. Another advantage of propofol is its antiemetic properties, which make it a good choice for patients at risk of postoperative nausea and vomiting. The propofol emulsion contains egg phospholipids and is contraindicated in patients with known hypersensitivity. This white emulsion is facetiously termed "milk of amnesia." Thiopental and propofol are the two commonly used intravenous anesthetics. Etomidate, as with propofol, has a rapid onset and

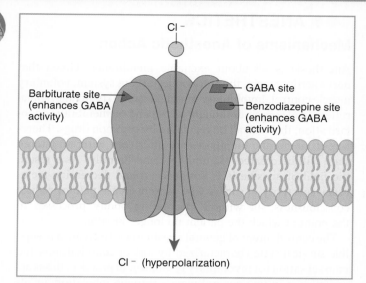

Figure 13-2. γ-Aminobutyric acid (*GABA*)-stimulated Cl⁻ channel. The GABA receptor is a ligand-gated Cl⁻ channel. Stimulation of this receptor leads to opening of the channel and the subsequent rush of Cl⁻ into the cell. This flow of Cl⁻ down its concentration gradient (into the cell) causes hyperpolarization of the cell and inhibits cell firing. In addition to a GABA binding site, the GABA receptor contains a benzodiazepine binding site as well as an independent binding site for barbiturate. Indeed, current thinking suggests a direct interaction between ethanol and the GABA receptor. Given the central importance of GABA as a central nervous system inhibitory neurotransmitter, it is not surprising that regulation of the GABA receptor is a key therapeutic strategy (anxiolytics, sedative-hypnotics, anesthetics, antiepileptics).

short duration; however, it *increases* blood pressure, making it useful for patients at risk for hypotension.

Unlike the parenteral agents that stimulate GABA receptors, ketamine is a dissociative anesthetic that binds to the phencyclidine (PCP) binding site on the NMDA-type glutamate receptor. Ketamine blocks (antagonizes) this stimulatory ion channel receptor. Indeed, ketamine is a version of

TABLE 13-3. Parenteral Anesthetics

DRUG	MECHANISM OF ACTION	SIDE EFFECT AND COMMENTS
Thiopental	Barbiturate ↑ GABA receptor activity	In common use ↓ Cerebral metabolic rate ↓ BP and respiration
Methohexital	Barbiturate ↑ GABA receptor activity	↓ Cerebral metabolic rate ↓ BP and respiration
Propofol	Nonbarbiturate ↑ GABA activity ↓ Glutamate activity	In common use Rapid onset and recovery Antiemetic
Etomidate	↑ GABA receptor activity	↑ BP (choice for patients at risk for hypotension) Ultra short acting
Ketamine	Blocks glutamate (NMDA receptor)	Selected pediatric uses Delirium during postoperative recovery (dissociative anesthetic)

GABA, γ-aminobutyric acid; *BP*, blood pressure; *NMDA*, N-methyl-ᴅ-aspartate.

PCP ("angel dust") and can elicit delirium (hallucinations) and vivid dreams during recovery. It also has a strong amnesic effect. Ketamine causes less respiratory depression than do other general anesthetics and stimulates heart rate, blood pressure, and cardiac output by sympathomimetic actions. These properties are useful in patients at risk for hypotension but not for the patient at risk of myocardial infarction. Ketamine also is advantageous because of its inherent analgesic properties. Ketamine has significant abuse potential. Ketamine also is frequently used for its anesthetic and analgesic effects on dogs, cats, rabbits, and other small animals.

Local (Regional) Anesthesia

Benzocaine, Bupivacaine, Cocaine, and Lidocaine

Local anesthesia is accomplished through agents such as lidocaine, bupivacaine, and cocaine by administration directly to the site where the action is needed. They act via direct interactions with voltage-gated Na^+ channels responsible for action potentials. In fact, one of their key characteristics is that they are readily ionizable compounds (weak bases) that cross cell membranes in the uncharged state, become protonated (and stuck) inside the cells, and interact with an intracellular component of Na^+ channels. Thus local anesthetics reversibly block action potentials responsible for nerve conduction. Although lidocaine and bupivacaine are the two most widely used clinical agents, other local anesthetics have unique characteristics. Indeed, cocaine remains a commonly used drug for nasal surgery because of its anesthetic and vasoconstrictive effects. Benzocaine is a prototypical over-the-counter local anesthetic that is used for such varied applications as hemorrhoidal itching and oral pain (toothache or teething).

●●● MUSCLE RELAXANTS

A key problem in general anesthesia is achieving a *depth* of anesthesia that not only removes consciousness but also prevents reflex muscle responses (reflex twitching) during surgery. Unfortunately, this muscle paralysis is one of the last effects achieved by general anesthesia and can require doses approaching toxic levels. To address these concerns, muscle relaxants (neuromuscular blockers) are used as adjuvants to anesthesia. This permits the use of lower (and safer) concentrations of general anesthetic during surgery. Similarly, these agents may be used to achieve flaccid paralysis in cases of assisted ventilation.

Neuromuscular Blockers

Atracurium, Mivacurium, Pancuronium, Succinylcholine, Tubocurarine, and Vecuronium

Recall from Chapter 6 that the neuromuscular junction (NMJ) is controlled by the somatic nervous system and acetylcholine-releasing nerves. In fact, as previously discussed, the nicotinic acetylcholine receptor at the NMJ is amenable to selective pharmacologic manipulation.

Surgical paralysis can be achieved through two approaches: competitive inhibition with NMJ nicotinic receptor antagonists (tubocurarine, atracurium, and vecuronium) or depolarization blockade with succinylcholine (Table 13-4). The first approach uses curare derivatives. Curare is a mixture of plant alkaloids containing the prototypical compound D-tubocurarine. These paralytic drugs work by competitive antagonism of the NMJ nicotinic receptor. Because of the side effects associated with first-generation drugs, they have largely been replaced by short-acting versions (atracurium and vecuronium).

The second approach to adjuvant paralysis makes use of succinylcholine. This agent is actually an agonist that leads to depolarization blockade and paralysis. This counterintuitive concept is worthy of brief discussion. As with acetylcholine, succinylcholine binds to the NMJ nicotinic receptor and stimulates muscle contraction. However, unlike acetylcholine, it is not degraded as rapidly and so remains in the synapse and *overstimulates* the receptor. The NMJ nicotinic receptor is unique in that it is exquisitely sensitive to overstimulation and responds by desensitizing—essentially shutting down as the receptors desensitize. Therefore the succinylcholine agonist provides a short-term phase I activation of the NMJ that can lead to muscle fasciculations. This is rapidly followed by a phase II desensitization characterized by flaccid paralysis. The advantage of this approach is that it is short acting and readily reversed. This is another example of the importance of receptor theory (receptor desensitization; see Chapter 2) having direct clinical relevance.

TABLE 13-4. Neuromuscular Blockade

DRUG	MECHANISM OF ACTION	COMMENT
Succinylcholine	Depolarization blockade; phases I and II	Fundamentally different mechanism of action (compared with curare-like drugs)—overstimulates receptor first, then desensitizes the receptor Very short duration
Atracurium	Competitive nicotinic blockade	Short duration of action
Pancuronium	Competitive nicotinic blockade	Long duration
Vecuronium	Competitive nicotinic blockade	Long duration
Mivacurium	Competitive nicotinic blockade	Very short duration

Spasmolytics

Baclofen, Dantrolene, and Diazepam

An important aspect of anesthesia involves the need for spasmolytics—agents to block muscle contraction directly—in the case of malignant hyperthermia. Malignant hyperthermia is a genetic defect that is uncovered during inhalant anesthesia (it was particularly problematic with halothane, an agent that has now largely been supplanted by other agents). It appears to lead to a situation in which Ca^{++} is released from the sarcoplasmic reticulum and not sequestered. Therefore the muscle cannot stop contracting. This leads to very high O_2 consumption and a lethal elevation in body temperature. Because it is not mediated by nerve signals, it cannot be prevented by classic NMJ blockade. Therefore it requires the use of an agent that acts directly on muscle—dantrolene. Dantrolene blocks the release of Ca^{++} from the sarcoplasmic reticulum and thereby prevents the malignant hyperthermia. Other agents that can be used as spasmolytics include diazepam (a $GABA_A$ agonist) and baclofen (a $GABA_B$ agonist). As a word of caution, dantrolene is extremely hepatotoxic. Another common clinical indication for antispasmodics is the use of botulinum toxin for cosmetic purposes (antiwrinkle) and spasticity associated with multiple sclerosis, cerebral palsy, and dystonias. In this case, botulinum toxin works by poisoning the nerves and disrupting acetylcholine release (by blocking vesicle trafficking to the plasma membrane).

●●● ANTICONVULSANTS

Underlying Pathophysiology of Epilepsy

Epilepsy is a disorder of the cerebral cortex characterized by intermittent, unpredictable, and repeated seizures. The seizure is an uncontrollable coordinated firing of neurons. In fact, the seizure is the physical manifestation of abnormal electrical activity in the brain. This activity can be manifested in a variety of ways but is most commonly thought of—by the general patient population, at least—as the tonic-clonic twitching of a grand mal episode. Interestingly, certain types of medications may contribute to seizures by lowering the seizure threshold, including antipsychotics, antidepressants, analgesics, some antibiotics, and bowel preparations that alter electrolyte balance.

Treatment of Seizure Disorders

Carbamazepine, Clonazepam, Diazepam, Ethosuximide, Gabapentin, Lacosamide, Lamotrigine, Levetiracetam, Oxcarbazepine, Phenobarbital, Phenytoin, Pregabalin, Rufinamide, Tiagabine, Topiramate, Valproic Acid, Vigabatrin, and Zonisamide

Epilepsy is treated with four general approaches that all work by inhibiting neuronal firing. The difficulty is controlling unregulated impulses without generating the types of inhibitions that produce anesthesia. Current therapeutic approaches focus on (1) blocking Na^+ channels, (2) blocking Ca^{++} channels, (3) antagonizing excitatory glutamate receptors, and (4) enhancing GABA activity. However, the precise mechanisms of action vary among the drugs (Figure 13-3). In fact, some compounds undoubtedly act in multiple ways.

Most of the first-line antiepileptic drugs act by slowing channel function. Notably, carbamazepine, lacosamide, lamotrigine, oxcarbazepine, phenytoin, rufinamide, topiramate, valproic acid, and zonisamide work by slowing the reversal of Na^+ channel inactivation (after depolarization). This effectively hyperpolarizes cells and slows their activity.

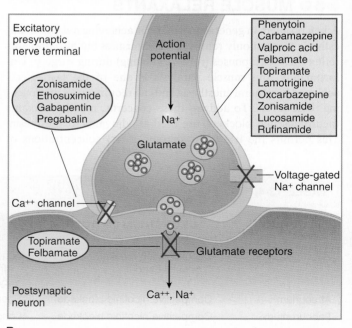

A   B

Figure 13-3. Mechanisms for antiepileptic drugs. Note that many of these drugs are thought to have multiple mechanisms of action. *GAD*, glutamic acid decarboxylase. *GABA*, γ-aminobutyric acid.

Carbamazepine has some unique pharmacokinetic properties that are noteworthy given its widespread use. Food enhances its bioavailability, and absorption is variable. In addition, it is not only rapidly metabolized by hepatic P450 enzymes to an active metabolite, oxcarbazepine, but it is also a hepatic P450 auto-inducer—that is, it induces its own metabolism. Drug interactions are frequent, and side effects are numerous. Phenytoin, in spite of a similar mechanism of action, has unique characteristics. Dissolution is the primary rate-limiting step, and absorption varies by manufacturer and formulation. It has a variable metabolism because it is metabolized by zero-order kinetics—as with alcohol, a constant amount of drug is metabolized per unit time—the concept of half-life ($t_{1/2}$) cannot be applied. When the dose of phenytoin increases, the time for drug elimination increases proportionally. Predictable dose-dependent side effects include nystagmus, ataxia, and altered mental status. Idiosyncratic side effects include drowsiness, lethargy, acne, and peripheral neuropathies. A signature side effect is gingival hyperplasia, the overgrowth of tissues of the gums. Drug interactions are also common. Lamotrigine antagonizes glutamate excitatory neurotransmitter activity (by blocking Na^+ channels). This decreases the excitatory tone in the CNS. The largest drawback to lamotrigine is a potentially fatal rash (Stevens-Johnson syndrome).

CLINICAL MEDICINE

Seizures

Seizures are more than the prototypical grand mal episode. For instance, seizures are categorized as *partial* (originating from a single part of the cortex) and *generalized* (involving widespread parts of the brain in both hemispheres). The hallmark of the partial seizure is that it does not include loss of consciousness. Within this categorization scheme are a number of types of seizures. These include the tonic-clonic grand mal and petit mal or absence seizures (generalized). In addition, more discrete disorders include simple and complex partial seizures (focal disturbances—motor, sensory, speech, or affective disorders).

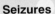

Topiramate and valproate not only block Na^+ channels but also facilitate GABA activity. Topiramate can cause CNS side effects at high doses (ataxia, confusion) and can produce kidney stones (careful hydration is required) as well as myopia and glaucoma. Valproate is confusing because it has multiple sites of action; it is reported to be an inhibitor of the GABA transaminase (increasing GABAergic tone), a blocker of Na^+ channels, as well as a potential inhibitor of Ca^{++} channels. Pharmacologically, valproate is important because it is an inhibitor of hepatic P450 enzymes. This may lead to potential severe drug interactions. It also has certain gastrointestinal and CNS effects on its own.

Ethosuximide, zonisamide, and, to a lesser extent, valproic acid block Ca^{++} channels (T currents) in the thalamus. Thalamic activity is thought to contribute in a substantive way to absence seizures. Note that the dual-channel activity of valproic acid (Na^+ and Ca^{++} channels) may explain its broad spectrum of activity (Table 13-5). Ethosuximide is a

CLINICAL MEDICINE

Treatment for Epilepsy

Many health issues should be addressed in patients taking antiepileptic drugs. Bone density may be reduced in drugs that induce hepatic P450 microsomal enzymes (carbamazepine, phenytoin, phenobarbital, oxcarbazepine, topiramate). Patients, especially women, taking these drugs should take calcium and vitamin D supplements because some antiepileptic drugs interfere with vitamin D metabolism. In addition, antiepileptic drugs that induce cytochrome P450s reduce the efficacy of many other drugs, including oral contraceptives. Combinations of antiepilepsy medications often are required to suppress seizures.

drug of choice for absence seizures. Zonisamide may cause serious rashes, kidney stones, and hyperthermia. It is also contraindicated in patients with known sensitivity to sulfa drugs.

Finally, as discussed in "Sedative-Hypnotic and Anxiolytic Agents" below, the primary inhibitory system in the brain is mediated by GABA. Therefore drugs that enhance GABA activity tend to suppress seizure activity. Prototypical agents are the barbiturates (e.g., phenobarbital) and benzodiazepines (e.g., diazepam, clonazepam) that enhance GABA receptor activity (they are allosteric activators of the GABA receptor). These actions increase Cl^- conductance and hyperpolarize neurons. In addition, newer agents such as gabapentin and tiagabine work by enhancing GABA activity. Gabapentin is well tolerated with few drug interactions and is also used for many other approved and unlabeled indications: to treat nerve pain, as a mood stabilizer, for migraine prevention, and for preventing menopausal hot flashes. A structural analog of gabapentin, pregabalin, has been approved for treatment of partial seizures and neuropathic pain. Tiagabine inhibits reuptake of GABA, thereby enhancing synaptic inhibitory activity. As with gabapentin, tiagabine is well tolerated; unlike gabapentin, it is sensitive to drugs that induce P450 enzymes as well as to displacement by drugs that are highly protein bound. An additional therapeutic target is GABA transaminase—the enzyme responsible for destroying GABA. This enzyme is inhibited by both valproic acid and vigabatrin. Vigabatrin is a structural analog of GABA and, through GABA transaminase inhibition, blocks GABA metabolism. As a result, levels of the inhibitory GABA neurotransmitter are increased.

Levetiracetam has a fundamentally different mechanism of action from any of the other antiepilepsy medications. This drug does not modulate any known inhibitory (GABAergic) or excitatory (Na^+ channel, glutamate) systems. Although its mechanism of action is unknown, it does bind to a novel presynaptic protein that may be involved in vesicle trafficking. Lacosamide, in addition to its ability to slow Na^+ channels, exhibits another novel mechanism of action. By binding to collapsin response mediator protein-2, a phosphoprotein involved in neuronal differentiation and axonal growth, lacosamide may be an alternative to patients who do not tolerate or respond to other antiepileptics.

TABLE 13-5. Antiepileptic Drugs

DRUG	MECHANISM OF ACTION	INDICATION	SIDE EFFECTS/NOTES
Carbamazepine	Blocks Na$^+$ channel	Partial and generalized seizures	CNS depression; teratogenic; hepatotoxic; P450 inducer
Oxcarbazepine	Blocks Na$^+$ channel; metabolite of carbamazepine	Partial seizures	Less induction of P450s compared with carbamazepine; hyponatremia
Valproic acid	Blocks Na$^+$ channel Blocks GABA transaminase May block Ca^{++} channel	Widely used; broad range of clinical indications	GI distress; hepatotoxicity; teratogenic; inhibits drug metabolism
Vigabatrin	Analog of GABA that irreversibly inhibits GABA transaminase, thereby slowing GABA degradation	Partial seizures and infantile spasms	Vision impairment/loss; only available through specialized program
Rufinamide	Blocks Na$^+$ channel	Broad spectrum seizures associated with Lennox-Gastaut syndrome in children	CNS depression (somnolence, fatigue, coordination difficulties), shortening of QT interval, multiorgan hypersensitivity
Ethosuximide	Blocks Ca^{++} channel	Absence seizures	GI distress
Phenobarbital	Potentiates GABA activity	Generalized and partial seizures	CNS depression; induces P450s; abuse potential
Phenytoin	Blocks Na$^+$ channel	Psychomotor and generalized seizures	CNS depression; hepatotoxicity; gingival hyperplasia; teratogenic; induces P450s
Gabapentin	Potentiates GABA activity	Partial seizures	Sedation
Pregabalin	Analog of gabapentin	Partial seizures and neuropathic pain	
Lamotrigine	Blocks Na$^+$ channel Blocks glutamate release	Generalized and partial seizures	Sedation; hepatotoxicity; severe rash
Topiramate	Blocks glutamate receptor Blocks Na$^+$ channel Enhances GABA activity	Partial and generalized seizures	Sedation; nervousness; ocular effects; hyperthermia (children); metabolic acidosis
Tiagabine	Potentiates GABA activity by blocking GABA reuptake	Partial seizures	Dizziness; tremor
Zonisamide	Blocks Na$^+$ and Ca^{++} channels	Partial seizures	Well tolerated; somnolence; ataxia; hyperthermia (children); contraindicated in sulfonamide allergies
Levetiracetam	Unknown MOA but binds to a presynaptic vesicle protein	Partial seizures	Well tolerated; lack of energy; behavioral problems
Lacosamide	Block Na$^+$ channel and CRMP-2	Partial seizures	Dizziness, ataxia, euphoria-type reactions, prolonged PR interval on electrocardiograms, delayed multi-organ hypersensitivity, psychologic dependence

CNS, central nervous system; *GABA*, γ-aminobutyric acid; *GI*, gastrointestinal; *MOA*, mechanism of action; *CRMP*, collapsin response mediator protein-2.

●●● ANTIDEPRESSANTS AND TREATMENT OF BIPOLAR DISORDER

Biogenic Amine Theory of Affective Disorder

On the basis of current effective treatments (tricyclic antidepressants and selective serotonin reuptake inhibitors), the biogenic amine theory of affective disorders has been developed. The basic concept is that decreases in norepinephrine and serotonin activities within the CNS are responsible for the psychiatric disorder. The theory is noteworthy because most effective therapies for depression *do not* modulate dopamine activity. This is in contrast to the antipsychotic agents that focus on dopamine (discussed later).

CLINICAL MEDICINE

Mood Disorders

Affective (mood) disorders include mania and depression (anxiety is covered in a separate section). *Depression*, by itself, is characterized by an altered state with decreased mood (melancholy, despondency) or inability to derive pleasure in everyday activities (anhedonia). This can also include, among other things, decreased appetite, feelings of worthlessness,

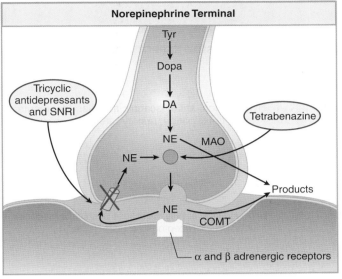

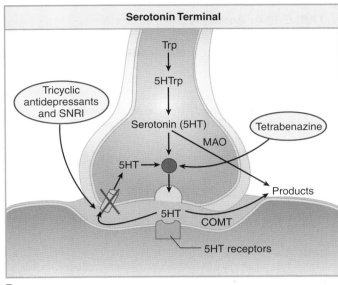

A

B

Figure 13-4. Biogenic amine reuptake inhibitors. Antidepressants (and selected psychomotor stimulants) act by blocking reuptake of biogenic amines (serotonin[*5HT*], norepinephrine[*NE*], and dopamine[*DA*]) into the nerve terminal. This increases the levels of synaptic neurotransmitter and enhances neuronal activity. The tricyclic antidepressants block both norepinephrine and serotonin transporters, while the selective serotonin reuptake inhibitors; (*SSRIs*) show a preference for serotonin transporter. Stimulants such as cocaine and amphetamine work on all biogenic amine transporters (dopamine, norepinephrine/epinephrine, and serotonin transporters) but exert their reinforcing effects by blocking the dopamine transporter or reversing this transporter to allow the passive flow of dopamine from the cell, respectively. Other centrally acting drugs (anti-Parkinson drugs) work by inhibiting the metabolism of the biogenic amines by monoamine oxidase [*MAO*] and catechol-*O*-methyltransferase (*COMT*). *dopa*, dihydroxyphenylalanine; *5HTrp*, 5-hydroxytryptophan; *Trp*, tryptophan; *Tyr*, tyrosine; *SNRI*, selective norepinephrine reuptake inhibitor.

and suicidal ideation. On the other hand, *mania* is characterized by a combination of euphoric mood, uncontrolled speech, and psychomotor agitation. This can also include inflated self-esteem, lack of intellectual and cognitive focus, and wild flights of fancy. In keeping with the notion that mania and depression seem to be at opposite ends of a behavioral spectrum, there is a clinical disease, known as *bipolar disorder*, in which a single patient cycles between the two states.

Tricyclic Antidepressants

Amitriptyline, Amoxapine, Desipramine, Doxepin, Imipramine, Maprotiline, Nortriptyline, and Trazodone

Given the prevailing biogenic amine hypothesis for depression, all effective therapeutics modulate the metabolism of dopamine, norepinephrine, and serotonin (Fig. 13-4). Historically, first-generation antidepressants were the tricyclics—so-named for their common three-ringed chemical structures (Table 13-6). (Be aware that there are also tricyclic antipsychotic drugs such as the phenothiazines [e.g., chlorpromazine, thioridazine]. This unfortunate dual nomenclature can lead to confusion, although the term *tricyclic* is most commonly reserved for antidepressants.)

BIOCHEMISTRY

Biogenic Amines

Recall from Chapter 6 that the catecholamines (dopamine, norepinephrine, and epinephrine) are all derived from the same precursor—the amino acid tyrosine. Therefore different cells in the CNS express different aspects of the biosynthetic pathway and can be characterized as either dopaminergic, noradrenergic (norepinephrine containing), or adrenergic. In a related biosynthetic pathway, another aromatic amino acid, tryptophan, can be used to synthesize the neurotransmitter serotonin. Collectively, these neurotransmitters (along with histamine) are known as the *biogenic amines*.

The prototype tricyclic antidepressant is imipramine. This compound acts by blocking the reuptake of norepinephrine and serotonin into their respective nerve terminals. As a result, the actions of the neurotransmitters are prolonged within the synapse. Related therapeutic agents are amitriptyline, amoxapine, desipramine, doxepin, maprotiline, and nortriptyline. The tricyclic antidepressants are important pharmacotherapeutics for several reasons. First, they are beneficial treatments for major depression. Second, tricyclic antidepressants are useful for many other conditions, including nerve pain, headache, panic disorders, eating disorders, and enuresis. Third, they have marked side

TABLE 13-6. Antidepressant Drugs

DRUG	MECHANISM OF ACTION	INDICATION	SIDE EFFECTS/COMMENT
Tertiary Amine			
Imipramine (desipramine is a metabolic product) Amitriptyline (nortriptyline is a metabolic product) Doxepin	Tricyclic antidepressant; blocks amine reuptake	Depression	Hypotension, antimuscarinic activities (dry mouth/eyes, constipation, urinary retention, nausea)
Triazolopyridine			
Trazodone	Blocks amine reuptake	Depression	No muscarinic activity; can cause priapism; antagonist at histamine receptor so causes sedation
SSRIs			
Citalopram (escitalopram is a metabolic product)	Inhibit serotonin reuptake	Depression	Generally safer than tricyclics; nausea, vomiting, sexual dysfunction
Fluoxetine		Depression	
Sertraline		Depression	
Fluvoxamine		OCD	
Paroxetine			
NE/serotonin selective			
Duloxetine Venlafaxine	Inhibit NE and serotonin reuptake	Depression Neuropathic pain	Increases blood pressure; hepatitis, cholestatic jaundice
Desvenlafaxine			Increases blood pressure
Aminoketone			
Bupropion	Inhibit NE and DA (no serotonin) reuptake	Depression	Lowest incidence of sexual side effects; agitation, anorexia, insomnia; lowers seizure threshold
MAO Inhibitor			
Phenelzine	MAO inhibitor	Depression	Risk of hypertensive crisis with tyramine-containing foods, dizziness, drowsiness, agitation, nausea

SSRI, selective serotonin reuptake inhibitor; *OCD*, obsessive-compulsive disorder; *NE*, norepinephrine; *DA*, dopamine; *MAO*, monoamine oxidase.

effects because of their mechanisms of action. Because they have a broad binding spectrum (most have antimuscarinic activities in addition to their reuptake blockade profile), as well as the potential to block norepinephrine reuptake in the peripheral (sympathetic) nervous system (see Chapter 6), they can elicit unwanted autonomic effects. In fact, the side effects represent a major obstacle to patient compliance. Potential adverse effects include (among the most severe) orthostatic hypotension, Na^+ channel blockade (cardiac conduction delays), tachycardia, palpitations, seizures, and sedation. There are also many minor side effects (anticholinergic side effects) associated with blockade of muscarinic receptors. Moreover, the tricyclic antidepressants have strong—and predictable—interactions with a variety of other pharmacotherapeutic agents. Because they block the reuptake of neurotransmitters, they work synergistically with noradrenergic and serotonergic agents (direct agonists) and with modulators of biogenic

amine metabolism (see "Monoamine Oxidase Inhibitors" below). In addition, there are additive adverse effects with other drugs that exhibit pharmacologically similar properties (e.g., sedation, cardiac conduction blockade). In spite of these concerns, the drugs remain efficacious. Although the tricyclic antidepressants have similar therapeutic efficacy, they have differing pharmacokinetic characteristics that make each uniquely valuable for individual patients.

Another commonly used antidepressant with a mechanism similar to the tricyclics but whose chemical structure is markedly distinct is trazodone. In addition to inhibiting norepinephrine and serotonin reuptake, trazodone also acts as an antagonist at histamine receptors. This property causes sedation and is useful for treating depression with an anxiety component. As an adverse effect, trazodone may cause priapism (painful and persistent erection of the penis).

Selective Serotonin Reuptake Inhibitors and Serotonin and Norepinephrine Reuptake Inhibitors

Citalopram, Desvenlafaxine, Duloxetine, Escitalopram, Fluoxetine, Fluvoxamine, Milnacipran, Paroxetine, Sertraline, Venlafaxine, and Bupropion (a Dopamine and Norepinephrine Uptake Inhibitor)

Unlike the tricyclic antidepressants, which block norepinephrine and serotonin uptake, selective serotonin reuptake inhibitors (SSRIs) block serotonin reuptake (see Fig. 13-4) with essentially no activity toward norepinephrine and dopamine. As a result, they have few side effects and a favorable therapeutic index. Related compounds in this family of SSRIs are fluoxetine, citalopram, escitalopram, venlafaxine, desvenlafaxine, sertraline, fluvoxamine, and paroxetine (see Table 13-6). They all share the favorable features of fluoxetine with varying pharmacokinetic profiles. An unexplained feature of antidepressants is the observation that it can take 2 to 3 weeks to obtain effective treatment of the depression. Although the reasons for this remain obscure, they surely involve an adaptation or remodeling of neuronal activity. SSRIs are no more efficacious than tricyclic antidepressants; however, SSRIs are generally safer and have fewer side effects. It is important, though, to slowly taper SSRIs to avoid withdrawal symptoms that can worsen underlying depression or cause mania to emerge. Withdrawal symptoms are most likely to occur after rapid discontinuation of short-acting SSRIs (i.e., paroxetine) and often resemble influenza (Box 13-1).

Of note, serotonin is not the complete story; later generation molecules (e.g., venlafaxine, duloxetine, desvenlafaxine) are aimed at inhibiting both serotonin and norepinephrine, subsequently termed serotonin and norepinephrine reuptake inhibitors. Although venlafaxine displays some selectivity for serotonin, duloxetine is almost equally balanced between the two neurotransmitters. Desvenlafaxine, the latest addition to this class, is the major active metabolite of venlafaxine and displays similar efficacy and potency compared with its parent compound. Adverse effects include nausea, insomnia, sexual dysfunction, fatigue, and elevated blood pressure.

Indeed, in terms of the serotonin role, it is now clear that the antidepressant bupropion has little activity at the serotonin transporter and relatively weak activity at the norepinephrine and dopamine transporters. Bupropion has few significant drug interactions, may be efficacious in patients who have not responded to SSRIs, and is not associated with sexual dysfunction.

However, bupropion lowers the seizure threshold and should not be used when there is a history of recent head injury or epilepsy. As an aside, bupropion is an example of a drug that was "repackaged" by the pharmaceutical industry for a different clinical indication. In this case, bupropion is also used to reduce craving in patients attempting to stop smoking.

In addition, a handful of antidepressants have shown benefit in patients with fibromyalgia and were "repackaged" for that indication as well. Duloxetine has a Food and Drug Administration–approved indication for pain associated with fibromyalgia, although fluoxetine, venlafaxine, and amitriptyline are also used off-label for this condition. A new drug released exclusively for fibromyalgia, milnacipran, is actually a selective norepinephrine reuptake inhibitor with a three times greater selectivity for norepinephrine reuptake inhibition over serotonin reuptake inhibition. Given its mechanism, milnacipran acts similarly to antidepressants, although the drug does not have Food and Drug Administration approval for this latter use in the United States. It is, however, approved for use in fibromyalgia.

Monoamine Oxidase Inhibitors

Phenelzine and Tranylcypromine

As noted in Chapter 6 and Figure 13-4, the primary mechanism for intracellular degradation of catecholamines (dopamine, norepinephrine, and epinephrine) and serotonin is accomplished through the activity of monoamine oxidase (MAO; primarily the MAO-A isoform in the case of norepinephrine and serotonin in the CNS). (Note that the MAO-B isoform, a dopamine-selective enzyme, is a pharmacotherapeutic target in Parkinson disease—through the use of selegiline.) Irreversible inhibition of the MAO-A enzyme by phenelzine leads to an increase in intracellular concentrations of primarily norepinephrine and serotonin. This can then "leak" out of the nerve terminal and increase synaptic concentrations of neurotransmitter. These drugs are not first-line therapies because MAO-A is also needed to break down other compounds, most notably tyramine. Tyramine is found in cheeses, red wines, avocados, chocolate, and many other foods (Box 13-2). Ingestion of these foods leads to a dramatic rise in tyramine (which is metabolized into a norepinephrine-like molecule), and indirectly produces sympathomimetic symptoms (e.g., hypertension, tachycardia, stroke). Numerous foods are contraindicated in patients taking MAO inhibitors because of the risk of tyramine-induced hypertensive crisis. In addition, there are numerous medication restrictions for patients taking MAO

Box 13-1. SYMPTOMS ASSOCIATED WITH RAPID WITHDRAWAL OF SELECTIVE SEROTONIN REUPTAKE INHIBITORS (MNEMONIC: FLUSH)

Flulike symptoms: fatigue, diarrhea, nausea, diaphoresis
Lightheadedness
Uneasiness, restlessness
Sleep, sensory disturbances
Headache

Box 13-2. FOODS CONTAINING TYRAMINE

Fermented foods (e.g., cheese, yogurt, sour cream, sauerkraut)
Wine and beer
Chocolate and coffee
Preserved fish (sardines, anchovies, herring)
Dried fruits
Avocado

Box 13-3. DRUGS CONTRAINDICATED WHILE TAKING MONOAMINE OXIDASE INHIBITORS

Amphetamines	Levodopa
Appetite suppressants	Local anesthetics containing
Asthma inhalants	sympathomimetic
Buspirone	vasoconstrictors
Cocaine	Meperidine
Cyclobenzaprine	Methyldopa
Decongestants	Methylphenidate
Dextromethorphan	Other antidepressants
Dopamine	Reserpine
Ephedrine	Stimulants
Epinephrine	Sympathomimetics
Guanethidine	Tryptophan

inhibitors because any drug that enhances central activity of norepinephrine, dopamine, or serotonin may cause hypertensive crisis or serotonin syndrome (Box 13-3).

CLINICAL MEDICINE

Serotonin Syndrome

Serotonin syndrome is a hyperserotonergic state that is potentially fatal and is caused by serotonin-enhancing drugs (generally a combination of two or more drugs). The syndrome manifests with a variety of psychiatric and nonpsychiatric symptoms, including euphoria, drowsiness, rapid eye movements, hyperreflexia, clumsiness, restlessness, feeling drunk and dizzy, contraction and relaxation of the jaw, sweating, intoxication, muscle twitching, rigidity, high body temperature, mental status changes, shivering, diarrhea, loss of consciousness, and death.

Treatment of Mania and Bipolar Disorder

Lithium

Lithium is given for mood *stabilization*. Bipolar disorder is characterized by mood swings—mania to depression. Treatment with traditional antidepressants is not effective (and is contraindicated) because it can trigger hypermania. Fortuitously, it was discovered that treatment with lithium salts (mainly lithium carbonate) is efficacious in managing mood swings. Until recently, lithium's mechanism of action was obscure, but it is now known that it blocks the key bioactive lipid second messenger inositol trisphosphate (IP_3). Specifically, it blocks the dephosphorylation of inositol monophosphate, which is an obligatory step in regenerating the precursor to IP_3 (Fig. 13-5).

Cleavage of phosphatidylinositol bisphosphate is triggered by G-protein–coupled receptors coupled to phospholipase C, such as those found throughout the brain. Therefore inhibition of IP_3 metabolism would be expected to have widespread effects on numerous systems (including neuronal activity). How this stabilizes mood is unknown, but it is clear that lithium has a narrow therapeutic window with a wide range of side effects. Early and usually transient adverse effects include vomiting, diarrhea,

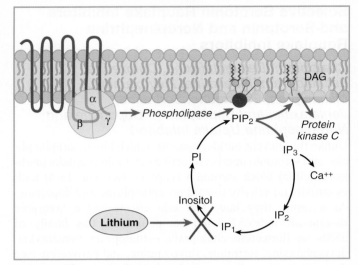

Figure 13-5. Site of action of lithium.

tremor, muscle weakness, and lethargy. Long-term adverse effects include diabetes insipidus, hypothyroidism, and cardiac abnormalities. Lithium is also the subject of many drug-drug interactions and is teratogenic. Because the therapeutic index of lithium is so narrow, its concentrations in the blood must be monitored to achieve optimal steady-state concentration. Likewise, thyroid function, complete blood count, creatinine, and cardiac function should be checked at baseline and monitored periodically.

BIOCHEMISTRY

Phosphatidylinositol Bisphosphate

The cleavage of phosphatidylinositol bisphosphate by phospholipase C yields diacylglycerol and IP_3. IP_3 triggers the release of Ca^{++}, which activates Ca^{++}-dependent protein kinases—calcium/calmodulin-dependent protein kinase II. Diacylglycerol is a regulator of lipid-dependent protein kinases (known as *PKCs*).

Interestingly, the mixed-function antipsychotic, aripiprazole (dopamine D_2 antagonist, serotonin $5HT_2$ antagonist, and partial agonist at D_2 and $5HT_{1A}$; described in detail in the following section), has been approved for treatment of the manic phase of bipolar disorder. This agent has been described as being "functionally selective" because it has varying activities depending on the specific cell it is acting upon. Because of this variability, it may be beneficial in patients who have not responded to other therapeutic approaches.

●●● ANTIPSYCHOTICS

Psychoses are mental disturbances of perceived reality, cognition, and diminished mood. *Schizophrenia* is the prototypical disorder that has positive and negative attributes—these represent gain or loss of function, respectively, rather than desirable or undesirable traits. Positive symptoms include hallucinations, bizarre behaviors, and delusions. Negative symptoms include diminished speech, blunted affect, and anhedonia (lack of interest in pleasurable activities). It is important to realize, however, that all psychoses are not schizophrenia and aspects of this disorder can be observed in drug abuse as well as in Alzheimer disease.

Dopamine Hypothesis of Schizophrenia

Based on the pharmacologic profiles of first-generation treatments for psychoses (the neuroleptic tricyclic antipsychotics such as chlorpromazine and thioridazine), the hypothesis was developed that schizophrenia is the outward manifestation of an overactive dopamine system, possibly overactivity within the mesolimbic or mesocortical regions of the brain (Table 13-7 and Fig. 13-6). Dopamine receptors are represented by five gene products, D_1 through D_5. However, they are classified into two functional groups: the D_1 class (D_1 and D_5) and the D_2 class (D_2, D_3, and D_4). In particular, agents that antagonize or block dopamine receptors (particularly the D_2 receptor class—D_2, D_3, and D_4) are effective treatments for this disorder (Table 13-8). In addition, agents that stimulate dopamine receptors or otherwise enhance its actions (e.g., cocaine) can lead to psychotic symptoms or exacerbate schizophrenic symptoms. Although this notion certainly has merit, it is clearly simplistic in its scope. Newer generation drugs target serotonergic receptors (particularly the $5HT_2$ receptor) and are clinically efficacious. The older term *neuroleptic* refers to the ability of these drugs to reduce spontaneous activity and excessive behaviors. In addition, the ability of these agents to reduce initiative, diminish emotion, and blunt affect also resulted in their early classification as *tranquilizers*. It is now clear, however, given their range of activities, that these drugs are more appropriately referred to as *antipsychotics*.

Antipsychotic Therapeutics

Aripiprazole, Asenapine, Chlorpromazine, Clozapine, Fluphenazine, Haloperidol, Iloperidone, Olanzapine, Paliperidone, Prochlorperazine, Quetiapine, Risperidone, Thioridazine, and Ziprasidone

First-generation antipsychotic compounds are essentially drugs that block dopamine D_2-type receptors. Prototypes include haloperidol and the phenothiazines (chlorpromazine, fluphenazine, prochlorperazine, and thioridazine; also known as *tricyclic antipsychotic drugs*). As previously mentioned, however, newer, "atypical" antipsychotics (clozapine, olanzapine, risperidone, ziprasidone, and quetiapine) display less antidopaminergic activity and exhibit preference for serotonin 2A ($5HT_{2A}$; 5-hydroxytryptamine 2A) receptor antagonism.

Typical antipsychotic drugs tend to be effective in reducing the positive symptoms of schizophrenia. That is, they blunt some of the "gained" symptoms such as hallucinations and delusions. Although this helps the patient return to societal relationships, it may not alleviate the anhedonia (inability to feel pleasure) and depression-like characteristics of the negative symptoms. The *atypical* antipsychotics, on the other hand, are more effective for alleviating both the positive and the negative symptoms of schizophrenia. Antipsychotics, like antidepressants, can require weeks before clinical efficacy is achieved. Antagonists such as the traditional first-generation phenothiazines and haloperidol antagonists can have profound side effects (see Table 13-8). On the dopamine side, antagonism blocks essential nigrostriatal communications and can lead to extrapyramidal side effects similar to symptoms of Parkinson disease (see "Neurodegeneration and Movement Disorders"). Extrapyramidal reactions—dystonias (trismus, glossospasm, oculogyric crisis,

TABLE 13-7. Actions of Central Dopamine Pathways

DOPAMINE TRACT	ORIGIN	INNERVATION	FUNCTION	DOPAMINE ANTAGONIST EFFECTS
Nigrostriatal	Substantia nigra	Basal ganglia	Extrapyramidal system movement	Movement disorders (parkinsonism, tardive dyskinesia, extrapyramidal reactions)
Mesolimbic	Ventral tegmental area	Limbic areas Amygdala, olfactory tubercle	Arousal, memory Stimulus processing	Antipsychotic
		Septal nuclei, cingulate gyrus	Motivational behavior	
Mesocortical	Ventral tegmental area	Frontal and prefrontal cortex	Cognition, communication, social function, response to stress	Antipsychotic
Tuberoinfundibular	Arcuate nucleus of the hypothalamus	Dopamine acts on cells in the anterior pituitary	Regulates prolactin release	Increased prolactin release (galactorrhea, menstrual disorders)

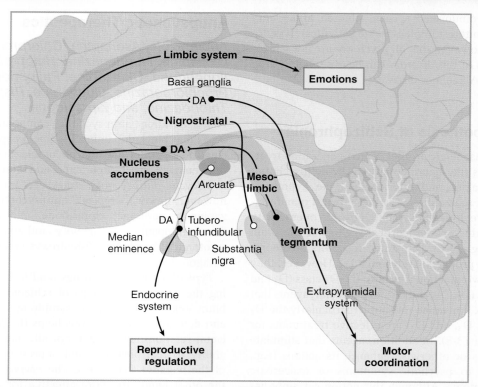

Figure 13-6. Dopaminergic pathways in the brain. The mesolimbic pathway is thought to be disrupted in schizophrenia. However, pharmacologic manipulations of the mesolimbic pathway can result in adverse effects within the nigrostriatal pathway (extrapyramidal movements) and the tuberoinfundibular pathway (galactorrhea, menstrual irregularities).

torticollis), paresthesias, pseudoparkinsonism, and even irreversible tardive dyskinesia—may occur as a result of the supersensitivity of blocked dopamine receptors. With the exception of tardive dyskinesia, most extrapyramidal side effects usually can be managed with antimuscarinics and antihistamines. Table 13-8 also details problems encountered with typical antipsychotics because of the "dirty" and nonselective nature of these compounds: antihistamine-like symptoms (sedation), atropine-like antimuscarinic actions (dry eyes/mouth, blurred vision, constipation, urinary retention), α-adrenergic blockade–induced orthostatic hypotension, and sedation.

Fortunately, newer *atypical* antipsychotics do not routinely cause movement disorders. However, these drugs come with their own unique adverse effects. Clozapine may cause agranulocytosis and therefore requires biweekly blood counts. All the atypical antipsychotic drugs (e.g., risperidone) are associated with stroke when used in the elderly (especially those with dementia). At high doses, risperidone has caused extrapyramidal effects; however, tardive dyskinesia has not proved to be a problem. Warnings have been added to the atypical antipsychotics concerning weight gain, development of diabetes, and unfavorable lipid profiles. Risperidone's major active metabolite paliperidone, which has been released as a drug in its own right, has been linked to QT prolongation but comes with a more tolerable metabolic profile than some of the other atypical antipsychotics. Similarly, ziprasidone prolongs the QT interval on electrocardiograms, but causes less

weight gain than other atypical antipsychotics. The newest additions to the antipsychotic armamentarium are iloperidone and asenapine. Iloperidone has less extrapyramidal effects compared with earlier agents but is associated with short-term weight gain and QT prolongation. Asenapine exhibits little to no effect on weight gain, diabetes risk, or dyslipidemias. Asenapine is available as a sublingual tablet and may be an option for patients with difficulty swallowing, although this formulation can cause a local anesthetic effect.

Aripiprazole, a drug said to be a "dopamine stabilizer," has a sufficiently different mechanism of action that it may be effective in some patients who have not responded to other therapies. Specifically, aripiprazole is a partial agonist at D_2 dopamine receptors and 5-HT_{1A} receptors but is an antagonist at 5-HT_2 receptors. In addition, aripiprazole is unlikely to prolong the QT interval substantially on electrocardiograms. It also produces little weight gain, dyslipidemia, or diabetes risk.

NEURODEGENERATION AND MOVEMENT DISORDERS

These disorders represent tremendous unmet medical needs. In the case of Parkinson disease, Huntington chorea, multiple sclerosis, and Alzheimer disease, partially effective therapies are available for treating symptoms, but the conditions cannot be cured.

TABLE 13-8. Antipsychotic Drugs

DRUG	MECHANISM OF ACTION*	INDICATION	SIDE EFFECTS/NOTES
Typical antipsychotics			
Butyrophenone			
Haloperidol	D_2	For all antipsychotics: Schizophrenia Acute psychotic illness (delirium) Severe agitation	All typical antipsychotics exhibit extrapyramidal side effects: acute dystonias, parkinsonism, neuroleptic malignant syndrome, tardive dyskinesia, motor restlessness, long-acting intramuscular injections available
Phenothiazines			
Chlorpromazine	$D2/5HT_2$		Less severe extrapyramidal side effects, antimuscarinic side effects, sedation, hypotension
Prochlorperazine	D_2	Effective for nausea and vomiting	Mild side effects, drowsiness
Fluphenazine	D_2		See haloperidol
Thioridazine	D_2		Less severe extrapyramidal side effects, antimuscarinic side effects, sedation, hypotension
Thioxanthene			
Thiothixene	D_2		Also used to treat intractable hiccups
Atypical antipsychotics			
Clozapine	$5HT_2/D_4$		Less severe extrapyramidal side effects, antimuscarinic side effects, sedation, hypotension, agranulocytosis, metabolic syndrome (weight gain, diabetes, lipid imbalances)
Olanzapine	$5HT_2/D_2$		Less severe extrapyramidal side effects, antimuscarinic side effects, elevates blood glucose, causes weight gain
Risperidone	$5HT_2/D_2$		Less severe extrapyramidal side effects
Ziprasidone	$5HT_2/D_2$		Less severe extrapyramidal side effects, sedation, rare increase in the cardiac QT interval, less weight gain than other atypical drugs
Quetiapine	$D_2 = 5HT_2$		Less severe extrapyramidal side effects, sedation, hypotension, cataracts
Aripiprazole	$D_2 = 5HT_{1A}$ agonist/$5HT_2$ antagonist		Hypotension, somnolence
Paliperidone	$D_2 = 5HT_2$		Less severe extrapyramidal side effects, somnolence, hyperprolactinemia, less metabolic effects
Iloperidone	$5HT_2/D_2$		Less severe extrapyramidal side effects, somnolence, dizziness, potential QT prolongation
Asenapine	$D_2 = 5HT_2$		Less severe extrapyramidal side effects, somnolence, oral hypoesthesia

*The order of the receptors reflects the drug's relative preference (the first receptor has the stronger affinity). All are receptor antagonists (except aripiprazole).
$5HT_2$, Serotonin.

Parkinson Disease

Apomorphine, Benztropine, Bromocriptine, Entacapone, Levodopa, Pergolide, Pramipexole, Rasagiline, Ropinirole, Rotigotine, Selegiline, Tolcapone, and Trihexyphenidyl

Parkinson disease is characterized by loss of dopaminergic neurons (Fig. 13-7) in the basal ganglia. The mainline treatments (Table 13-9) are based on the following actions:

- Replacing the lost dopamine with an excess of precursor (levodopa)
- Directly stimulating dopamine receptors with an agonist (bromocriptine, pergolide, ropinirole, pramipexole, rotigotine)
- Inhibiting dopamine breakdown (selegiline, rasagiline, tolcapone, entacapone)
- Blocking muscarinic activity (trihexyphenidyl, benztropine)

The logical treatment for Parkinson disease would be to administer dopamine. Unfortunately, dopamine does not cross the blood-brain barrier. Levodopa, however, does enter the brain and is the immediate precursor of dopamine synthesis (see Chapter 6). When administered, levodopa therefore increases dopamine content in surviving nigrostriatal neurons and alleviates the symptoms of lost neurons. However, levodopa has several significant problems. First, it is rapidly metabolized in the periphery by the amino acid decarboxylase. Therefore it is administered as a combination therapy with carbidopa—a potent decarboxylase inhibitor that does not cross the blood-brain barrier and does not affect CNS metabolism. Carbidopa prevents peripheral breakdown (or degradation) of levodopa, permitting more of it to enter the CNS. Second, levodopa exhibits a short $t_{1/2}$. This causes patients to cycle between normal and parkinsonian states (the so-called *on-off phenomenon*). Third, levodopa therapy has a limited lifetime of effectiveness (generally less than 5 years). This is probably due to continuing loss of nigrostriatal neurons to the point where there is no remaining neuronal infrastructure for converting levodopa to dopamine and subsequently releasing the neurotransmitter. It has been hypothesized that the degradation of dopamine generates free radicals that may contribute to oxidative damage and neuronal loss in the nigrostriatal regions. Dose-limiting toxicities include dyskinesia (aberrant and uncontrollable movements), nausea, and psychosis (hallucinations and confusion).

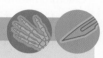

ANATOMY & PATHOLOGY

Parkinson Disease

Parkinson disease is characterized by a specific loss of dopaminergic neurons originating in the substantia nigra. The etiology of the disease is unknown but is believed to involve oxidative stress (perhaps caused by reactive O_2 species originating from the breakdown of dopamine) as well as environmental factors. These neurons, projecting to the corpus striatum, are responsible for modulating movement (in a tonic fashion). Sadly, disease symptoms do not occur until more than 80% of neurons have died, limiting treatment options and long-term prognosis.

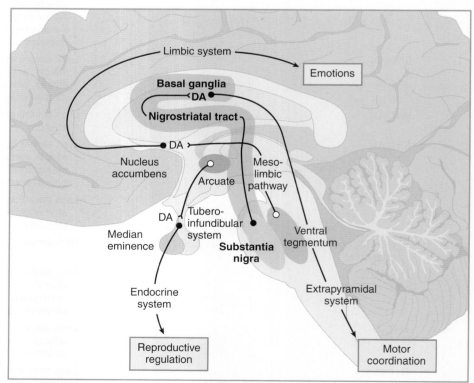

Figure 13-7. Dopaminergic (*DA*) pathways disrupted in Parkinson disease. Drugs that treat Parkinson disease facilitate actions of dopamine in the nigrostriatal tract. Adverse effects of these drugs are due to their nonspecific actions in the mesolimbic/mesocortical pathways (psychosis, hallucinations).

TABLE 13-9. Drugs for Treatment of Parkinson Disease

DRUG	MECHANISM OF ACTION	SIDE EFFECTS/COMMENT
Levodopa	DA precursor	Administered in combination with peripheral decarboxylase inhibitor (carbidopa); fluctuations in clinical response, nausea, hallucinations and confusion in the elderly
Bromocriptine	Partial DA agonist	Hypertension, nausea, fatigue
Pergolide	DA agonist (D_1/D_2)	Hypertension, nausea, fatigue
Ropinirole	DA agonist (D_2-selective)	Well tolerated, nausea, fatigue
Pramipexole	DA agonist (D_2-selective)	Well tolerated, nausea, fatigue
Rotigotine	DA agonist (D_2-selective)	Well tolerated, nausea, fatigue
Selegiline	MAO-B inhibitor	May enhance adverse levodopa reactions in patients with advanced disease; anxiety, insomnia
Rasagiline	MAO-B inhibitor	May enhance adverse levodopa reactions in patients with advanced disease; anxiety, insomnia
Entacapone/tolcapone	COMT inhibitors	Rare but severe liver problems with tolcapone; nausea, dizziness, drowsiness
Trihexyphenidyl	Muscarinic receptor antagonist	Limited utility; antimuscarinic side effects, sedation, mental confusion
Benztropine	Muscarinic receptor antagonist	Limited utility, antimuscarinic side effects, sedation, mental confusion

DA, dopamine; *MAO*, monoamine oxidase; *COMT*, catechol-*O*-methyltransferase.

The direct dopamine agonists offer an alternative to levodopa therapy for maintaining dopaminergic tone. Bromocriptine and pergolide are prototypical agents. Bromocriptine is a D_2 receptor agonist and a partial D_1 agonist. Because partial agonists do not elicit a full biologic response (they have reduced efficacy), they antagonize the full agonist potential of the endogenous dopamine. Pergolide is an agonist at both the D_1 and D_2 receptor subtypes. The later-generation agents ropinirole, pramipexole, and rotigotine are more selective for D_2 receptor subtypes. Because their duration of action is longer than that of levodopa, dopamine agonists may be beneficial for patients experiencing the "on-off" symptoms of levodopa. All these dopamine receptor agonists have troubling psychotic side effects, nausea, and fatigue as well as orthostatic hypertension. Recall that the antipsychotic agents work by blocking excess dopaminergic activity. Therefore it is not surprising that dopamine agonists can lead to psychotic side effects. The newer drugs (pramipexole, ropinirole, and rotigotine) exhibit more rapid onset kinetics and less gastrointestinal disturbance. They are limited, however, by the risk of producing sleep disorders (sudden sleep attacks). Pergolide may also cause damage to cardiac valves related to its cumulative dosage and duration of use.

The latest addition to clinical therapy for Parkinson disease is apomorphine. This drug, a dopamine receptor agonist, is said to be a rescue drug. It is used to treat "off" periods in patients who have been using standard dopamine agonist therapy for 3 to 5 years. Apomorphine is administered as a subcutaneous injection and works quickly—within 5 to 10 minutes. The drug is hampered by substantial nausea and vomiting as well as severe hypotension.

Inhibitors of dopamine metabolism are another potential treatment for Parkinson disease. Just as carbidopa inhibits levodopa metabolism, tolcapone and entacapone (inhibitors of catechol-*O*-methyltransferase) and selegiline and rasagiline (MAO-B inhibitors) block the degradative metabolism of dopamine (see Fig. 13-4). These drugs, then, increase the $t_{1/2}$ of the neurotransmitter in synapses. The side effects for tolcapone are similar to the levodopa/carbidopa combination: nausea, orthostatic hypertension, and psychotic episodes. Tolcapone is noteworthy for causing hepatotoxicity, an adverse event that is much less problematic with entacapone. Selegiline targets the dopamine-selective MAO-B and may have neuroprotective antioxidant effects. Importantly, selegiline and rasagiline lack the peripheral side effects of the MAO-A inhibitors (MAO-A selectively breaks down serotonin, epinephrine, and norepinephrine, so its inhibition is associated with serotonin syndrome and/or hypertensive crisis). Taken together, all the drugs that prevent dopamine breakdown are used to extend the actions of levodopa to prevent the end-of-dose wearing-off effect and lower the levodopa dose.

Finally, Parkinson disease can be treated with anticholinergic agents. The rationale is that symptoms of the disease are manifested when the loss of dopaminergic neurons creates unopposed cholinergic activity within the striatum. Therefore some therapies target this cholinergic activity with anticholinergics such as trihexyphenidyl or benztropine. These compounds have modest clinical utility and are limited by considerable antimuscarinic side effects (sedation, urinary retention, blurred vision, and confusion). These therapies are effective for treating parkinsonian tremor, especially early in therapy when symptoms are mild. Although numerous drugs possess anticholinergic properties, only those that cross the blood-brain barrier are effective treatments for Parkinson disease.

As a clinical correlate, a number of drug therapies elicit Parkinson-like symptoms when administered in excessive concentrations. Noteworthy are typical antipsychotics, such as haloperidol and fluphenazine. As previously explained, typical antipsychotics work by blocking dopamine receptors (predominantly D_2). At sufficient concentrations, dopaminergic blockade begins to resemble the loss of neurons typical of Parkinson disease. Care, then, must be taken to monitor doses and side effects for patients receiving antipsychotic therapy.

Alzheimer Disease

Donepezil, Galantamine, Rivastigmine, and Tacrine (Acetylcholinesterase Inhibitors), and Memantine (NMDA Receptor Antagonist)

Alzheimer disease is characterized by a progressive loss of cognitive function. Neuropathologically, this disorder is defined by the deposition of insoluble extracellular protein deposits (plaques composed of aggregates of β-amyloid) and formation of intracellular neurofibrillary tangles composed of the filamentous tau (τ) protein. There are currently no effective treatments for Alzheimer disease. However, based on the observation that the earliest neurotransmitter lost appears to be acetylcholine, some therapies are aimed at increasing acetylcholine. Specifically, four inhibitors of acetylcholinesterase are approved for use in patients with Alzheimer disease: tacrine, donepezil, rivastigmine, and galantamine (Table 13-10). These drugs are relatively selective for the CNS form of acetylcholinesterase and are also used to improve cognitive function in patients with vascular dementia (e.g., for strokes or transient ischemic attacks). However, when these drugs do improve cognition in Alzheimer patients, they only modestly extend the period of independent living and treat the symptoms, not the underlying cause of the disease. Moreover, based on their mechanism (cholinesterase inhibition) they can elicit effects similar to SLUD syndrome (*s*alivation, *l*acrimation, *u*rination, and *d*efecation) discussed in Chapter 6. Of the group, tacrine is associated with hepatotoxicity and is rarely used.

Memantine is unique among the drugs used to manage Alzheimer disease in that it is an NMDA receptor antagonist. Because it has been postulated that overexcitation of glutamate may play a role in Alzheimer disease, memantine may prevent adverse effects associated with abnormal glutamate transmission. It has been beneficial for even advanced forms of Alzheimer disease and is better tolerated than cholinesterase inhibitors.

TABLE 13-10. Acetylcholinesterase Inhibitors for Treatment of Alzheimer Disease

DRUG	COMMENT
Donepezil	Nausea, vomiting, diarrhea, insomnia; however, best tolerated drug
Rivastigmine	Nausea, vomiting, diarrhea, insomnia
Galantamine	Nausea, vomiting, diarrhea, insomnia
Tacrine	Not widely used because of dose-limiting side effects: gastrointestinal disturbances, anorexia, nausea, vomiting, diarrhea, potential hepatotoxicity

Multiple Sclerosis

Interferon-β, Glatiramer, and Natalizumab

Multiple sclerosis is an autoimmune disease characterized by loss of the myelin sheath (inflammatory demyelination) that surrounds axons in the CNS. Demyelination disrupts transmission of nerve impulses, leading to a host of symptoms, including weakness in the limbs, abnormal gait, and incoordination. Therapies are limited. During acute attacks, corticosteroids may be used.

To prevent relapses and progression of the disease, three different immunomodulatory drugs may be used: interferon-β_{1a}/interferon-β_{1b}, glatiramer, or natalizumab. These drug types are administered subcutaneously or intramuscularly. Although the precise mechanism of the interferons is unknown, numerous immunomodulatory actions have been suggested. Adverse effects of interferons resemble flulike symptoms (fever, chills, myalgias), which can be minimized by pretreatment with acetaminophen. Shortness of breath and tachycardia may also occur. Unfortunately, neutralizing antibodies to the interferons develop quickly and may negate their benefit. Glatiramer is an intriguing compound in that it is a synthetic polypeptide composed of the precise amino acid sequence of myelin basic protein targeted by the immune system of patients with multiple sclerosis. This creates a situation in which the pharmacologic therapy mimics the antigenic properties of myelin basic protein; therefore, in the presence of the drug, the immune system attacks the pharmacologic agent rather than the body. Adverse effects usually consist of irritation at the injection site, but systemic reactions (chest tightness, flushing, palpitations, dyspnea) may occur transiently within a few minutes postinjection. Neither of these therapies offers a cure, and benefits are relatively modest. Natalizumab is a new monoclonal antibody (humanized) directed against α_4-integrin, a cell surface protein that mediates adhesion of leukocytes to specific targets and facilitates white blood cell entry into the CNS. Although it is an attractive new approach, natalizumab carries a black box warning for its potential to cause progressive multifocal leukoencephalopathy.

Because multiple sclerosis takes its toll on numerous organ systems, pharmacologic therapies used to manage the many secondary symptoms of multiple sclerosis are shown in Table 13-11.

Huntington Chorea

Tetrabenazine

In 2008, tetrabenazine became the first drug approved for treating Huntington chorea. Huntington chorea is a rare inherited disorder characterized by disturbances of mood, memory, and jerky involuntary movements. The syndrome appears to be caused by excessive dopamine activity. Tetrabenazine reversibly inhibits the human vesicular monoamine transporter-2, resulting in depletion of the monoamines (including dopamine). Because of its effects on monoamines, tetrabenazine may increase the risk of depression and suicidality.

TABLE 13-11. Treatments for Conditions Associated with Multiple Sclerosis

SYMPTOM	DRUGS
Spasticity, gait difficulty	Baclofen, diazepam, dantrolene
Overactive bladder	Oxybutynin, tolterodine, desmopressin
Overactive bowel	Dicyclomine
Constipation	Fiber, fluids
Depression	Antidepressants
Paresthesias	Tricyclic antidepressants, carbamazepine

GENETICS

Huntington Chorea

Huntington chorea is a genetic disorder characterized by choreiform movements—abnormal voluntary movements (jerky motor incoordination). It is caused by the inheritance, in non-Mendelian fashion, of trinucleotide repeats in the protein Huntingtin. For reasons that remain obscure, this trinucleotide expansion (long tracts of glutamine residues) leads to selective loss of medium spiny neurons that project from the striatum to the globus pallidus. This leads to a loss of inhibitory activity and increased excitatory drive that promotes uncontrolled movements. Unfortunately, no drugs slow progression of this disease (death occurs within 15 to 20 years). In addition, only one drug effectively treats the movement symptoms because the loss of neurons is so selective that global treatments produce too many side effects. Tetrabenazine (a vesicular monoamine transporter inhibitor) has recently been approved to treat the movement symptoms associated with the disease. Huntington disease is invariably accompanied by depression with occasional paranoia and psychosis. These symptoms are treated with standard antidepressants or antipsychotics.

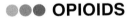

●●● OPIOIDS

Endogenous Opioid System and Pain Management

Opioid analgesics are used primarily to treat severe pain, although they may also be used to treat cough (hydrocodone, dextromethorphan), diarrhea (diphenoxylate), or for anesthetic purposes. Specifically, opiates are plant alkaloids derived from the opium poppy. Opioids are chemically related compounds. These compounds, like many drugs, work by binding to receptors for natural neurotransmitters within the body. In this case, it appears that the endogenous opioids (endorphins, dynorphins, and enkephalins) are peptides found in regions of the nervous system involved in transmitting, organizing, and perceiving pain. The opioid receptors are categorized into three families: mu (μ), kappa (κ), and delta (δ). The major player for pain management is the μ receptor, with κ also playing a significant role in spinal transmission of pain.

The opioid receptors work through inhibitory G-protein signaling (decreasing cyclic adenosine monophosphate synthesis) that results in decreased firing of presynaptic neurons in the spinal cord or postsynaptic firing of neurons in the CNS. In the former case, this occurs through decreases in Ca^{++} influx, whereas the latter is mediated primarily through increases in Na^+ outflow and a resulting hyperpolarization of neurons. In each case, the pain signal is either blocked or diminished or is not *perceived* as noxious ("dulled").

Opioid Analgesics

Butorphanol, Codeine, Dextromethorphan, Diphenoxylate, Fentanyl, Hydrocodone, Hydromorphone, Meperidine, Methadone, Morphine, Nalbuphine, Oxycodone, and Pentazocine
Naloxone and Naltrexone (Antidotes)

The opioid analgesics are categorized as strong, moderate, or weak agonists (Table 13-12). The prototypical strong opioid agonists are morphine (a precursor of heroin), hydromorphone, meperidine, methadone, and fentanyl. This designation as "strong" reflects not only their analgesic characteristics but also their abuse liability and their ability to cause respiratory depression. These drugs are used to treat moderate to severe pain. Because of abuse potential, most opioid agonists are classified as controlled substances by the U.S. Drug Enforcement Administration. Morphine is the prototypical compound to which other opioids/opiates are compared.

Methadone has a very long $t_{1/2}$ that causes the drug to accumulate. This prolonged duration of activity is ideal for using methadone to wean heroin addicts from the illicit substance because withdrawal symptoms occur later and are less severe with methadone compared with heroin. This is an example of using a drug with *cross-tolerance* but more favorable pharmacokinetics (longer $t_{1/2}$). There is concern that methadone may cause cardiac arrhythmias (including torsades de pointes) by delaying myocardial repolarization.

At the opposite end of the spectrum, meperidine has a short duration of action, necessitating frequent dosing. Because of its short $t_{1/2}$, meperidine is often used during labor because its short duration of activity produces less respiratory depression in infants. One of the metabolites of meperidine metabolism may accumulate in patients with renal failure, causing seizures, dysphoria, and agitation. An additional short-acting opioid is fentanyl, which is often used as a surgical anesthetic adjunct. Fentanyl may also be used for pain relief for regional (intrathecal) anesthesia. Unique dose forms of fentanyl include long-acting transdermal patches and short-acting lollipops. Note, however, that these alternative fentanyl dose forms could be deadly to an opioid-naive child.

Moderate opioid agents include codeine and hydrocodone. These drugs are usually the first to be tried when nonsteroidal antiinflammatory drugs are insufficient to control pain. Another moderately effective therapeutic is oxycodone, although this drug has a high potential for abuse. The abuse potential relates to the relatively high doses in which it is

TABLE 13-12. Opioid Analgesic Drugs

DRUG	MECHANISM OF ACTION	INDICATION	SIDE EFFECTS/COMMENT
Morphine	Strong opiate; μ agonist	Analgesic	Poorly bioavailable Side effects shared by most opioid drugs: respiratory depression, nausea, vomiting, dizziness, confusion, constipation, abuse potential
Meperidine	Strong opiate; μ agonist	Analgesic	Treatment for postoperative shivering
Methadone	Strong opiate; μ agonist	Analgesic, heroin recovery	Used in maintenance therapy for recovering opiate addicts because it has a long $t_{1/2}$
Fentanyl	Strong opiate; μ agonist	Analgesic	100 times more potent than morphine
Oxycodone	Moderate μ agonist	Analgesic	Excellent bioavailability; significant abuse liability
Codeine	Moderate μ agonist	Cough suppressant, analgesic	Frequently combined with aspirin or acetaminophen
Pentazocine	κ agonist and partial μ agonist	Analgesic	Lower abuse potential than others
Buprenorphine	Partial μ agonist and weak κ agonist	Analgesia and treatment for opiate addiction	Partial agonist with weak analgesic activity; alleviates symptoms of opiate withdrawal

packaged and the discovery that alternative routes of administration (intranasal ["snorting"] or intravenous) produce a rapid "high."

Weak opioid analgesics include nalbuphine, butorphanol, and pentazocine. These drugs have mixed effects, with full agonist activity at κ receptors and partial agonist activity at μ receptors. Recall that a partial agonist competes with the endogenous opioid (with a smaller effect) leading to an overall antagonist effect. These pharmacologic actions permit pain relief with minimal risk of respiratory depression and less likelihood for abuse.

Side effects after opioid administration are significant. In addition to respiratory depression (the predominant cause of death in overdose victims), there is miosis (a defining characteristic), cough suppression (an indication for the moderate μ agonists codeine and hydrocodone), emesis, constipation from slowed gastrointestinal motility (diphenoxylate is prescribed as an antidiarrheal), urinary retention and reduced uterine tone (prolongs labor) because of effects on smooth muscles, and histamine release (specific to morphine). Additional adverse effects are included in Box 13-4.

In the event of opioid/opiate overdose, two antagonists at μ and κ receptors, naloxone and naltrexone, can be administered to reverse life-threatening respiratory depression or hypotension. Of course, administration of these drugs also precipitates withdrawal symptoms in patients who are physically dependent on opioids/opiates (Table 13-13).

New classes of nonopiate analgesics have also been developed. These other analgesics include tramadol and ziconotide. Tramadol binds weakly to μ receptors but also inhibits reuptake of norepinephrine and serotonin. Thus this drug may

Box 13-4. ADVERSE EFFECTS OF OPIOID ANALGESICS

Miosis	Postural hypotension
Respiratory depression	Constipation
Cough suppression	Urinary retention
Emesis	Itching, urticaria
Elevated intracranial pressure	

TABLE 13-13. Opioid Withdrawal Signs and Symptoms

SYMPTOMS	SIGNS
Regular Withdrawal	
Anxiety	Diarrhea
Dysphoric mood	Fever
Increased pain sensitivity	Increased blood pressure
Insomnia	Piloerection (goosebumps)
Irritability	Pupillary dilation
Muscle aches	Sweating
Nausea, cramps	Tachycardia
Opioid craving	Vomiting
Restlessness	Yawning
Protracted Withdrawal (Relapse Liability)	
Anxiety	Cyclic change in weight, pupil size, respiratory center sensitivity
Drug craving	
Insomnia	

Note that a symptom is reported by the patient, whereas a sign is something measured or observed.

modulate the emotional aspects of pain. Tramadol lowers the seizure threshold and may cause seizures in patients who are predisposed. Ziconotide is the first in a new class of nonopiate pain relievers. The drug—a 25 amino acid peptide derived from a snail conotoxin—blocks N-type Ca^{++} channels, preventing the release of neurotransmitters involved with pain transmission. Ziconotide is administered only intrathecally and may cause psychosis, cognitive impairment, hallucinations, or changes in mood or consciousness.

Management of Migraine Headache Pain

Almotriptan, Eletriptan, Frovatriptan, Naratriptan, Rizatriptan, Sumatriptan, and Zolmitriptan

Note: These drugs end in "-triptan."

Certainly any of the analgesics (nonsteroidal antiinflammatory drugs, opioids/opiates) can be used to treat headaches, including migraines. The underlying etiology of migraine headaches is thought to involve dilation of cerebral and cranial arteries mediated at least in part by release of substance P, prostaglandins, leukotrienes, and bradykinins—all of which propagate pain responses. The "triptans" have found a unique niche in pharmacotherapy as a result of their ability to block neurogenic inflammation. Triptans are drugs that act as selective agonists at serotonin 1B and 1D receptor subtypes. Overall, triptans prevent release of vasoactive substances, block inflammation, and constrict arteries.

Sumatriptan is the prototypical agent to which the others are compared. Differences among agents primarily are either pharmacokinetic (oral rizatriptan and zolmitriptan nasal spray are fast acting; frovatriptan has the longest duration of activity), are related to adverse effects (naratriptan and almotriptan are usually the best tolerated), or pertain to compatibility with other drugs (eletriptan may have less adverse interaction with MAO inhibitors).

Because of vasoconstrictive effects, triptans are contraindicated in patients with ischemic heart disease, a history of myocardial infarction, uncontrolled hypertension, arrhythmias, asthma, or pregnancy. The drugs are commonly associated with chest tightness or pressure; sensations of warmth, tingling, or burning; hypertension; tachycardia; and a bad taste in the mouth.

●●● SEDATIVE-HYPNOTIC AND ANXIOLYTIC AGENTS

GABA Receptor Modulators

The sedative-hypnotic and anxiolytic agents generally are barbiturates and benzodiazepines, which are both GABA receptor modulators. *Sedation* refers to a calming effect that decreases excitement and moderates hyperexcitability. *Hypnosis*, in the pharmacologic sense, refers to drowsiness and the promotion and maintenance of sleep. Anxiety disorders are a large family of clinical problems that were previously known as *psychoneuroses*. These include various phobias, social anxiety disorder, generalized anxiety disorder, obsessive-

compulsive disorder, and posttraumatic stress disorder. Just as agents that activate or potentiate GABA (the most common inhibitory neurotransmitter in the brain) are effective in calming the overactivity of epilepsy, they also are effective as anxiolytics and sedative-hypnotics. Barbiturates and benzodiazepines are useful in the treatment of panic attacks and generalized anxiety, various phobias, insomnia, and as discussed previously, epilepsy and spasticity. Furthermore, they are used adjunctively for general anesthesia (Table 13-14).

Benzodiazepines

Alprazolam, Clonazepam, Diazepam, Lorazepam, Temazepam, Triazolam, and Flumazenil (Antidote)

Most of these drugs end in "-olam" or "-epam."

The $GABA_A$ receptor is a pentameric ligand-gated Cl^- channel (see Fig. 13-2). (In contrast, the $GABA_B$ receptor is a 7-transmembrane, G-protein–coupled receptor with a different pharmacologic profile.) The prototypical benzodiazepine for anxiolysis is diazepam, which acts by binding to $GABA_A$ receptors to enhance the actions of GABA; in other words, it acts as an allosteric modulator of GABA receptors. Specifically, benzodiazepines increase the *frequency* of Cl^- channel opening. Clinically useful benzodiazepine anxiolytics include alprazolam, clonazepam, and lorazepam. Benzodiazepines may be used primarily for their hypnotic effects to facilitate sleep in patients with insomnia. Examples include temazepam and triazolam.

Benzodiazepines differ from each other pharmacokinetically, primarily with respect to their onset of activity and their duration of action. Diazepam acts very quickly and has a long $t_{1/2}$. This prolonged duration of action can cause "hangover" effects. Benzodiazepines are classified as controlled substances by the Drug Enforcement Administration because of their potential for abuse. Benzodiazepines cannot be discontinued abruptly or withdrawal symptoms will occur (Box 13-5). After long-term use of benzodiazepines, it is wise to switch patients to diazepam, a benzodiazepine with a long $t_{1/2}$.

Adverse effects associated with benzodiazepines are primarily related to CNS depression (drowsiness, dizziness, incoordination), although respiratory depression is a concern if other CNS depressants are used simultaneously. In cases of benzodiazepine overdose, the $GABA_A$ receptor antagonist flumazenil can be administered. Compared with barbiturates, benzodiazepines have a superior safety profile, with CNS depression reaching a plateau before achieving a comatose state (Fig. 13-8).

Nonbenzodiazepine GABA_A Receptor Modulators

Eszopiclone, Zaleplon, and Zolpidem

Several nonbenzodiazepine compounds also interact with the $GABA_A$ receptors but have not been associated with tolerance. These drugs include zolpidem, zaleplon, and

TABLE 13-14. Sedative-Hypnotic/Anxiolytic Drugs

DRUG	MECHANISM OF ACTION	INDICATION	SIDE EFFECTS/COMMENT
Diazepam	Benzodiazepine	Anxiety disorders, status epilepticus, anesthetic premedication, muscle relaxant	Relatively safe drug Produces cognitive impairment, increased reaction time, lightheadedness, nausea, vomiting
Alprazolam	Benzodiazepine	Anxiety disorders, phobias	See diazepam
Midazolam	Benzodiazepine	Anesthesia adjuvant	See diazepam
Triazolam	Benzodiazepine	Insomnia	See diazepam
Zolpidem	Nonbenzodiazepine agonist at the GABA receptor	Insomnia	Dizziness, confusion
Phenobarbital	Barbiturate	Seizure disorders, status epilepticus, sedation	Induction of P450 metabolic enzymes; respiratory depression, drowsiness, vertigo, nausea, vomiting, diarrhea
Secobarbital	Barbiturate	Insomnia, sedation, seizure disorders (acute)	Induction of P450 metabolic enzymes; respiratory depression, drowsiness, vertigo, nausea, vomiting, diarrhea
Ethanol	Unknown but thought to interact with GABA receptor	Used as an intoxicant and for its sedative-hypnotic effects	Dysphoria, sedation, vomiting, coma, respiratory depression

GABA, γ-aminobutyric acid.

eszopiclone. Zaleplon's claim to fame is that it has a quick onset of action and its actions are terminated in 4 hours. This short duration of action makes zaleplon ideal for patients who wake up in the middle of the night and cannot fall back to sleep, because as long as there are at least 4 hours until the patient must awaken, no hangover effects are experienced.

Barbiturates

Phenobarbital and Secobarbital
Although the benzodiazepines act by enhancing the action of GABA (serving to increase the frequency of Cl⁻ channel opening), the barbiturates also bind to the $GABA_A$ receptor at a distinct site and enhance GABA activity by facilitating the *duration* of time that the receptor Cl⁻ channel remains open. Phenobarbital and secobarbital are prototypical barbiturates. Because of their abuse liability and potential for overdose, the barbiturates are not as widely prescribed as the benzodiazepines. They do serve as a valuable tool in the treatment of seizure disorders, as previously described.

Other Anxiolytics

Buspirone
Finally, buspirone, a partial agonist at serotonin 1A receptors ($5HT_{1A}$), is an effective treatment for generalized anxiety. Unlike benzodiazepines and barbiturates, however, it takes several weeks for maximal effects to be seen.

Box 13-5. SYMPTOMS OF BENZODIAZEPINE WITHDRAWAL

After Moderate Drug Use

Anxiety, agitation
Increased sensitivity to light and sound
Paresthesias, strange sensations
Muscle cramps
Myoclonic jerks
Sleep disturbance
Dizziness

After High-Dose or Long-Term Use

Seizures
Delirium

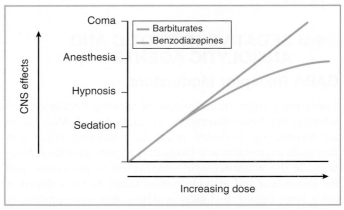

Figure 13-8. Relative safety of benzodiazepines compared with barbiturates. *CNS*, central nervous system.

TABLE 13-15. Tolerance and Dependence Potential of Commonly Abused Drugs

	DYNAMIC TOLERANCE	PHYSICAL DEPENDENCE	PSYCHOLOGIC DEPENDENCE	WITHDRAWAL SYNDROME
THC	+	—	+	—
Morphine	++++	++++	++++	++++
Ethanol	++	++++	+++	++++
Barbiturates	++	++++	+++	++++
Amphetamines	++++	+	+++	+
Cocaine	+	+	+++	+
LSD	+++	—	++	—
PCP	++	—	+	—
Nicotine	++	++	++	++
Caffeine	++	+	+	+

++++, Pronounced effect; +++, moderate effect; ++, low effect; +, slight effect; —, no effect; *THC*, tetrahydrocannabinol; *LSD*, lysergic acid diethylamide; *PCP*, parachlorophenate.

Alcohol

Ethanol is noteworthy because there is growing evidence that it exerts its sedative-hypnotic effects by binding to the GABA$_A$ receptor. Therefore, in many respects, it resembles the benzodiazepines and is synergistic with (and potentiates) both the pharmacologic and toxicologic effects of the benzodiazepines and barbiturates. For this reason, it can be viewed, in many cases, as a *natural* form of self-medication (i.e., calms the nerves). As seen in the following section, however, this is a simplistic and dangerous view of this abused drug.

⬤⬤⬤ ABUSED RECREATIONAL DRUGS

Abused Drugs as False Messengers

Drugs of abuse (e.g., alcohol, nicotine, heroin, cannabinoids, cocaine) are generally natural products that serve as false messengers at endogenous receptor systems. They basically bind to receptor systems and mimic natural neurotransmitters but generally with much greater potency (Table 13-15).

Alcohol

As discussed in the preceding section, ethanol (ethyl alcohol) exerts many of its effects on the GABA$_A$ receptor. It is not as simple of a drug as benzodiazepines because of its other behavioral effects. At low doses, ethanol produces social disinhibition, feelings of pleasure, and even euphoria. At escalating doses, however, it interferes with motor control and produces dysphoria, sedation, vomiting, coma, and even death (through respiratory depression). The reinforcing nature of the drug and perhaps the seat of its abuse liability is due to activation of the mesolimbic dopamine pathway. As with the opiates, after long-term use, ethanol produces behavioral and physiologic tolerance and physical dependence. Hence, withdrawal from severe alcohol dependence produces strong physiologic effects, including seizures

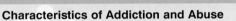

CLINICAL MEDICINE

Characteristics of Addiction and Abuse

Potent opioid full agonists are the most effective analgesics, but they are accompanied by strong abuse liability. This is because opioid agonists can produce euphoria. With long-term use, however, the body develops tolerance and dependence, requiring more drug to produce the high, and the body simultaneously depends on the drug to maintain homeostasis. This is a dangerous behavioral combination that leads to the unique physical and psychologic dependence that underlies addiction. These characteristics render the strong opioid agonists (along with nicotine and alcohol) the most addictive drugs. Unfortunately, because of this, some patients suffer because physicians are reluctant to prescribe opioids for pain. The fear of addiction is largely unfounded in patients with legitimate pain. Proper administration of opioids to alleviate pain has a low risk of addiction, although physical dependence will occur. The medication must be slowly tapered in these patients after therapeutic treatment of the pain.

(Box 13-6; see also Table 13-15). Such acute withdrawal effects are treated with benzodiazepines such as diazepam. In fact, there is cross-tolerance between ethanol and the benzodiazepines. This means that, for certain physiologic effects, one will substitute for the other—not because they are structurally similar but because they interact with the same molecular target: the GABA-stimulated Cl⁻ channel. Long-term use of alcohol adversely affects nearly every organ system in the body. Long-term alcohol abuse is treated with other pharmacologic agents that produce aversive effects by interfering with ethanol metabolism (disulfiram) or by modulating endogenous serotonin, opiate, or GABAergic systems (ondansetron, naltrexone, or acamprosate, respectively).

NEUROSCIENCE

Differentiating Tolerance, Dependence, and Addiction

Tolerance occurs when larger doses of drug are required to produce the same effect. Tolerance can occur for numerous reasons: innate tolerance is genetically determined, pharmacokinetic tolerance results from changes in drug metabolism, and pharmacodynamic tolerance is caused by adaptive changes in receptor density or second messenger characteristics. Cross-tolerance is sometimes used pharmacologically during detoxification to allow one drug to substitute for another.

Dependence can be either *physical* or *psychologic*. Psychologic dependence is manifested by cravings for a drug—probably the major cause of relapse. Physical dependence is virtually synonymous with *withdrawal*. Cessation of use of drugs that cause physical dependence will result in withdrawal symptoms. Importantly, tolerance and dependence are biologic phenomena and *do not imply drug abuse*.

Abuse or *addiction* denotes an overwhelming compulsion and preoccupation with obtaining and using a drug. Not all drugs of abuse are associated with the same propensity to cause tolerance or dependence.

Cocaine and Psychomotor Stimulants

Cocaine and the psychomotor stimulants (amphetamine and methamphetamine) work directly through antagonizing dopamine reuptake and storage in the CNS. Cocaine blocks dopamine reuptake (and, to lesser extent, norepinephrine and serotonin) through antagonism of reuptake transporter pumps. As a result, cocaine enhances dopamine activity within the nigrostriatal track (activating motor behavior). Simultaneously, cocaine acts directly on the mesolimbic dopamine pathway to serve as a behavioral reinforcer. Through

other pathways, it produces euphoria. Interestingly, in keeping with the dopamine theory of affective disorders, high doses of cocaine can produce manic behavior and acute psychoses. The drugs within the amphetamine family (amphetamine, methamphetamine, and methylenedioxymethamphetamine) have similar mechanisms of action and act by releasing intracellular pools of dopamine and reversing the dopamine transporter to pump neurotransmitter into the synapse. Methylenedioxymethamphetamine is important because it has 5HT activities and causes hallucinogenic effects as well. These compounds, in addition to their addictive liability, have significant, even fatal, side effects because of their potent peripheral sympathomimetic activities (see Chapter 6).

ANATOMY

Mesolimbic Dopamine Pathway

In nearly every case, administration of abused substances activates the mesolimbic dopamine pathway. This pathway (considered to be a ventral extension of the nigrostriatal tract) originates in the ventral tegmental area (A10 nucleus) and projects to the nucleus accumbens. The mesolimbic pathway appears to serve as the reinforcement circuit for the brain. That is, things that are generally good for the health and welfare of the individual and species (eating, drinking, sex) elicit its activity, which drives the behavior to be repeated. Abused substances—whether or not they have a dopaminergic mechanism—also activate the mesolimbic pathway. The difference is that they do so to a much greater extent. This may account for why there is such a strong drive to abuse many illicit drugs.

Attention Deficit Disorder/Attention Deficit–Hyperactivity Disorder

Also of note, stimulants such as amphetamine, methylphenidate, dextroamphetamine, and lisdexamphetamine, although controlled substances with dependence/abuse liability, are widely used to treat behavioral disorders such as attention deficit disorder, attention deficit–hyperactivity disorder, and narcolepsy in both children and adults. Lisdexamphetamine is interesting in that it has a lysine amino acid residue affixed to the stimulant that is removed in the gut. This prevents abuse because the lysine prevents the "high" associated with crushing and snorting the tablet material. The newer nonstimulant atomoxetine, a drug that selectively inhibits reuptake of norepinephrine, is also commonly used for attention deficit disorder behavioral conditions because it is not associated with a potential for abuse. It has, however, been associated with hepatotoxicity.

Cannabinoids (Dronabinol and Marijuana)

Cannabis is the most widely used illicit drug in the United States. Smoking the cannabis plant volatilizes many plant alkaloids including the active ingredient, Δ^9-tetrahydrocannabinol (Δ^9THC). This compound interacts with high affinity at an endogenous receptor of unknown function—the cannabinoid receptor (for which there are central and peripheral nervous system forms). The natural ligand for these receptors is believed to be a derivative of arachidonic acid, anandamide. Use of cannabis produces a "high" that is distinct from that of alcohol, stimulants, or opiates. It is accompanied by impairment of short-term cognitive function, memory, reaction time, and perception (especially of time). Clinically, Δ^9THC is used as the prescription drug dronabinol to manage chemotherapy-associated nausea and vomiting and in AIDS-related anorexia. Moreover, given its ability to stimulate appetite (the "munchies"), it is also used to counteract the cachexia associated with cancer.

Nicotine

Nicotine dependence contributes to the foremost preventable cause of death today—smoking. Besides the fact that the drug—a stimulant (a direct agonist at nicotinic acetylcholine receptors)—is reinforcing, its pattern of administration probably significantly contributes to its addictive nature. Each puff produces a small reinforcing effect, repeated many times over the course of a day. Combined with the fact that it is associated with pleasurable social activities, nicotine's pharmacology and the psychosocial behaviors associated with its use combine to create, for some individuals, the ultimate physical and psychologic dependence. Withdrawal from nicotine, although unpleasant, is not life-threatening (Box 13-7). Nicotine is readily absorbed across membranes (skin, lung epithelium, oral membranes), and a variety of approaches to treating nicotine dependence are available, including nicotine gums, lozenges, inhalers, and transdermal patches. In addition, the antidepressant bupropion appears to reduce nicotine craving. Most recently, varenicline, a partial nicotinic agonist (at α_4/β_2 receptors), has been approved for smoking cessation. This compound decreases craving and reduces the pleasure of smoking by occupying receptors with only a partial effect.

●●● COMPLEMENTARY AND ALTERNATIVE MEDICINE

St. John's Wort

Some patients use St. John's wort to treat depression. The product appears to be more effective than placebo and in some clinical studies was as effective as tricyclic antidepressants or SSRIs for treating mild to moderate depression. St. John's wort may inhibit serotonin reuptake, which would explain its antidepressant activity.

Box 13-7. SYMPTOMS OF NICOTINE WITHDRAWAL

Irritability
Anxiety
Dysphoric or depressed mood
Difficulty concentrating
Restlessness
Decreased heart rate
Increased appetite or weight gain

Typically, St. John's wort is well tolerated. The biggest concerns with this natural product are related to drug-drug interactions. St. John's wort induces hepatic microsomal CYP P450 enzymes, altering the metabolism of many drugs and possibly rendering them ineffective. In addition, St. John's wort decreases the effectiveness of oral anticoagulants. This supplement should never be used with other medications that alter serotonergic neurotransmission (i.e., triptans, prescription antidepressants, opioids, *MAO* inhibitors) because of the risk of serotonin syndrome.

Melatonin

Melatonin is often used by people who have difficulty sleeping, especially if their insomnia is related to jet lag or shift work. Melatonin is synthesized endogenously in the pineal gland. Its primary role seems to be regulation of circadian rhythm, endocrine secretions, and sleep patterns. Light inhibits melatonin secretion; dark stimulates its secretion. For many years, dietary supplements containing melatonin have been used to treat insomnia (especially by travelers to counteract jet lag). Ramelteon is structurally related to melatonin and is the first drug approved for insomnia that is not a CNS depressant. It is an agonist at the melatonin MT1 and MT2 receptors. It has minimal abuse liability and a short duration of action, so it is less likely to cause daytime sedation.

Patients should not drive or operate heavy machinery for 4 to 5 hours after using melatonin. Although usually well tolerated, supplements have been reported to cause transient drowsiness, headache, dizziness, depression, and mild anxiety. Melatonin may increase the risk of bleeding in patients taking oral anticoagulants. In addition, sedation may be exacerbated by concomitant use of other CNS depressants (e.g., alcohol, benzodiazepines, antihistamines). Although speculative, melatonin may increase blood glucose in patients with diabetes, exacerbate seizure disorders in susceptible individuals, and worsen hypertension in some patients.

Kava

Kava, a popular social drink in Pacific Island countries, is sometimes used as a supplement to treat anxiety disorders. Although a variety of pharmacologic effects have been noted with kava, including anxiolytic, sedative, anticonvulsant, local anesthetic, spasmolytic, antiinflammatory, and analgesic activities, the mechanisms for these effects are unknown and do not appear to be mediated via known pathways.

When used orally, kava can cause gastrointestinal disturbances, headache, dizziness, drowsiness, miosis, and extrapyramidal effects. Hepatotoxicity is also a concern with kava. Kava may inhibit hepatic P450 enzymes, and it exacerbates CNS sedation when used with other CNS depressants. Owing to the hepatic toxicity, the Food and Drug Administration is in the process of banning kava in the United States; several other countries have already done so.

●●● TOP FIVE LIST

1. Anesthetics, antiepileptics, and sedative hypnotic drugs generally work by modulating ion channels (primarily GABA-stimulated Cl^- channels, but also Na^+ and Ca^{++} channels).
2. Antidepressants work by blocking biogenic amine reuptake (inhibiting norepinephrine and/or serotonin transporters).
3. Antipsychotic agents are antagonists of dopamine (or serotonin) receptors.
4. Neurodegenerative diseases are targeted by agents that treat symptoms (increasing dopamine activity for Parkinson disease; increasing acetylcholine activity for Alzheimer disease); however, cure is not currently possible.
5. The opioids stimulate (and simulate) natural analgesic systems in the CNS (endorphins and enkephalins).

Self-assessment questions can be accessed at www. StudentConsult.com.

Case Studies

CASE STUDY 1

A 54-year-old homeless male, who admits to smoking cigarettes all his adult life, is admitted to the hospital with evidence of tuberculosis. This gentleman weighs 65 kg and says he was diagnosed with chronic heart failure and asthma "many years ago." For the past 15 years, he has been obtaining theophylline samples from a physician who volunteers at the local homeless shelter, so you decide to continue the drug while he is hospitalized. In the hospital, the patient has been receiving 100 mg theophylline every 12 hours. However, you realize that theophylline is metabolized by P450 microsomal enzymes, and you've placed the patient on several medications that alter the metabolism of theophylline, including ciprofloxacin, which is known to increase theophylline levels, and rifampin, which is known to induce the P450 enzymes, thus reducing theophylline levels. You decide that it is best to obtain laboratory data to determine what the patient's plasma levels of theophylline are because of these potential drug interactions. The laboratory report indicates that the patient's plasma concentration of theophylline is 3.6 mg/L (target range is 5 to 15 mg/L).

1. Knowing that the published value of volume of distribution (Vd) for theophylline is 0.48 L/kg, calculate this man's Vd for theophylline.

2. Knowing that the published half-life ($t_{1/2}$) for theophylline in a smoker is 4.5 hours, what is the rate at which theophylline is cleared in this patient?

3. What loading dose should this patient be given to quickly increase his theophylline plasma level to 10 mg/L?

CASE STUDY 2

A 68-year-old patient is transferred to your practice. She is concerned because she has been taking the same medication for 60 years for her asthma, but it does not seem to be working very well lately. She says that she has taken the same dose of theophylline all her life—ever since she was 8 years old—and she wanted her previous doctor to increase the dose, but he did not. She is certain that the reason her asthma has been under poor control for the past few months is because her doctor refuses to prescribe more. (In actuality, her previous doctor had suggested discontinuing the theophylline entirely and switching her to a long-acting corticosteroid/β_2-agonist combination because theophylline requires careful monitoring and has numerous drug interactions and severe toxicities. However, she refused because she had heard that steroids are "bad for you.")

"Theophylline has worked for my entire life. When it stopped working recently, my doctor refused to increase the dose. Why would a drug I've taken my whole life suddenly stop working?"

You review her medications and find that she is also taking cimetidine for gastroesophageal reflux and rifampin for a severe staphylococcal bone infection. You check her serum theophylline levels and find that they are 4.0 mg/L (target range is 5 to 15 mg/L).

1. What are some of the considerations for dosing a drug with a narrow therapeutic index (e.g., theophylline) throughout the lifespan of a patient?

2. Are there any pharmacokinetic interactions between rifampin and theophylline that could affect this woman's theophylline plasma levels?

3. Are there any pharmacokinetic interactions between cimetidine and theophylline that could affect this woman's theophylline plasma levels?

CASE STUDY 3

A 16-year-old female comes to the emergency department with severe abdominal cramps. She is sweaty and appears feverish. On workup, she becomes nauseated and vomits pill fragments. She reports that she ingested "a hundred pills, but I don't remember the type." On examination, her temperature is 101.2° F, her blood pressure is 128/72 mm Hg, her pulse is 120 beats/min, and her respirations are 34 breaths/min.

1. What is your initial management strategy for this patient after addressing the ABCs (airway, breathing, circulation)?

2. What over-the-counter medicine could be responsible for the initial symptoms?

3. Initial arterial blood gas levels are drawn (pH, 7.64; pCO_2, 16 mm Hg; pO_2, 98 mm Hg). What are potential mechanisms underlying this alkalosis?

4. Repeat laboratory measurements are taken 2 hours after the patient receives 2 L normal saline. The results are now pH, 7.27; pCO_2, 16 mm Hg; and pO_2, 103 mm Hg. What are potential mechanisms leading to the secondary acidosis?

5. The patient's condition continues to worsen. What is the next course of treatment?

CASE STUDY 4

A 33-year-old female is brought to the emergency department by her husband one Saturday morning. She reports such a severe headache that she cannot open her eyes. Her oral temperature is 104.1° F. Her husband mentions, "My wife has a rash on the back of her head."

According to the woman's husband, she was previously in good health. On the previous day, the woman rose early in the morning to complete her exercise routine and remarked to her husband about what a great workout she had. However, as the day progressed, she noted a "large painful lump" on the back of her head. By evening, she noticed additional lumps and was concerned because the lumps were beginning to spread down the back of her head and neck. She also began having diarrhea that evening. Although the woman had been seen by her family doctor "after hours" the previous evening, no definitive diagnosis had been made, and she was sent home. Throughout the night, the woman had severe diarrhea and vomiting.

Almost as soon as the patient arrived in the emergency department, she began complaining of an irregular heartbeat. An electrocardiogram revealed premature ventricular contractions; the woman denied a prior history of cardiovascular problems. On examination of the patient's head, the "rash" on the back of her head appeared to be spreading down her neck and across her face. At the emergency department, an astute attending physician correctly diagnosed the woman as having erysipelas. The patient has no history of drug allergies.

1. What is erysipelas, and which microorganisms are the most likely culprits?

2. What is the most likely cause of the patient's cardiac arrhythmias?

3. A scab is identified on the patient's scalp, and both group A streptococci and staphylococci are isolated and cultured. Blood cultures are negative, which is common with erysipelas (blood cultures are positive in only 5% of cases). Discuss an antimicrobial that is appropriate for this patient.

4. After 5 days of receiving an intravenous antibiotic, her fever finally subsided and she was discharged with a prescription for 10 additional days of therapy with oral dicloxacillin. In addition, at the time of discharge, a first-year resident informed the patient that the laboratory had just called with results of a stool culture that had been conducted during admission because the patient's abdominal pain and diarrhea had worsened while she was hospitalized. *Clostridium difficile* toxins were identified in the patient's stool culture. What is the source of this gastrointestinal microorganism, and how is this secondary infection treated?

CASE STUDY 5

A 70-year-old man with a history of long-standing hypertension and recently diagnosed type 2 diabetes mellitus comes to the oncology clinic. He has just found out the gastric pain that he attributed to a "flare-up" of his peptic ulcer disease is actually giant large-cell lymphoma, an aggressive neoplasm. As the director of the oncology clinic, you tell the patient that he will be receiving six to eight cycles of a chemotherapeutic regimen known as CHOP, followed by consolidative radiation therapy to his stomach and lymph nodes. The patient asks for additional information about the CHOP regimen, and you explain that this is a combination of four different drugs: cyclophosphamide, doxorubicin, vincristine, and prednisone.

1. When explaining the long-term complications of doxorubicin to the patient, what do you warn him about and what can be done to prevent or minimize the drug's effects?

2. When explaining long-term complications associated with vincristine, of what do you warn the patient?

3. What long-term complications are associated with cyclophosphamide, and how can they be prevented?

CASE STUDY 6

A clinical study is conducted in which a healthy volunteer is administered norepinephrine, epinephrine, and isoproterenol. Blood pressure, total peripheral resistance, and heart rate are monitored during drug infusions. The results of this study are depicted in the accompanying figure.

1. Explain the widely disparate results for these three adrenergic agonists. Specifically address the receptors responsible for the various hemodynamic changes.

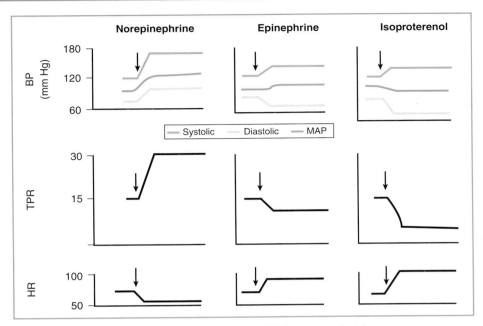

HR, heart rate; *TPR,* total peripheral resistance; *BP,* blood pressure; *MAP,* mean arterial pressure.

CASE STUDY 7

A 75-year-old male complains of "stomach pain" and massive rectal bleeding when passing stools. He is also gingerly holding his left shoulder. On questioning, he tells you that last week, he slipped on the ice and fell while shoveling snow. He was prescribed celecoxib by his family doctor for persistent shoulder pain and swelling. When the pain failed to resolve after a few days, this man scheduled a second appointment with his family physician. This time, his regular doctor was out of town, so he was seen instead by another partner in the practice, who prescribed ibuprofen. The pain has persisted for several weeks and during this time, he has been taking both celecoxib and ibuprofen regularly. In the middle of the night, the man was brought to the emergency department when he filled the toilet bowl with bloody stools twice. He was feeling faint and had nearly passed out before his wife was able to summon an ambulance. His medical history includes hypertension and peptic ulcer disease. The hypertension is controlled with medication, and there have been no ulcers in more than a decade. The following are the patient's pertinent laboratory values from his complete blood count, with normal values shown in parentheses:

Hemoglobin = 11.9 g/dL (13.8 to 17.2 g/dL)
Hematocrit = 34% (40.7 to 50.3%)
Mean corpuscular volume = 75.9 μm³ (80.0 to 97.6 μm³)
Mean corpuscular hemoglobin = 24.0 pg/cell (26.7 to 33/7 pg/cell)
Mean corpuscular hemoglobin concentration = 30.0 g/dL (32.7 to 35.5 g/dL)

1. **You suspect that because of his massive gastrointestinal bleeding, the patient is iron-deficient. What other tests might you order to confirm your diagnosis?**

2. **What do you suppose contributed to patient's loss of iron?**

3. **Ultimately, surgical intervention was needed to halt the severe gastrointestinal bleeding, and the patient was discharged home with a prescription for iron supplements. What might you tell the patient and note in his chart regarding this iron therapy?**

CASE STUDY 8

A 45-year-old man enters a clinic for the first time. He tells the doctor, "I feel fine, but the nurse at work took my blood pressure. It was 150/100 mm Hg and 160/102 mm Hg on two different days. She says I need a checkup."

Despite a thorough examination to determine an identifiable cause for his hypertension, none was found, and the patient was given a diagnosis of stage 2 essential hypertension. The patient was instructed on lifestyle changes including (a) smoking cessation, (b) regular exercise, (c) alcohol limitations (no more than two beers per day), and (d) a low-fat, low-cholesterol, low-salt diet.

The patient was motivated to initiate these lifestyle modifications, so the physician prescribed only hydrochlorothiazide initially and scheduled a follow-up examination for 2 months later. The patient returned 2 weeks later with a painful, swollen, red big toe joint. His potassium level was 3.2 mEq/L (normal, 3.5 to 5.0 mEq/L), and his uric acid level was 11.9 mg/dL (normal, 3 to 8 mg/dL).

1. **Account for the patient's painful toe and his abnormal laboratory values.**

2. **The patient's pharmacologic therapy was changed to atenolol. Although the patient's blood pressure had lowered to 132/94 mm Hg with atenolol, his heart rate was**

only 50 beats/min. The patient reported easy fatigability and a reduction in exercise tolerance. Explain how atenolol causes these adverse effects.

3. Because the patient reported other adverse effects associated with the β-blocker (e.g., reduced libido, sleep disturbances), it was decided that instead of lowering the dose, a drug from a different class would be tried. Atenolol was gradually tapered over a period of 1 week. Why was the dose of atenolol tapered slowly?

4. The patient was started on lisinopril. How does lisinopril work, and what adverse effects might the patient experience?

CASE STUDY 9

A 60-year-white male weighing 170 pounds is brought to the emergency department by his wife because his "ankles are swollen." You view the patient's extremities and note that he has stage 4 pitting edema in his ankles. The patient tells you that he has a history of poorly controlled hypertension. Before prescribing any medications, you ask the laboratory to check his Na^+, K^+, and serum creatinine. Pertinent laboratory values are:

K^+: 3.5 (3.3 to 4.9 mmol/L)
Na^+: 140 mmol/L (135 to 145 mmol/L)
Creatinine: 2.5 mg/dL (0.5 to 1.7 mg/dL)

1. What is this patient's creatinine clearance?

2. What is the best choice of medication to reduce this patient's edema on an outpatient basis?

3. At your suggestion, the patient follows up with the internal medicine department. In addition to having hypertension, he also finds out that he has type 2 diabetes. The internist gives the patient an additional prescription. Unfortunately, you see the patient again in the emergency department 2 weeks after his appointment with internal medicine. This time, he is reporting an irregular heartbeat. An electrocardiogram reveals that the patient has a prolonged P-R interval and QRS duration, atrioventricular conduction delays, and a loss of P waves. Laboratory work reveals that his potassium level is elevated at 5.7 mEq/L. Which class of medication did the internist most likely prescribe for the patient's hypertension?

CASE STUDY 10

An 8-year-old boy with asthma has recently developed a nonproductive cough. His asthma has been well controlled over the past 3 years since he started allergy desensitization immunotherapy (allergy shots). He is presently taking cromolyn (four puffs per day) as well as albuterol (two puffs) when needed or before exercise. He demonstrates good inhaler technique

and uses a spacer. During your workup, you discover that the family has just "adopted" a puppy and the boy's asthma symptoms have been flaring up. His peak flow rates have been falling, and he has been having more nocturnal symptoms.

1. What is your plan to minimize and manage the child's asthma symptoms, given that the puppy remains in the household?

2. What adverse effects are especially of concern in a young child using inhaled corticosteroids?

CASE STUDY 11

A 49-year-old male has been given a diagnosis of hyperreactive airway disease and asthma. After a bout with influenza, he developed a recurrent cough that interferes with his job and active lifestyle. The cough and associated tight chest are unresponsive to over-the-counter cold and flu medications. The patient is somewhat surprised when you start working him up for gastroesophageal reflux disease (GERD). He states that his stomach is fine and he has never had heartburn.

1. What is the connection between asthma and GERD?

2. What agents can be given to the patient to treat his GERD symptoms?

CASE STUDY 12

A. A 41-year-old woman is admitted for severe chest pains. She appears as a thin, flushed, nervous woman. Her complaints include nervousness, palpitations, weight loss despite strong appetite, and unexplained bruising. She states she is being treated for deep vein thrombosis with warfarin 5 mg/day. Physical examination reveals a blood pressure of 190/95 mm Hg, pulse of 125 beats/min, and temperature of 102.6° F. Your exam also reveals droopy eyes, decreased visual acuity, an enlarged thyroid, atrial fibrillation, pitting edema, and tremor.

1. What is your initial diagnosis, and how would you treat the patient?

B. A 37-year-old female wants to breastfeed her first child. She requests information on contraception choices before leaving the hospital. She has a strong family history of cardiovascular disease and is presently a two-pack-per-day smoker. She previously had a conventional intrauterine device that was removed because of severe bleeding. She also states that spermicidal foams and condoms cause her itching and burning.

2. What type of contraception would you recommend to the patient?

Case Study Answers

CASE STUDY 1

1. Using the published value for Vd and the patient's weight, the patient's specific Vd is calculated at:

$$Vd = (0.48 \text{ L/kg})(65 \text{ kg}) = 31.2 \text{ L}$$

2. Smokers are known to metabolize theophylline more rapidly than nonsmokers. A commonly accepted $t_{1/2}$ is used when dosing theophylline in cigarette smokers. Using this value (4.5 hours) and the patient's estimated Vd (which was calculated in the previous question), clearance for this patient is calculated as:

$$Cl = \frac{0.693 \text{ (Vd)}}{t_{1/2}} = \frac{0.693 \text{ (31.2 L)}}{4.5 \text{ hr}} = 48 \text{ L/hr or 80 mL/min}$$

3. Because the patient's plasma levels of theophylline are lower than the target values, give him a loading dose to quickly boost his theophylline values back into the target range. The following equation allows achieves this:

$$\text{Loading dose} = \frac{(Vd)(Cp \text{ desired} - Cp \text{ initial})}{F}$$

$$\text{Loading dose} = \frac{31.2 \text{ L} (10 \text{ mg/L} - 3.6 \text{ mg/L})}{1}$$

$$= 200 \text{ mg theophylline}$$

CASE STUDY 2

1. It is not uncommon for children to require higher theophylline dosages than adults, so it is not entirely surprising that this woman has taken the same theophylline dose since she was a small child. There probably are two pharmacokinetic reasons for this. One has to do with volume of distribution, the other with hepatic metabolism. Recall that when clinicians dose theophylline, they are aiming for theophylline levels between 5 and 15 mg/L in the serum. Theophylline's volume of distribution is relatively restricted; it does not distribute into fatty tissue. In childhood, a larger percentage of the body is composed of water versus adipose tissue. This water, in essence, "dilutes" theophylline, so even though a child weighs less than an adult, there is more total body water in a child in which the theophylline is diluted. Children are routinely given larger mg/kg doses of theophylline than adults are.

Second, during early childhood, the metabolic capacity of the liver reaches its peak level. After approximately 9 years of age, the liver's metabolic capacity begins a slow decline. Therefore, children hepatically metabolize theophylline faster than adults do, often necessitating larger doses than for adults.

Although she weighs more now than she did as a child, her body composition is composed of less water (and more fat) and her hepatic metabolic capability declined with age (even in the absence of overt hepatic disease); therefore she may actually require less drug on a mg/kg basis than she did as a child to maintain theophylline levels within the 5 to 15 mg/L target range. In spite of these factors (favoring effectiveness), the drug is currently ineffective. Something else is going on.

2. Rifampin is a potent inducer of P450 hepatic enzymes. Because theophylline is metabolized by these same enzymes, rifampin could decrease theophylline levels, rendering theophylline less effective. This probably is what has occurred and probably is the reason this woman is having more breathing difficulties recently.

3. Cimetidine is a potent inhibitor of P450 hepatic enzymes. Because theophylline is metabolized by these same enzymes, cimetidine could increase theophylline levels, leading to theophylline-related toxicities.

CASE STUDY 3

1. After the ABCs are addressed (airway, breathing, circulation), the D component (decontamination) of toxicology management should be initiated. Orogastric lavage should be initiated, followed by ingestion of activated charcoal. Activated charcoal binds the toxic substance, preventing absorption. The patient is usually put into a left side (left lateral; decubitus), head down (Trendelenburg) position to protect the airway from emesis and to limit transit of gastric contents into the small intestine.

2. Aspirin (salicylate) poisoning is consistent with the patient's initial symptoms. Salicylates directly stimulate the respiratory center in the medulla to cause hyperpnea and tachypnea. This rapid deep breathing leads to an initial respiratory alkalosis. The elevation in body temperature is consistent with salicylate uncoupling of oxidative phosphorylation. Salicylates are gastric irritants and trigger vomiting and cramps.

3. Salicylates directly stimulate the respiratory center in the medulla to cause hyperpnea and tachypnea. This rapid deep breathing leads to an initial respiratory alkalosis. The increased respiration rate results in increased CO_2 removal at the lung, which decreases H^+ ion concentration in plasma. Remember that $CO_2 + H_2O = H_2CO_3 = H^+ + HCO_3^-$.

4. Compensation for the initial respiratory alkalosis is achieved by increased renal excretion of HCO_3^-, accompanied by a decrease in renal bicarbonate reabsorption. This mechanism explains the low bicarbonate levels in the plasma of the first blood sample. By uncoupling oxidative phosphorylation, plasma CO_2 levels increase faster than CO_2 can be removed by enhanced respiration (now driven by acidosis), further exacerbating acidosis. In addition, derangement of carbohydrate metabolism leads to accumulation of lactic acid and pyruvate, and impaired renal function leads to accumulation of sulfuric and phosphoric acids. As metabolic acidosis worsens and urine acidifies, excretion of weak acid salicylate metabolites will decrease.

5. To reduce the metabolic acidosis, an intravenous bolus of sodium bicarbonate or addition of sodium bicarbonate to 5% dextrose in water should be initiated. Additional, oral activated charcoal can be administered. To correct for low K^+ plasma levels (increased excretion of K^+ is an indirect result of diminished reabsorption of bicarbonate), intravenous potassium can be delivered. In extreme cases, hemodialysis can be started to remove salicylate metabolites. In the case of salicylate-induced seizures, phenobarbital may be administered.

CASE STUDY 4

1. Erysipelas is an infection of subcutaneous tissues. Patients often have a fever and dermatologic findings. Muscle and joint pains, nausea, headache, and skin discomfort often are noted as well. A defect in the skin barrier permits the infection to occur (e.g., trauma, abrasion, skin ulcer, insect bite, eczema, psoriatic lesions). Group A streptococci are the most common organisms responsible for erysipelas, followed by groups G, C, and B streptococci or staphylococci.

2. Because the patient has no prior history of cardiovascular disease but has a high fever and has been having episodes of diarrhea and vomiting for more than 12 hours, her cardiac arrhythmias are probably related to electrolyte disturbances, especially hypokalemia.

3. Although it is possible that streptococci or staphylococci isolated from a scab on the patient's scalp are simply normal flora, you cannot rule out the possibility that either one (or both) of these microorganisms might be the cause of her current infection. Most of the penicillins will provide adequate coverage against streptococcal organisms; however, whenever staphylococci are isolated, it must be assumed that the organisms make β-lactamases. Therefore a penicillinase-resistant penicillin is the most appropriate drug of choice for this patient. Because the patient was quite ill by the time she came to the emergency department, it is appropriate to admit her and initiate intravenous nafcillin.

4. *Clostridium difficile* may be part of a patient's normal gastrointestinal flora, but this bacterium often overgrows under opportune conditions, such as during or immediately after antibacterial therapy. Alternatively, the organism may have been acquired at the hospital because many institutions report difficulties controlling the spread of this bacterium from patient to patient, probably as a result of poor handwashing techniques on the part of the staff. Typically, metronidazole is the first-choice antibiotic used to treat *C. difficile* infections; however, patients should be warned that strict avoidance of alcohol is imperative. Vancomycin is another antibiotic reliably used to treat infections caused by *C. difficile*. Although most patients initially respond to treatment with metronidazole or vancomycin, as many as 3% to 5% of patients continually relapse. Use of probiotics may be considered because it addresses the real issue underlying *C. difficile* diarrhea, which is not the mere presence of the microorganism in the gastrointestinal tract but rather an absence of "healthy" bacteria that can keep clostridial growth in check. Probiotic therapies replace some of the missing "healthy" bacterial species and have even been used successfully in patients who were refractory to treatment with metronidazole and vancomycin.

CASE STUDY 5

1. Doxorubicin is associated with cardiotoxicity that may be life-threatening. The likelihood of cardiotoxicity and its severity are related to the cumulative dose received. Because of the patient's history of hypertension, he is already at risk of cardiotoxicity. Other risk factors include preexisting cardiac disease, prior thoracic radiation therapy, and very young or very old age. A technitium-99 based multiple-gated acquisition scan (MUGA scan) should be obtained before initiating therapy to evaluate ejection fraction. Doxorubicin therapy is often discontinued if left ventricular ejection fraction falls to less than 45% because additional therapy could lead to irreversible heart failure. The drug dezrazoxane, a chelating agent, is used as a pretreatment to prevent anthracycline-induced cardiomyopathy.

2. Vincristine is associated with dose-limiting neurotoxicity, especially peripheral neuropathy. Those with existing neurologic diseases and the elderly are most susceptible. Typically, neurotoxicity is a cumulative effect that occurs only after several treatments. As a result, patients should be given a neurologic assessment at baseline and before each treatment. If the patient has a history of long-standing diabetes mellitus with accompanying peripheral neuropathies, vincristine could aggravate them.

3. Cyclophosphamide is associated with secondary myeloproliferative and lymphoproliferative malignancies, bladder fibrosis and bladder cancer, and sterility. Bladder problems may be prevented by maintaining adequate hydration and administering mesna therapy. (Mesna stands for sodium 2-mercaptoethane sulfonate, an agent that reacts with acrolein and other urotoxic metabolites of cyclophosphamide or ifosfamide to form stable, nonurotoxic compounds. Mesna does not have any antitumor activity, nor does it appear to interfere with the antitumor activity of antineoplastic drugs.)

CASE STUDY 6

In this clinical study, intravenous infusion of norepinephrine produces a rise in both systolic and diastolic blood pressure. Stimulation of α-receptors (norepinephrine favors a (greek symbol "alpha") receptors), accompanying vasoconstriction, and the increase in total peripheral resistance (TPR) (see the middle tracing) are responsible for the rise in blood pressure.

However, when administering adrenergic agents, do not forget about the baroreceptors. Because of reflex actions of baroreceptors, heart rate actually declines. Therefore, despite the fact that norepinephrine also stimulates β-receptors on the heart, because of the reflex activity of baroreceptors there may actually be a decline in pulse rate as sympathetic outflow is blocked and vagal (parasympathetic) tone temporarily predominates.

A common misconception is to consider epinephrine and norepinephrine as having the same pharmacologic actions. Compare the results of norepinephrine infusion with the results of epinephrine infusion. After infusion of epinephrine, there is a rise in systolic pressure with a fall in diastolic pressure. This is counterintuitive and arises specifically because of stimulation of β_2-receptors in the vasculature.

Under normal conditions, the body is under the control of sympathetic norepinephrine-releasing nerves. These nerves "talk" directly to α_1-receptors and lead to vasoconstriction and increased TPR. This is the minute-to-minute regulation of blood pressure that prevents postural hypotension.

However, under conditions of fight-or-flight, cardiac output must increase, and increased perfusion of skeletal muscles also is necessary. This is accomplished through mechanisms that produce the physiologic tracings shown for epinephrine. Epinephrine stimulates α- and β-receptors. When epinephrine stimulates β_2-receptors in the vasculature, the typical α effect is overridden, leading to vasodilation and accompanying decrease in TPR (thereby increasing blood flow to the muscle). Therefore diastolic pressure falls. Simultaneously, stimulation of β_1-receptors within the heart produces a dramatic increase in heart rate and contractility. There is a corresponding increase in systolic pressure with a modest change or no change in mean arterial pressure.

The effect of epinephrine is most dramatically illustrated by comparison with infusion of isoproterenol, a β-selective agonist. Here, there is a dramatic drop in TPR because the β_2 response is unopposed by any α_1 effect. In addition, systolic pressure rises because of the increased blood pressure that results from stimulation of myocardial β_1-receptors. The foregoing discussion is of great importance because of the tendency to lump all adrenergic agonists into one large class of stimulatory agents. Based on their roles in the integrated physiology of the autonomic nervous system, there is tremendous diversity in pharmacologic responses to these agents.

CASE STUDY 7

1. Perhaps the best indicators of iron deficiency anemia are a decrease in serum ferritin level and an elevated total iron-binding capacity. In addition, a peripheral blood smear might be performed, which would be expected to reveal hypochromic microcytic red blood cells if your suspicion is correct.

2. The patient has a history of peptic ulcer disease. Despite that history, two different physicians prescribed nonsteroidal antiinflammatories for him, and the second doctor failed to tell the patient to stop taking the celecoxib when the ibuprofen was recommended. Although celecoxib is COX-2 specific, gastrointestinal bleeding may still occur, even when it is used alone, and this patient was taking celecoxib concomitantly with ibuprofen. Use of the nonsteroidal antiinflammatory drugs caused the gastrointestinal bleeding, which in turn caused the iron deficiency.

3. Iron may cause constipation, but this can be prevented with a stool softener. Iron may also cause stools to darken in color. Iron therapy will most likely be continued for 3 to 6 months to ensure saturation of all iron stores. Serum ferritin will be the best predictor to monitor iron stores after correction of hemoglobin and hematocrit.

CASE STUDY 8

1. Hydrochlorothiazide, a first-line antihypertensive drug for most patients, may cause hyperuricemia and hypokalemia. In this patient, hyperuricemia precipitated an acute gout attack—thus the reason for the painful, swollen, red toe.

   Patients need to have potassium levels monitored with both thiazide and loop diuretics. Unless a sufficient amount of K^+ is obtained from dietary sources (e.g., bananas, orange juice), a potassium supplement is often necessary.

2. Atenolol is a β_1-selective antagonist; that is, the drug prevents norepinephrine from interacting with β_1-receptors. When β_1-receptors in the myocardium are blocked, both resting heart rate and exercise-induced heart rates are slowed. β-Blockers can precipitate atrioventricular blockade as well.

3. During therapy with β-blockers, there is up-regulation of β-receptors. Rapid discontinuation of β-blockers can promote a hyperadrenergic state, leading to tachycardia.

4. Lisinopril is an angiotensin-converting enzyme (ACE) inhibitor. ACE inhibitors prevent conversion of angiotensin I to angiotensin II. Because angiotensin II is a potent vasoconstrictor in the arteries and veins, lisinopril will lower total peripheral resistance by acting in a balanced fashion throughout the vasculature. In addition, because angiotensin II stimulates aldosterone release, this drug will prevent Na^+ and fluid retention that is mediated by the renin-angiotensin-aldosterone system.

   ACE inhibitors may cause hyperkalemia, and up to 40% of patients may experience a dry cough, thought to result from bradykinin accumulation. Angioedema of lips and tongue may also occur. In the event of a persistent cough, the patient can be switched to an angiotensin receptor blocker.

CASE STUDY 9

1. Creatinine clearance is calculated according to the following formula:

$$\text{CrCl (mL/min)} = \frac{[(140 - \text{Age})(\text{Body weight in kg})]}{(\text{Serum creatinine})(72)}$$

1 pound = 2.2 kg, so the patient weighs 77 kg. We know the patient's age and we know his serum creatinine measurement, so we can calculate creatinine clearance.

For this patient,

$$\text{CrCl (mL/min)} = \frac{[(140 - 60)(77 \text{ kg})]}{(2.5)(72)} = 34 \text{ mL/min}$$

2. Because of their action in the loop of Henle (the region of the nephron with the greatest potential for sodium reabsorption), loop diuretics such as furosemide are the best choices for reducing this patient's fluid overload. Spironolactone is rarely used in men because of its antiandrogenic side effects. Thiazides cannot eliminate large amounts of fluid. In addition, given the patient's declining kidney function, furosemide is a superior choice to hydrochlorothiazide, because most thiazides are ineffective at low glomerular filtration rates. Mannitol is used only intravenously, so it is not appropriate for outpatient management of edema. A potassium supplement is often prescribed along with furosemide to counteract the loss of K^+ associated with the use of loop diuretics.

3. The patient's electrocardiogram findings are consistent with hyperkalemia. ACE inhibitors such as enalapril, as well as angiotensin receptor blockers (ARBs), elevate serum potassium levels by interfering with the downstream actions of aldosterone in the kidneys. Because the patient was already taking potassium supplements, the addition of an ACE inhibitor or an ARB caused his potassium levels to rise to dangerously high levels, despite the loop diuretic that he was taking.

Periodic monitoring of K^+ levels is imperative when combining medications such as diuretics, K^+ supplements, ACE inhibitors, or ARBs, which can alter potassium levels. In addition, patients should be cautioned about eating certain foods that contain large amounts of K^+ such as bananas, orange juice, and K^+-containing salt substitutes while taking prescription potassium supplements or K^+-retaining medications.

CASE STUDY 10

1. The boy should be reassessed for allergy to dog dander. (A common misconception is that allergies to dogs are caused by dog hair; pet allergies are caused by pet dander.) The puppy should be barred from the second floor, where the child's room is located (trigger avoidance). Carpeting in the child's bedroom should be replaced with wood or rubberized flooring to minimize accumulation of pet dander in the bedroom. The house should be dusted and vacuumed regularly with a vacuum that has a high-quality filtration system (preferably one that is vented outdoors). Electrostatic filters can also be placed over air vents in the house. Regular bathing of the puppy may help.

If additional pharmacotherapy is needed, cromolyn can be discontinued and replaced with inhaled corticosteroids. In addition, montelukast, a leukotriene receptor antagonist, might be added to the treatment regimen. If necessary, a long-acting β_2-agonist may also be added. In essence, stepwise therapy might be instituted until the child's symptoms are brought under control.

2. Corticosteroids cause linear growth suppression. This is seen even with inhaled corticosteroids. There is an average height difference of 1 cm per year between children treated with inhaled corticosteroids and controls. However, the risks of not adequately controlling asthma are more dangerous than the growth suppression.

As for all patients using inhaled corticosteroids, the child should rinse his mouth with water after using the inhaled corticosteroid to prevent thrush (an oral fungal infection).

CASE STUDY 11

1. Airway constriction occurs in response to refluxed gastric acids. Results from some studies suggest that as many as 63% of children with asthma may have GERD.

2. A proton pump inhibitor, such as omeprazole, may be added to the patient's other medications, which include nasal and orally inhaled glucocorticoids as well as a leukotriene receptor antagonist.

CASE STUDY 12

1. You suspect that the patient is experiencing life-threatening thyrotoxicosis (thyroid storm). As you are ordering thyroid tests to confirm your diagnosis, you aggressively manage cardiac events and fever with β-blockers and aspirin. To stabilize the patient before thyroid surgery, you use a combination of thionamide and iodide to suppress the overactive thyroid gland.

2. You might suggest a progestin-only "mini-pill" during the period that she is breastfeeding. Estrogen-containing formulations may suppress lactation. However, you will caution her that this type of contraception requires a commitment to take the pill at the same time each day to achieve maximal efficacy. Another option would be medroxyprogesterone injection every 3 months. However, you must warn her of the possibility of bone loss, a recently identified complication of depot medroxyprogesterone. After she finishes breastfeeding her child, you may switch her to a low-dose estrogen/progestin formulation. You might counsel her that smoking and estrogen contraception places her at high risk for thromboembolic events.

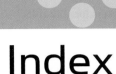

Index

Note: Page numbers followed by *b* indicate boxes, *f* indicate figures and *t* indicate tables.

A

Abacavir, 74, 74*b*
Abatacept, 171*t*, 172
Abciximab, 119
Absorption, 1–7
 bioavailability with, 14–15, 14*f*
 dosage form and, 3, 4*f*
 first-pass effect and, 4, 4*b*, 4*f*
 ionization in, 2–3, 2*b*, 3*b*
 molecular weight in, 3
 routes of administration in, 3–7, 4*b*
Abuse. *See* Drug abuse
ABVD treatment, 85*b*
Acarbose, 185
ACE inhibitors. *See* Angiotensin-converting enzyme inhibitors
Acebutolol, 106*t*, 107*f*, 108, 128–130, 129*t*
Acetaminophen, 36, 36*f*, 36*t*, 37*t*, 165
Acetazolamide, 156–157, 156*f*
Acetylcholine (ACh), 91–92, 95*b*, 99*t*, 202*t*.
  See also Cholinergic systems
Acetylcholinesterase (AChE), 95, 95*b*
Acetylcholinesterase (AChE) inhibitors, 101, 218, 218*t*
N-Acetylcysteine, 36, 36*f*, 36*t*, 37*t*
ACh. *See* Acetylcholine
AChE. *See* Acetylcholinesterase
Acne, 167, 168*t*, 169*b*
Activated charcoal, 29
Acyclovir, 72–73, 73*t*
Adalimumab, 171*t*, 172
Addiction, 223*b*, 224*b*
Addison disease, 183–185, 184*b*
Adefovir dipivoxil, 72–73, 73*t*
Adenosine, 146
Adenosine diphosphate inhibitors, 118–119
Adrenal gland, 181–185, 181*b*, 182*f*, 182*t*, 183*b*, 183*f*, 185*b*
 Addison disease and, 183–185, 184*b*
 Cushing syndrome and, 181–183, 184*f*
 hirsutism and, 185
 steroid-mediated signal transduction and, 185*b*, 185*f*
Adrenal insufficiency, 183–185, 184*b*
α-Adrenergic agonists, 104–106, 104*f*, 106*t*, 107*f*
 α₂, 133–134, 133*f*, 134*f*

β-Adrenergic agonists, 103*f*, 104*f*, 106*t*, 107*f*, 108
 β₂, 189–190
α-Adrenergic antagonists, 106–107, 106*t*, 107*f*
 α₁, 132, 196
β-Adrenergic antagonists (β-Blockers), 20, 104*f*, 106*t*, 107*f*, 108
 for arrhythmias, 145
 for heart failure, 138, 140*b*
 for hypertension, 128–130, 128*f*, 129*t*, 130*b*
Adrenergic systems, 94*t*, 101–104
 biochemistry of, 101–102, 102*f*, 103*f*
 drugs affecting, 103*f*, 104–108, 104*f*, 106*t*, 107*f*
 receptor subtypes of, 92–93, 94*t*, 103–104, 104*f*
  α, 103–104, 103*f*, 104*f*, 105*f*, 105*t*, 106*t*
  β, 104, 104*f*, 105*t*, 106*f*
Affective disorders, 208–209, 208*b*.
  See also Antidepressants
Affinity, 17, 18*t*
Aging, pharmacokinetic changes with, 12–13
Agonist, 17, 19–20, 20*f*
Albuterol, 106*t*, 107*f*, 108
Alcohol. *See* Ethanol
Aldosterone, 183*b*, 183*f*
Aldosterone receptor antagonists, 132
Alemtuzumab, 85–86, 86*t*
Alfuzosin, 106–107, 196
Alginic acid, 173–174
Aliskiren, 127*f*, 132
Alkylating agents, 80*t*, 81–83, 82*f*
Allergies. *See* Hypersensitivity reactions
Allopurinol, 169, 170*f*
Almotriptan, 221
Alprazolam, 221, 222*t*
Alteplase, 119, 120*t*
Alternative medicine. *See* Complementary and alternative medicine
Altretamine, 81–83
Alzheimer disease, 218, 218*t*
Amantadine, 71*f*, 72
Ambenonium, 101
Amikacin, 53–55
Amiloride, 158–159, 158*f*
Amino acids, neurotransmitters synthesized from, 95*b*

γ-Aminobutyric acid (GABA), 202*t*, 204*f*, 221–222, 222*t*
γ-Aminobutyric acid (GABA)-activated receptor, 24, 26*f*
Aminoglutethimide, 181–183
Aminoglycosides, 53–55, 54*t*, 55*t*
Aminopenicillins, 46, 47*t*
Amiodarone, 145–146
Amitriptyline, 209–210, 210*t*
Amlodipine, 132–133
Amoxapine, 209–210
Amoxicillin, 46, 47*t*
Amphetamine, 209*f*, 224
Amphotericin B, 65–66, 66*b*
Ampicillin, 46, 47*t*
Amprenavir, 75
Amyl nitrate, 38
Anakinra, 171*t*, 172, 172*b*
Analgesics, opioid, 219–221, 220*b*, 220*t*, 223*b*
Anaphylactic shock, 167*b*
Andropause, 195
Anemia, 120–122, 121*t*
 hematopoietic stimulating factors for, 122
 supplementation for, 120–122, 121*b*, 121*t*, 123*b*
Anesthetics, 203–205, 204*b*
 inhalation, 203–204, 203*t*
 intravenous, 204–205, 204*f*, 204*t*
 local, 205
 mechanisms of, 202*f*, 203
Angiogenesis, 81*b*
Angiotensin, 183*b*, 183*f*
Angiotensin receptor blockers (ARBs), 131–132
Angiotensin-converting enzyme (ACE) inhibitors
 for heart failure, 138, 140*b*
 for hypertension, 130–131, 130*f*, 131*f*
Anidulafungin, 67–68
Anion gap, 30*b*
ANS. *See* Autonomic nervous system
Antacids, 173, 174*t*
Antagonist, 17, 20, 20*f*
Anterior pituitary hormones, 181–188
 adrenal gland disorders, 181–185, 181*b*, 182*f*, 182*t*, 183*b*, 183*f*, 184*b*, 184*f*, 185*b*, 185*f*

Anterior pituitary hormones (*Continued*)
  growth-related disorders, 187–188, 188*f*
  prolactin disorders, 188
  thyroid disorders, 185–187, 186*f*, 187*b*, 187*t*
Antibacterials, 42–63, 45*f*, 45*t*
  aminoglycosides, 53–55, 54*t*, 55*t*
  carbapenems, 51, 52*t*
  cell wall synthesis inhibitors, 43–53, 53*t*
  cephalosporins, 12, 48–53, 48*b*, 49*t*, 51*b*,
    52*t*
  chloramphenicol, 56–57, 56*f*, 56*t*
  cycloserine, 52
  DNA/RNA synthesis inhibitors, 62–63
  folic acid synthesis inhibitors, 60–62, 60*f*
  lincosamides, 56*f*, 57, 57*t*
  linezolid, 60
  lipopeptides, 63
  macrolides, 57–59, 57*b*, 58*b*, 58*t*
  metronidazole, 63
  monobactams, 51–52, 52*t*
  mupirocin, 59
  nitrofurantoin, 53
  penicillins, 12, 43–46, 45*f*, 47*t*, 48, 48*b*,
    52*t*, 154*b*
  polymyxin B, 53
  protein synthesis inhibitors, 53–60, 54*f*
  retapamulin, 59
  rifaximin, 63
  streptogramins, 60
  sulfonamides, 60–61, 60*f*, 61*b*, 61*t*
  tetracyclines, 55–56, 55*f*, 55*t*, 56*t*
  trimethoprim, 60*f*, 61–62
  vancomycin, 52, 53*t*
Antibiotic-associated diarrhea, 76
Antibiotics, cytotoxic, 80*t*, 82*f*, 83–84
Anticholinergics, 31, 32*t*.
    See also Cholinergic systems
Anticholinesterases.
    See Acetylcholinesterase inhibitors
Anticoagulant drugs, 111–116
  direct thrombin inhibitors, 114
  heparins, 111*b*, 112–114, 112*b*
  vitamin K antagonists, 114–116, 114*t*,
    115*b*, 115*t*
Anticonvulsants, 206–207
  epilepsy pathophysiology and, 206
  seizure disorder treatments, 206–207,
    206*f*, 207*b*, 208*t*
Antidepressants, 208–212
  biogenic amine theory of affective
    disorder, 208–209
  mania and bipolar disorder treatment, 212,
    212*f*
  monoamine oxidase inhibitors, 209*f*, 210*t*,
    211–212, 211*b*, 212*b*
  SSRIs and SNRIs, 209*f*, 210*t*, 211, 211*b*
  tricyclic, 209–210, 209*f*, 210*t*
Antidiuretic hormone. *See* Vasopressin
    analogs
Antiepileptic drugs, 206–207
  epilepsy pathophysiology and, 206
  seizure disorder treatments, 206–207,
    206*f*, 207*b*, 208*t*

Antifungals, 65–68, 65*f*
  azoles, 65*f*, 66–67, 66*t*, 67*b*, 67*t*
  caspofungin, 65*f*, 67–68
  ciclopirox, 65*f*, 68
  flucytosine, 65*f*, 68
  griseofulvin, 65*f*, 68
  polyenes, 65–66, 65*f*, 66*b*
  terbinafine, 65*f*, 68
Antihelmintics, 70, 70*t*
Antihistamine drugs, 161–163, 162*f*, 162*t*,
    178*t*
  H₁ antagonists, 162, 162*b*
  H₂ blockers, 163, 163*t*
Antiinfective agents, 41, 42*b*, 43*t*, 76–78, 77*t*
Antiinflammatory drugs
  NSAIDs
    for inflammatory disorders, 163–167,
      163*t*, 164*f*, 166*t*
    peptic ulcer disease and, 176, 176*b*
    for rheumatoid arthritis, 170–172
  steroidal, 163–167, 163*t*, 164*f*
Antimalarials, 68–70, 69*t*
Antimetabolites, 82*f*, 83, 84*f*
Antimicrobials, 41, 42*b*
Antimuscarinic drugs, 100–101, 178*t*
Antimycobacterials, 64–65
  clofazimine, 65
  ethambutol, 64–65
  isoniazid, 64
  pyrazinamide, 64
  rifampin, 64
Antineoplastic therapy. *See* Cancer therapy
Antiparasitics, 68–71
  antihelmintics, 70, 70*t*
  antimalarials, 68–70, 69*t*
  head lice medications, 70–71
Anti-Parkinson drugs, 209*f*, 216–218, 216*f*,
    217*t*
Antiplatelet drugs, 116–119, 117*f*, 117*t*
  adenosine diphosphate inhibitors, 118–119
  glycoprotein IIb/IIIa inhibitors, 119
  phosphodiesterase inhibitors, 118
  salicylates, 117–118, 117*f*, 118*f*
Antipseudomonal penicillins, 47*t*, 48
Antipsychotics, 212–214
  dopamine hypothesis of schizophrenia,
    213, 213*t*, 214*f*, 215*t*
  therapeutics, 213–214, 215*t*
Antivirals, 71–74, 71*f*
  host cell penetration interference, 71*f*, 73
  for HPV, 73–74
  integrase inhibition, 71–72, 71*f*
  intracellular synthesis inhibition, 72–73,
    73*t*
  viral neuraminidase inhibition, 72
  viral uncoating inhibition, 71*f*, 72
Anxiolytic agents. *See* Sedative-hypnotics
Apomorphine, 216–218
Arachidonic acid, 23
Arachidonophobia, 23–24, 25*f*
ARBs. *See* Angiotensin receptor blockers
Ardeparin, 112–113, 112*b*
Aripiprazole, 212, 213–214, 215*t*

Arrhythmias, 142–146, 142*b*, 143*t*
  β-blockers for, 145
  calcium channel blockers for, 146
  potassium channel blockers for, 145–146,
    145*f*, 146*b*
  sodium channel blockers for, 142–145,
    143*f*, 143*t*
Arsenic, 37–38, 37*t*
Artemether, 69
Arthritis. *See* Rheumatoid arthritis
Asenapine, 213–214, 215*t*
Aspirin, 30*b*, 117–118, 117*f*, 118*f*, 164*f*, 165,
    166*t*, 167*b*
Asthma, 167–169, 168*b*, 170*t*
Atazanavir, 75
Atenolol, 106*t*, 107*f*, 128–130, 129*t*
Atherosclerotic lesions, 148*b*
Atorvastatin, 147–148
Atovaquone-proguanil, 69
Atracurium, 98–100, 205, 205*t*
Atropine, 100–101
Attention deficit disorder, 224
Attention deficit–hyperactivity disorder, 224
Autonomic nervous system (ANS), 91–109.
      See also Parasympathetic nervous
      system; Sympathetic nervous system
  adrenergic systems of, 94*t*, 101–104
    biochemistry of, 101–102, 102*f*, 103*f*
    drugs affecting, 103*f*, 104–108, 104*f*,
      106*t*, 107*f*
    receptor subtypes of, 92–93, 94*t*,
      103–104, 103*f*, 104*f*, 105*f*, 105*t*, 106*f*,
      106*t*
  cholinergic systems of, 94–101, 94*t*
    acetylcholinesterase inhibitors affecting,
      101, 218, 218*t*
    biochemistry of, 94–95, 95*f*
    muscarinic drugs affecting, 99*t*,
      100–101
    nicotinic drugs affecting, 96–100, 101
    receptor subtypes of, 92–93, 92*f*, 93*t*,
      94*t*, 96, 97*f*, 97*t*, 98*f*, 99*f*, 99*t*
  indirect effectors of, 104*f*, 108–109,
    109*t*
  organization of, 91–94
    neurochemical, 91–92, 93*f*
    neuroreceptor, 92–93, 93*t*
    physiologic responses, 93–94, 94*t*
Azacitidine, 83
Azathioprine, 89
Azelastine, 162, 162*b*
Azithromycin, 57–59, 58*t*
Azoles, 65*f*, 66–67, 66*t*, 67*b*, 67*t*
Aztreonam, 51–52, 52*t*

B

Baclofen, 206
Bacteria, normal, 41, 42*t*
Barbiturates, 222, 222*f*, 222*t*
Basophilic stippling, 38, 38*b*
Beclomethasone, 166
Benazepril, 130–131

Bendamustine, 81–83
Benign prostatic hyperplasia, 196
Benzocaine, 205
Benzodiazepines, 221, 222*b*, 222*f*, 222*t*
 for serotonin syndrome, 32–33, 33*b*, 33*t*,
  34*t*
 toxicity of, 31, 32*t*
Benztropine, 100–101, 216–218, 217*t*
Benzyl alcohol, 71
Besifloxacin, 62–63
Betamethasone, 166–167
Betaxolol, 128–130, 129*t*
Bethanechol, 99*t*, 100, 175–176
Bevacizumab, 85–86, 86*t*
Biguanides, 197–198
Bile acid sequestrants, for hyperlipidemia,
 149, 149*b*, 150*b*
Bioavailability (F), 14–15, 14*b*, 14*f*
Biogenic amines, 208–209, 209*b*.
  See also Antidepressants
Biologics, 24–27, 26*t*, 85–87, 85*f*, 172*b*
Biotransformation. *See* Metabolism
Bipolar disorder, 208*b*, 212, 212*f*
Bismuth subsalicylate, 176
Bisoprolol, 128–130, 129*t*
Bisphosphonates, 193–195
Bleeding disorders, 120
Bleomycin, 83–84
β-Blockers. *See* β-Adrenergic antagonists
Blood-brain barrier, 8, 8*b*, 8*f*
Bretylium, 145–146
Bromocriptine, 216–218, 217*t*
Bronchodilators, 167–169
Budesonide, 166, 176–177
Bumetanide, 157, 157*f*
Bupivacaine, 205
Bupropion, 210*t*, 211
Buspirone, 19, 222
Busulfan, 81–83
Butorphanol, 219–221

C
C1 inhibitor, 123
CA. *See* Carbonic anhydrase
Calcitonin, 193–195, 194*t*
Calcium channel blockers, 132–133, 133*f*,
 146
Calcium supplements, 193–195, 194*t*
Cancer therapy, 79–90
 adverse effects of, 80*t*
 biologics, 85–87, 85*f*
 complementary and alternative medicine,
  89–90
 cytotoxic, 80–85, 80*f*, 82*f*
  alkylating agents, 80*t*, 81–83, 82*f*
  antibiotics in, 80*t*, 82*f*, 83–84
  antimetabolites, 82*f*, 83, 84*f*
  mitotic inhibitors, 82*f*, 84–85
 endocrine therapy, 87, 87*t*
 monoclonal antibodies, 85–86, 86*t*
 resistance to, 79–80, 80*t*
 signal transduction inhibitors, 86–87

Candesartan, 131–132
Cannabinoids, 224–225
Capecitabine, 83
Captopril, 130–131
Carbachol, 99*t*, 100
Carbamazepine, 206–207, 206*f*, 208*t*
Carbapenems, 51, 52*t*
Carbenicillin, 47*t*, 48
Carbidopa, 216–217
Carbon monoxide (CO), 34, 35*t*
Carbonic anhydrase (CA), 156–157, 156*b*,
 156*f*, 160*t*
Carboplatin, 81–83
Carcinoid syndrome, 33*b*
Cardiac output, 125
Cardiotoxicity, 34–35
 carbon monoxide, 34, 35*t*
 hematologic and cardiovascular
  toxidromes, 34–35, 35*t*
Cardiovascular system, 125–151
 arrhythmias, 142–146, 142*b*, 143*t*
 complementary and alternative medicine
  for, 150–151
 heart failure, 138–142, 138*f*, 138*t*, 139*f*,
  139*t*, 140*b*, 140*t*
 hyperlipidemia, 146–150, 147*f*, 147*t*
 hypertension, 125–135, 126*b*, 126*f*, 127*f*,
  128*t*, 135*t*
 pulmonary arterial hypertension,
  135–136, 136*f*
 stable angina, 136–137, 136*b*, 137*b*, 137*t*
Cardiovascular toxidromes, 34–35, 35*t*
Carmustine, 81–83
Carteolol, 128–130, 129*t*
Carvedilol, 108, 128–130, 129*t*
Caspofungin, 65*f*, 67–68
Catecholamines. *See* Autonomic nervous
  system
Cefaclor, 49*t*, 51
Cefadroxil, 49*t*, 50–51
Cefazolin, 49*t*, 50–51
Cefdinir, 49*t*, 51
Cefditoren, 49*t*, 51
Cefepime, 49*t*, 51
Cefixime, 49*t*, 51
Cefotaxime, 49*t*, 51
Cefotetan, 49*t*, 51
Cefoxitin, 49*t*, 51
Cefpodoxime, 49*t*, 51
Cefprozil, 49*t*, 51
Ceftazidime, 49*t*, 51
Ceftibuten, 49*t*, 51
Ceftizoxime, 49*t*, 51
Ceftriaxone, 49*t*, 51
Cefuroxime, 49*t*, 51
Ceiling effect, 17–18
Celecoxib, 165–166, 176
Cell cycle, 80*f*, 81*b*
Cell wall synthesis inhibitors, 43–53, 53*t*
Central nervous system (CNS), 201–226
 abused recreational drugs affecting,
  223–225, 223*t*, 224*b*, 225*b*
 anatomy of, 92*b*

Central nervous system (CNS) (*Continued*)
 anesthetics affecting, 202*f*, 203–205, 203*t*,
  204*b*, 204*f*, 204*t*
 anticonvulsants affecting, 206–207, 206*f*,
  207*b*, 208*t*
 antidepressants affecting, 208–212, 209*f*,
  210*t*, 211*b*, 212*b*, 212*f*
 antipsychotics affecting, 212–214, 213*t*,
  214*f*, 215*t*
 complementary and alternative medicine
  affecting, 225
 drugs that penetrate, 8, 8*b*
 muscle relaxants affecting, 205–206, 205*t*
 neurodegeneration and movement
  disorders in, 209*f*, 214–219, 216*b*,
  216*f*, 217*t*, 218*t*, 219*b*, 219*t*
 neurotransmitters of, 202*t*
 pain management in, 219, 220*b*, 220*t*,
  223*b*
 pharmacologic molecular targets in,
  201–202, 202*f*
 sedative-hypnotics and anxiolytic agents
  affecting, 221–223, 222*b*, 222*f*, 222*t*
Cephalexin, 49*t*, 50–51
Cephalosporins, 48–53, 48*b*, 52*t*
 elimination of, 12
 first-generation, 49*t*, 50–51
 prescribing, 51*b*
 second-generation, 49*t*, 51
 third-generation, 49*t*, 51
Cephapirin, 49*t*, 50–51
Cephradine, 49*t*, 50–51
Certolizumab pegol, 171*t*, 172
Cetirizine, 162
Cetuximab, 85–86, 86*t*
Charcoal, activated, 29
Checkpoint control, 81*b*
Chlorambucil, 81–83
Chloramphenicol, 56–57, 56*f*, 56*t*
Chloroquine, 69, 69*t*
Chlorpheniramine, 162
Chlorpromazine, 213–214, 215*t*
Chlorthalidone, 157–158, 158*f*
Cholesterol, 147, 147*f*, 150, 150*b*, 184*f*, 185*b*
Cholestyramine, 149
Cholinergic systems, 94–101, 94*t*
 acetylcholinesterase inhibitors affecting,
  101, 218, 218*t*
 biochemistry of, 94–95, 95*f*
 muscarinic drugs affecting, 99*t*, 100–101
 nicotinic drugs affecting, 96–100
 receptor subtypes of, 92*f*, 93*t*, 96
  muscarinic, 92–93, 94*t*, 96, 97*f*, 97*t*, 98*f*,
   99*f*, 99*t*
  nicotinic, 92–93, 94*t*, 96, 97*f*, 97*t*, 99*t*
Cholinesterase inhibitors.
  See Acetylcholinesterase inhibitors
Ciclesonide, 166
Ciclopirox, 65*f*, 68
Cilostazol, 118
Cimetidine, 12, 163, 174–175, 175*t*
Cinchonism, 144
Ciprofloxacin, 62–63

Cisplatin, 81–83
Citalopram, 210*t*, 211
Cladribine, 83
Clarithromycin, 57–59, 58*t*
Clemastine, 162
Clevidipine, 132–133
Clindamycin, 56*f*, 57, 57*t*
Clofarabine, 83
Clofazimine, 65
Clomifene, 189–190
Clonazepam, 206–207, 206*f*, 221
Clonidine, 104–106, 106*t*, 107*f*, 133–134
Clopidogrel, 118–119
Clozapine, 213–214, 215*t*
CNS. *See* Central nervous system
CO. *See* Carbon monoxide
Cocaine, 205, 209*f*, 224
Codeine, 219–221, 220*t*
Colchicine, 169
Colesevelam, 149
Colestipol, 149
Common cold, 76
Complementary and alternative medicine, 225
   for antibiotic-associated diarrhea, 76
   for cancer prevention, 89–90
   for cardiovascular system, 150–151
   for CNS, 225
   for common cold, 76
   for endocrine disorders, 199
   gastrointestinal, 179
   renal system and, 159–160, 160*b*
   toxicology of, 39
   for yeast infections, 76
Conivaptan, 159
Constipation, 177, 180*t*
Contraception, 190–192, 191*t*
Cooperativity, 20
Coronary stents, drug-eluting, 88*b*
Cortical diluting segment, 157
Corticosteroids, 163–169, 163*t*, 164*f*, 176–177, 181, 182*t*, 184*b*, 185*b*, 185*f*. *See also* Adrenal gland
Cortisol, 181–183, 184*f*
Crohn disease, 176–177
Cumulative frequency distribution, 18–19, 19*f*
Curare, 98–100
Cushing syndrome, 181–183, 184*f*
Cyanide poisoning, 38
Cyclooxygenase-2 inhibitors, 165–166
Cyclophosphamide, 81–83
Cycloserine, 52
Cyclosporine, 88–89, 89*f*
CYP450. *See* Microsomal P450 isoenzymes
Cyproheptadine, 32–33, 33*b*, 33*t*, 34*t*, 162
Cytarabine, 83
Cytochrome P450 (CYP450).
    See Microsomal P450 isoenzymes
Cytotoxic drugs, 80–85, 80*f*, 82*f*
   alkylating agents, 80*t*, 81–83, 82*f*
   antibiotics in, 80*t*, 82*f*, 83–84
   antimetabolites, 82*f*, 83, 84*f*
   mitotic inhibitors, 82*f*, 84–85

D
Dacarbazine, 81–83
Dactinomycin, 83–84
Dalfopristin, 60
Dalteparin, 112–113, 112*b*
Dantrolene, 206
Daptomycin, 63
Darbepoetin-α, 122
Darifenacin, 100–101
Darunavir, 75
Dasatinib, 86–87
Daunorubicin, 83–84
Decitabine, 83
Deferoxamine, 37*t*, 38
Delavirdine, 75
Demeclocycline, 55–56
Dependence, 224*b*
Depolarizing muscle relaxant, 100, 205
Depression, 208*b*. *See also* Antidepressants
Desensitization, 20
Desflurane, 203–204, 203*t*
Desipramine, 209–210
Desired drug level, 13–14, 14*f*
Desloratadine, 162
Desmopressin, 188–189, 189*b*, 189*f*
Desvenlafaxine, 210*t*, 211
Dexamethasone, 166
Dexlansoprazole, 175, 175*t*
Dexmedetomidine, 104–106, 106*t*, 107*f*
Dextromethorphan, 219–221
Diabetes mellitus, 196–199, 196*b*, 197*b*, 198*f*, 199*b*
Diabetic ketoacidosis, 199*b*
Diarrhea, 76, 177, 177*b*, 179*t*
Diazepam, 206–207, 206*f*, 221, 222*t*
Dicloxacillin, 46–48, 47*t*
Dicyclomine, 100–101
Didanosine, 74, 74*b*
Diffusion, passive, 2, 2*b*
Diftitox, 26–27
Digoxin, 139–142, 141*b*, 141*f*, 146
Dihydropyridines, 132–133
Diltiazem, 132–133, 146
Dimercaprol, 37–38, 37*t*
Dinoprostone, 189–190
Diphenhydramine, 162
Diphenoxylate, 219–221
Dipyridamole, 118
Direct thrombin inhibitors, 114
Disease-modifying antirheumatic drugs (DMARDs), 170–172, 171*t*
Disopyramide, 142–145, 143*f*, 143*t*
Distribution, 7–8, 8*b*
   plasma protein binding, 7–8, 7*t*, 8*b*
   selective, 8, 8*b*, 8*f*
Diuresis, ionized, 29–30, 30*b*, 30*t*
Diuretics
   carbonic anhydrase inhibitors, 156–157, 156*f*, 160*t*
   complementary and alternative medicine as, 159–160, 160*b*
   for hypertension, 128
   loop, 128, 157, 157*f*, 160*t*

Diuretics (*Continued*)
   major classes of, 160*t*
   osmotic, 155–156
   potassium-sparing, 158–159, 158*f*
   selection of, 160*t*
   thiazides, 157–158, 158*f*, 160*t*
DMARDs. *See* Disease-modifying antirheumatic drugs
DNA synthesis inhibitors, 62–63
Dobutamine, 106*t*, 107*f*, 108, 141
Docetaxel, 84–85
Docosanol, 71*f*, 73
Dofetilide, 145–146
Donepezil, 101, 218, 218*t*
Dopamine, 107*f*, 108, 202*t*
   antidepressants and, 209, 209*f*
   for heart failure, 142
   mesolimbic pathway, 224*b*
   in Parkinson disease, 216–218, 216*f*, 217*t*
   schizophrenia and, 213, 213*t*, 214*f*, 215*t*
Dopamine receptor agonists, 188
Dopamine receptor antagonists, 188
Doripenem, 51
Dorzolamide, 156–157, 156*f*
Dosage form, absorption and, 3, 4*f*
Dose-response curves, 17–19, 18*f*, 19*b*, 19*f*
Dose-response relationships, 17–19, 18*f*, 18*t*, 19*b*, 19*f*
Doxazosin, 106–107, 132, 196
Doxepin, 209–210, 210*t*
Doxorubicin, 83–84
Doxycycline, 55–56
Dronabinol, 224–225
Dronedarone, 145–146
Drug abuse, 223–225, 223*b*, 224*b*
   alcohol, 223–224, 223*t*, 224*b*
   cannabinoids, 224–225
   cocaine and psychomotor stimulants, 224
   as false messengers, 223–225, 223*t*
   nicotine, 225, 225*b*
Drug level, desired, 13–14, 14*f*
Drug-drug interactions, 11*b*
   absorption and, 3, 5*t*
   elimination and, 12, 13*t*
   mechanism for, 10–11
   protein binding and, 7–8
Drug-eluting coronary stents, 88*b*
Duloxetine, 210*t*, 211
Dutasteride, 196

E
Echinacea, 76
Echothiophate, 101
Eculizumab, 122–123
Eczema, 167
Edrophonium, 101
EDTA. *See* Ethylenediaminetetraacetic acid
Efavirenz, 75
Eicosanoids, 163, 163*t*
Electron transport chain, 37*b*
Eletriptan, 221

Elimination, 11–13, 13*b*, 13*f*, 13*t*
  bioavailability with, 14–15, 14*f*
  in renal system, 154–155, 155*b*, 155*f*
Eltrombopag, 123
Emtricitabine, 74, 74*b*
Enalapril, 130–131
Endocrine pharmacology, 181–199, 182*t*.
      See also Men's reproductive disorders;
      Women's reproductive disorders
  anterior pituitary hormones, 181–188
    adrenal gland disorders, 181–185, 181*b*,
        182*f*, 182*t*, 183*b*, 183*f*, 184*b*, 184*f*,
        185*b*, 185*f*
    growth-related disorders, 187–188, 188*f*
    prolactin disorders, 188
    thyroid disorders, 185–187, 186*f*, 187*b*,
        187*t*
  complementary and alternative medicine
      for, 199
  hypothalamic-pituitary axis and, 181,
      181*b*, 182*f*, 182*t*
  pancreatic disorders, 196–199, 196*b*,
      197*b*, 198*f*, 199*b*
  posterior pituitary hormones, 188–189
    oxytocin, 188–189
    vasopressin analogs, 188–189, 189*b*,
        189*f*
Endocrine therapy, for cancer, 87, 87*t*
Endometriosis, 192–193
Enfuvirtide, 75
Enoxaparin, 112–113, 112*b*
Entacapone, 216–218, 217*t*
Entecavir, 72–73, 73*t*
Entry inhibitors, 75–76
Enzyme replacement therapy, 26
Epigenetics, 87*b*
Epilepsy, 206–207, 206*f*, 207*b*, 208*t*
Epinastine, 162
Epinephrine, 91–94, 94*t*. *See also* Adrenergic
      systems
Epirubicin, 83–84
Eplerenone, 132
Epoetin-α, 122
Eprosartan, 131–132
Eptifibatide, 119
Erectile dysfunction, 195, 195*t*
Erlotinib, 86–87
Ertapenem, 51
Erythromycin base, 57–59
Erythromycin estolate, 57–59
Erythromycin ethylsuccinate, 57–59
Erythromycin stearate, 57–59
Erythropoietins, 122
Escitalopram, 211
Esmolol, 128–130, 129*t*, 145
Esomeprazole, 175, 175*t*
Estramustine, 81–83
Estrogen, 194*t*
  in contraceptives, 190–192, 191*t*
  in hormonal replacement therapy,
      192–193, 193*b*
Eszopiclone, 221–222
Etanercept, 89, 171*t*, 172

Ethacrynic acid, 157
Ethambutol, 64–65
Ethanol
  abuse of, 223–224, 223*t*, 224*b*
  for methanol poisoning, 33–34, 34*b*, 34*f*,
      35*t*
  as sedative-hypnotic, 222*t*, 223
Ethosuximide, 206–207, 206*f*, 208*t*
Ethylenediaminetetraacetic acid (EDTA),
      37*t*, 38
Etodolac, 165
Etomidate, 204, 204*t*
Etravirine, 75
Exenatide, 198–199
Ezetimibe, 149

F
F. *See* Bioavailability
Famciclovir, 72–73, 73*t*
Famotidine, 163, 174–175, 175*t*
Felodipine, 132–133
Fenofibrate, 148–149
Fentanyl, 219–221, 220*t*
Fesoterodine, 100–101
Fexofenadine, 162
Fibrates, 148–149, 149*b*
Fick's law of diffusion, 2*b*
Filgrastim, 122
Finasteride, 185, 196
First-pass effect, 4, 4*b*, 4*f*
Fish oil. *See* Omega-3-acid ethyl esters
Flecainide, 142–145, 143*f*, 143*t*
Floxuridine, 83
Fluconazole, 67, 67*b*
Flucytosine, 65*f*, 68
Fludarabine, 83
Fludrocortisone, 183–185, 184*b*
Flumazenil, 31, 32*t*, 221
Flunisolide, 166
Fluoroquinolones, 62–63, 62*t*, 63*b*
Fluorouracil, 83
Fluoxetine, 210*t*, 211
Fluphenazine, 213–214, 215*t*
Flutamide, 87, 185
Fluticasone, 166
Fluvastatin, 147–148
Fluvoxamine, 210*t*, 211
Folate, for anemia, 120–122, 121*b*, 123*b*
Folic acid synthesis inhibitors, 60–62,
      60*f*
Fomepizole, 33–34, 34*b*, 34*f*, 35*t*
Fondaparinux, 114
Food, drug absorption and, 4–5, 5*t*
Food and Drug Administration, pregnancy
      and, 190, 190*b*, 190*t*
Fosamprenavir, 75
Foscarnet, 72–73, 73*t*
Fosinopril, 130–131
Frank-Starling curve, 138, 138*f*
Frovatriptan, 221
Furosemide, 157, 157*f*
Fusion inhibitors, 75

G
GABA. *See* γ-Aminobutyric acid
GABA-activated receptor. *See* γ-
      Aminobutyric acid-activated receptor
Gabapentin, 206–207, 206*f*, 208*t*
Galantamine, 101, 218, 218*t*
Ganciclovir, 72–73, 73*t*
Gastric lavage, 29
Gastroesophageal reflux disease (GERD),
      173–176, 174*b*
  alginic acid for, 173–174
  antacids for, 173, 174*t*
  H_2 blockers for, 174–175, 175*b*, 175*t*
  PPIs for, 175, 175*b*, 175*t*
  prokinetic drugs for, 175–176
Gastrointestinal pharmacology, 173–180,
      174*f*
  complementary and alternative medicine,
      179
  for constipation, 177, 180*t*
  for diarrhea, 76, 177, 177*b*, 179*t*
  for GERD, 173–176, 174*b*, 174*t*, 175*b*,
      175*t*
  for IBD, 176–177, 176*t*
  for IBS, 177–179
  for nausea and vomiting, 177, 178*t*
  for peptic ulcer disease, 176, 176*b*
Gatifloxacin, 62–63
Gefitinib, 86–87
Gemcitabine, 83
Gemfibrozil, 148–149
Gemifloxacin, 62–63
Gemtuzumab, 85–86, 86*t*
Gemtuzumab ozogamicin, 26–27
Gene targeting, 27*b*
Gentamicin, 53–55
GERD. *See* Gastroesophageal reflux disease
Glatiramer, 218
Glomerulus, 153*b*, 154*b*
Glucocorticoids, 86*t*, 87, 88*t*, 89, 163–167,
      163*t*, 164*f*, 181, 182*t*, 185*b*, 185*f*.
      See also Adrenal gland
α-Glucosidase inhibitors, 198
Glutamate, 202*t*
Glycoprotein IIb/IIIa inhibitors, 119
Glycopyrrolate, 100–101
GnRH agonists. *See* Gonadotropin-releasing
      hormone agonists
Golimumab, 171*t*, 172
Gonadotropic hormones, 189–190
Gonadotropin-releasing hormone (GnRH)
      agonists, 192–193
Gout, 169, 170*f*
Gram staining, 42*b*
Granulocyte colony-stimulating factor, 122
Granulocyte-macrophage colony-stimulating
      factor, 122
Graves disease, 186–187
Griseofulvin, 65*f*, 68
Growth arrest, 81*b*
Growth-related disorders, 187–188, 188*f*
Guanosine triphosphate (GTP)-binding
      proteins, 21, 21*f*

H

H$_1$ antagonists, 162, 162b
H$_2$ blockers, 163, 163t, 174–175, 175b, 175t
Haloperidol, 213–214, 215t
HDLs. *See* High-density lipoproteins
Head lice medications, 70–71
Heart, normal conduction pathway of, 144b
Heart failure, 138–142, 138f, 139f, 139t, 140b, 140t
  ABCDs of managing, 138, 140t
  ACE inhibitors for, 138, 140b
  β-blockers for, 138, 140b
  dobutamine for, 141
  dopamine for, 142
  milrinone for, 141, 141f
  nesiritide for, 142
  positive inotropes for, 139–142, 141b, 141f
  precipitating factors for, 138t
  spironolactone for, 138, 140b
  vicious cycle of, 138, 139f
Heartburn. *See* Gastroesophageal reflux disease
Heavy metal poisons, 36–38, 37t
Hematologic toxidromes, 34–35, 35t
Hematology, 111–124, 112f, 113f
  anemia, 120–122, 121t
    hematopoietic stimulating factors for, 122
    supplementation for, 120–122, 121b, 121t, 123b
  anticoagulant drugs, 111–116
    direct thrombin inhibitors, 114
    heparins, 111b, 112–114, 112b, 116, 116t
    vitamin K antagonists, 114–116, 114t, 115b, 115t
  antiplatelet drugs, 116–119, 117f, 117t
    adenosine diphosphate inhibitors, 118–119
    glycoprotein IIb/IIIa inhibitors, 119
    phosphodiesterase inhibitors, 118
    salicylates, 117–118, 117f, 118f
  bleeding disorders, 120
  hereditary angioedema, 123
  hereditary tyrosinemia, 122
  immune thrombocytopenic purpura, 123
  paroxysmal nocturnal hemoglobinuria, 122–123
  phenylketonuria, 123
  thrombolytic drugs, 119
    first-generation, 119
    second-generation, 119, 120t
Hematopoietic stimulating factors, 122
Heparins, 112–114
  LMWHs, 112–113, 112b
  synthetic alternatives, 114
  unfractionated, 111b, 112–114
  warfarin v., 116, 116t
Hepatotoxicity, 36
Hereditary angioedema, 123
Hereditary tyrosinemia, 122
High-density lipoproteins (HDLs), 148b
Hirsutism, 159b, 185

HIV. *See* Human immunodeficiency virus
Hormonal replacement therapy, 192–195, 193b. *See also* Testosterone replacement therapy
Hormones. *See* Endocrine pharmacology
HPV. *See* Human papilloma virus
5HT3 antagonists. *See* Serotonin receptor antagonists
Human immunodeficiency virus (HIV), 74–76, 74b
Human papilloma virus (HPV), 73–74, 73b
Huntington chorea, 218–219, 219b
Hydrochlorothiazide, 157–158, 158f
Hydrocodone, 219–221
Hydrocortisone, 166–167, 183–185, 184b
Hydromorphone, 219–221
Hydrophilic drug, 2
Hydrophobic drug, 2
Hydroxocobalamin, 38
Hydroxychloroquine, 69, 69t
Hyoscyamine, 100–101
Hyperbaric oxygen, for CO poisoning, 34, 35t
Hypercortisolism, 181–183, 184f
Hyperlipidemia, 146–150, 147f, 147t
  bile acid sequestrants for, 149, 149b, 150b
  fibrates for, 148–149, 149b
  statins for, 147–148, 147f, 148b
Hypersensitivity reactions, 161b. *See also* Antihistamine drugs
Hypertension, 125–135, 126b, 126f, 127f, 128t, 135t
  ACE inhibitors for, 130–131, 130f, 131f
  aldosterone receptor antagonists for, 132
  ARBs for, 131–132
  β-blockers for, 128–130, 128f, 129t, 130b
  calcium channel blockers for, 132–133, 133f
  centrally acting α$_2$-agonists for, 133–134, 133f, 134f
  diuretics for, 128
  α$_1$-receptor blockers for, 132
  renin inhibitors for, 127f, 132
  vasodilators for, 134–135, 134f, 135b
Hyperthyroidism, 186–187, 187t
Hypogonadism, 195
Hyponatremia, 159
Hypothalamus, 181, 181b, 182f, 182t
Hypothyroidism, 187, 187b, 187t

I

IBD. *See* Inflammatory bowel disease
IBS. *See* Irritable bowel syndrome
Ibuprofen, 165
Ibutilide, 145–146
Idarubicin, 83–84
Ifosfamide, 81–83
Iloperidone, 213–214, 215t
Imatinib, 86–87
Imipenem/cilastatin, 51
Imipramine, 209–210, 210t

Imiquimod, 74
Immune thrombocytopenic purpura, 123
Immunopharmacology, 87–89, 88t
Immunosuppressive agents, 88–89, 89f
Incretin mimetics, 198–199
Indapamide, 157–158, 158f
Indinavir, 75
Indirect effectors of ANS function, 104f, 108–109, 109t
Indirect-acting cholinomimetics, 101
Indomethacin, 165
Inflammatory bowel disease (IBD), 176–177, 176t
Inflammatory disorders, 161–172. *See also* Antiinflammatory drugs
  antihistamine drugs for, 161–163, 162f, 162t, 178t
    H$_1$ antagonists, 162, 162b
    H$_2$ blockers, 163, 163t
  asthma, 167–169, 168b, 170t
  gout, 169, 170f
  rheumatoid arthritis, 170–172, 171t
  of skin, 167, 168t, 169b
Infliximab, 89, 171t, 172, 177
Inhalation administration, 6
Inhalation anesthetics, 203–204, 203t
Insulin, 196–197, 196b
Insulin secretogogues, 197, 198f
Integrase inhibition, 71–72, 71f, 76
Interferon-β, 218
International normalized ratio, 117b
Intestinal disease, drug absorption and, 4, 5t
Intracellular synthesis inhibition, 72–73, 73t
Intravenous administration, 6, 6b
Intravenous anesthetics, 204–205, 204f, 204t
Inverse agonists, 19–20
Ionization, absorption and, 2–3, 2b, 3b
Ionization constant (pK$_a$), 2, 3
Ionized diuresis, 29–30, 30b, 30t
Ipratropium, 100–101
Irbesartan, 131–132
Iron, 37t, 38, 120–122, 121b, 121t
Irritable bowel syndrome (IBS), 177–179
Isoflurane, 203–204, 203t
Isoniazid, 64
Isoproterenol, 106t, 107f, 108
Isosorbide dinitrate, 136–137
Isosorbide mononitrate, 136–137
Isradipine, 132–133
Itraconazole, 67
Ivermectin, 70
Ixabepilone, 84–85

K

Kanamycin, 53–55
Kava, 225
Ketamine, 204–205, 204t
Ketoconazole, 66, 66t, 67t, 181–183
Ketoprofen, 165
Ketorolac, 165
Ketotifen, 162, 162b
Kinetics, 9–10, 9b, 9f

L

Labetalol, 106*t*, 108, 128–130, 129*t*
Lacosamide, 206–207, 206*f*, 208*t*
β-Lactamase inhibitors, 48
Lamivudine, 74, 74*b*
Lamotrigine, 206–207, 206*f*, 208*t*
Lanreotide, 187–188
Lansoprazole, 175, 175*t*
Lapatinib, 86–87
LDLs. *See* Low-density lipoproteins
Lead, 37*t*, 38, 38*b*
Leukotriene receptor antagonists, 167–169
Leukotrienes, 163*t*, 164*f*
Levetiracetam, 206–207, 206*f*, 208*t*
Levocabastine, 162, 162*b*
Levodopa, 216–218, 217*t*
Levofloxacin, 62–63
Levothyroxine, 187, 187*b*
Lidocaine, 142–145, 143*f*, 143*t*, 205
Lincosamides, 56*f*, 57, 57*t*
Lindane, 70–71
Lines of Zahn, 111*b*
Linezolid, 60
Liothyronine, 187, 187*b*
Lipid soluble, 2
Lipopeptides, 63
Lipoproteins, 148*b*
Liraglutide, 198–199
Lisinopril, 130–131
Lithium, 212, 212*f*
LMWHs. *See* Low-molecular-weight heparins
Loading dose, 15
Local anesthetics, 205
Lomustine, 81–83
Loop diuretics, 128, 157, 157*f*, 160*t*
Loop of Henle, 153*b*
Lopinavir/ritonavir, 75
Loratadine, 162
Lorazepam, 221
Losartan, 131–132
Lovastatin, 147–148
Low-density lipoproteins (LDLs), 148*b*
Low-molecular-weight heparins (LMWHs), 112–113, 112*b*
Lumefantrine, 69

M

Macrolides, 57–59, 57*b*, 58*b*, 58*t*
Macula densa, 153*b*
Maintenance dose, 15
Malaria, 68, 69*b*, 69*t*
Mania, 208*b*, 212, 212*f*
Mannitol, 155–156
Maprotiline, 209–210
Maraviroc, 75–76
Marijuana, 224–225
Mast cell stabilizers, 167–169, 168*b*
Mebendazole, 70, 70*t*
Mecamylamine, 98–100
Mecasermin, 187–188

Mechlorethamine, 81–83
Meclizine, 162
Medroxyprogesterone, 192–193, 193*b*
Mefloquine, 69
Meglitinides, 197, 198*f*
Melatonin, 225
Meloxicam, 165
Melphalan, 81–83
Memantine, 218
Menopause, 192–193, 193*b*
Men's reproductive disorders, 195–196
    benign prostatic hyperplasia, 196
    erectile dysfunction, 195, 195*t*
    hypogonadism and andropause, 195
Menstrual disorders, 192–193, 192*t*
Meperidine, 219–221, 220*t*
Mercaptopurine, 83
Mercury, 37*t*, 38
Meropenem, 51
Mesalamine, 176, 176*t*
Mesangial cells, 153*b*
Mesolimbic dopamine pathway, 224*b*
Metabolism, 8–11
    bioavailability with, 14–15, 14*f*
    microsomal P450 isoenzymes, 10
        induction and inhibition of, 10–11, 12*b*, 12*t*
        phase I reactions, 10, 10*b*, 10*f*
        phase II reactions, 10, 10*f*
    rates of, 9–10, 9*b*, 9*f*
Metformin, 12, 197-198
Methacholine, 99*t*
Methadone, 219–221, 220*t*
Methamphetamine, 224
Methanol, 33–34, 34*b*, 34*f*, 35*t*
Methazolamide, 156–157, 156*f*
Methicillin, 46–48, 47*t*
Methimazole, 186–187
Methohexital, 204–205, 204*t*
Methotrexate, 83
Methoxamine, 104–106, 107*f*
Methyldopa, 133–134
Methylprednisolone, 166
Methylxanthines, 167–169
Metoclopramide, 32–33, 33*b*, 33*t*, 34*t*, 175–176
Metolazone, 157–158, 158*f*
Metoprolol, 106*t*, 107*f*, 108, 128–130, 129*t*
Metronidazole, 63
Metyrapone, 181–183
Mexiletine, 142–145, 143*f*, 143*t*
Mezlocillin, 47*t*, 48
Micafungin, 67–68
Microsomal P450 isoenzymes, 10
    induction and inhibition of, 10–11, 12*b*, 12*t*
        phase I reactions, 10, 10*b*, 10*f*
        phase II reactions, 10, 10*f*
Miglitol, 185
Milnacipran, 211
Milrinone, 141, 141*f*
Minocycline, 55–56

Minoxidil, 134–135
Misoprostol, 176, 189–190
Mitomycin, 81–84
Mitotane, 181–183
Mitotic inhibitors, 82*f*, 84–85
Mivacurium, 98–100, 205, 205*t*
Moexipril, 130–131
Mofetil, 89
Molecular weight, absorption and, 3
Mometasone, 166–167
Monoamine oxidase inhibitors, 209*f*, 210*t*, 211–212, 211*b*, 212*b*
Monobactams, 51–52, 52*t*
Monoclonal antibodies, 85–86, 86*t*
Montelukast, 164*f*, 168
Mood disorders. *See* Affective disorders
Morphine, 219–221, 220*t*
Movement disorders, 214–219
    Alzheimer disease, 218, 218*t*
    Huntington chorea, 218–219, 219*b*
    multiple sclerosis, 218, 219*t*
    Parkinson disease, 209*f*, 216–218, 216*b*, 216*f*, 217*t*
Moxifloxacin, 62–63
Mucous membrane administration, 6
Multiple sclerosis, 218, 219*t*
Mupirocin, 59
Muscarine, 99*t*, 100
Muscarinic drugs, 100–101
    agonists, 99*t*, 100
    antagonists, 100–101
    indirect-acting agonists, 101
Muscarinic receptors, 92–93, 94*t*, 96, 97*f*, 97*t*, 98*f*, 99*f*, 99*t*
Muscle relaxants, 205–206
    neuromuscular blockers, 205, 205*t*
    spasmolytics, 206
Mycophenolate, 89

N

Nadolol, 128–130, 129*t*
Nafcillin, 46–48, 47*t*
Nalbuphine, 219–221
Naloxone, 31–32, 32*t*, 219–221
Naltrexone, 219–221
Nanomedicine, 27
Naproxen, 165
Naratriptan, 221
Natalizumab, 177, 218
Natamycin, 65–66
Natural penicillins, 46, 47*t*
Nausea, 177, 178*t*
Nebivolol, 108, 128–130, 129*t*
Nelarabine, 83
Nelfinavir, 75
Neomycin, 53–55
Neostigmine, 101
Nephron, 153*b*
Nesiritide, 142
Netilmicin, 53–55
Neurochemical organization, of ANS, 91–92, 93*f*

Neurodegeneration, 214–219
  Alzheimer disease, 218, 218t
  Huntington chorea, 218–219, 219b
  multiple sclerosis, 218, 219t
  Parkinson disease, 209f, 216–218, 216b, 216f, 217t
Neuroleptics. See Antipsychotics
Neuromuscular blockers, 205, 205t
Neuroreceptor organization, of ANS, 92–93, 93t
Neurotoxicity, 30–34
  of anticholinergics, 31, 32t
  of benzodiazepines, 31, 32t
  of methanol, 33–34, 34b, 34f, 35t
  opioids, 31–32, 32t
  of organophosphates, 30–31, 31f, 31t
  serotonin syndrome, 32–33, 33b, 33t, 34t, 212b
Neurotransmitters, 91–92, 93f, 95b, 202t
Nevirapine, 75
Niacin, 149, 150b
Nicardine, 132–133
Nicotine, 96, 98, 225, 225b
Nicotinic drugs, 96–100
  agonists, 98
  antagonists, 98–100
  indirect-acting agonists, 101
Nicotinic receptors, 92–93, 94t, 96, 97f, 97t, 99t
Nifedipine, 132–133
Nilotinib, 86–87
Nimodipine, 132–133
Nisoldipine, 132–133
Nitazoxanide, 63
Nitisinone, 122
Nitrates, 136–137, 137b
Nitrofurantoin, 53
Nitroglycerin, 136–137
Nitrous oxide, 203–204
Nizatidine, 163, 174–175, 175t
NMDA receptor antagonists, 218
Nonbenzodiazepine GABA_A receptor modulators, 221–222, 222t
Non-nucleoside reverse transcriptase inhibitors, 75
Nonsteroidal antiinflammatory drugs (NSAIDs)
  for inflammatory disorders, 163–167, 163t, 164f, 166t
  peptic ulcer disease and, 176, 176b
  for rheumatoid arthritis, 170–172
Nonsynthetic reactions. See Phase I reactions
Norepinephrine, 91–92, 104–106, 202t. See also Adrenergic systems
  antidepressants and, 209, 209f
  autonomic receptors for, 92–93, 94t
Norfloxacin, 62–63
Nortriptyline, 209–210
NSAIDs. See Nonsteroidal antiinflammatory drugs
Nucleoside/nucleotide reverse transcriptase inhibitors, 74, 74b
Nystatin, 65–66

O
Octreotide, 187–188
Ofloxacin, 62–63
Olanzapine, 213–214, 215t
Olmesartan, 131–132
Olopatadine, 162, 162b
Omega-3-acid ethyl esters (fish oil), 150–151
Omeprazole, 175, 175t
Opioids, 219–221
  analgesics, 219–221, 220b, 220t, 223b
  endogenous, 219
  toxicity of, 31–32, 32t
Opioid receptor antagonists, 180t
Oral administration, 4–5, 5b, 5t, 6b
Oral contraceptives, 190–192, 191t
Organophosphate poisoning, 30–31, 31f, 31t
Orphan diseases, 172b
Oseltamivir, 71f, 72
Osmotic diuretics, 155–156
Osteoblasts, 193b
Osteoclasts, 193b
Osteoporosis, 193–195, 193b, 194t
Oxacillin, 46–48, 47t
Oxaliplatin, 81–83
Oxcarbazepine, 206–207, 206f, 208t
Oxybutynin, 100–101
Oxycodone, 219–221, 220t
Oxytetracycline, 55–56
Oxytocin, 188–190

P
Paclitaxel, 84–85
Pain management, 219
  for migraine headaches, 221
  with opioid analgesics, 219–221, 220b, 220t, 223b
Paliperidone, 213–214, 215t
Pancreatic disorders, 196–199, 196b, 197b, 198f, 199b
Pancuronium, 98–100, 205, 205t
Panitumumab, 85–86, 86t
Pantoprazole, 175, 175t
Parasympathetic nervous system, 91, 92b, 92f, 92t. See also Cholinergic systems
  neurotransmitters of, 91–92, 93f
  physiologic responses of, 93–94, 94t
  receptors of, 92–93, 93t
Parathyroid hormone (PTH), 158b, 194t, 195
Parenteral administration, 6, 6b, 6t
Parenteral anesthetics. See Intravenous anesthetics
Parkinson disease, 209f, 216–218, 216b, 216f, 217t
Paroxetine, 210t, 211
Paroxysmal nocturnal hemoglobinuria, 122–123
Partial agonists, 19, 20f
Partial fatty acid oxidation inhibitor, 137
Passive diffusion, 2, 2b
PCOS. See Polycystic ovary syndrome
Pegaptanib, 27

Pegfilgrastim, 122
Pegvisomant, 187–188
Pemetrexed, 83
Penbutolol, 128–130, 129t
Penciclovir, 72–73, 73t
Penicillamine, 37t, 38
Penicillins
  adverse effects of, 44–45, 52t
  β-lactamase inhibitors and, 48
  drug interactions with, 45–46
  elimination of, 12
  mechanism of action of, 43, 45f
  prescribing, 48b
  probenecid and, 154b
  resistance to, 43, 45f
  subclassification of, 46–48, 47t
    amino-, 46, 47t
    antipseudomonal, 47t, 48
    natural, 46, 47t
    penicillinase-resistant, 46–48, 47t
Penicillin G, 46, 47t
Penicillin V, 46, 47t
Penicillinase-resistant penicillins, 46–48, 47t
Pentazocine, 219–221, 220t
Pentostatin, 83
Peptic ulcer disease, 176, 176b
Pergolide, 216–218, 217t
Perindopril, 130–131
Permethrin, 71
pH, 2–3, 2b, 3b
Pharmacodynamics, 17–27, 18t
  agonists, 17, 19–20, 20f
  antagonists, 17, 20, 20f
  biologics, 24–27, 26f
  dose-response relationships, 17–19, 18f, 18t, 19b, 19f
  time-response relationships, 19, 19f
Pharmacokinetics, 1–15, 2t
  absorption, 1–7
    dosage form, 3, 4f
    ionization, 2–3, 2b, 3b
    molecular weight, 3
    routes of administration, 3–7, 4b
  changes with aging, 12–13
  in clinical practice, 13–15, 14b
    bioavailability, 14–15, 14f
    desired drug level, 13–14, 14f
    loading dose, 15
    maintenance dose, 15
  distribution, 7–8, 8b
    plasma protein binding, 7–8, 7t, 8b
    selective, 8, 8b, 8f
  drug factors affecting, 14–15, 14f
  elimination, 11–13, 13b, 13f, 13t
  metabolism, 8–11
    microsomal P450 isoenzymes, 10
    rates of, 9–10, 9b, 9f
Phase I reactions, 10, 10b, 10f
Phase II reactions, 10, 10f
Phenelzine, 210t, 211–212
Phenindamine, 162
Phenobarbital, 206–207, 206f, 208t, 222, 222t

Phenoxybenzamine, 106–107, 106t, 107f
Phentolamine, 106–107, 106t, 107f
Phenylephrine, 104–106, 106t, 107f
Phenylketonuria, 123
Phenytoin, 206–207, 206f, 208t
Phosphatidylinositol 4,5-bisphosphate (PIP$_2$), 22–23, 23f, 212b
Phosphodiesterase inhibitors, 118, 195, 195t
Physiologic responses, to ANS stimulation, 93–94, 94t
Physostigmine, 31, 32t, 101
Pilocarpine, 99t, 100
Pimecrolimus, 88–89
Pindolol, 108, 128–130, 129t
Pioglitazone, 198, 198f
PIP$_2$. See Phosphatidylinositol 4,5-bisphosphate
Piperacillin, 47t, 48
Piroxicam, 165
Pituitary gland, 181, 181b, 182f, 182t. See also Anterior pituitary hormones; Posterior pituitary hormones
pK$_a$. See Ionization constant
Placental barrier, 8
Plasma protein binding, 7–8, 7t, 8b
Plerixafor, 122
Podofilox, 74
Poisoning. See Toxicology
Polycystic ovary syndrome (PCOS), 159b
Polyenes, 65–66, 65f, 66b
Polymyxin B, 53
Posaconazole, 67
Positive inotropes, 139–142, 141b, 141f
Posterior pituitary hormones, 188–189
    oxytocin, 188–189
    vasopressin analogs, 188–189, 189b, 189f
Potassium channel blockers, 145–146, 145f, 146b
Potassium-sparing agents, 128, 158–159, 158f, 160t
Potency, 17, 18t
PPIs. See Proton pump inhibitors
Pralidoxime, 30–31, 31f, 31t, 101
Pramipexole, 216–218, 217t
Pramlintide, 198–199
Pravastatin, 147–148
Praziquantel, 70
Prazosin, 106–107, 106t, 107f, 132, 196
Prednisolone, 166
Prednisone, 166
Pregabalin, 206–207, 206f, 208t
Pregnancy, 189–190, 190b, 190t
Premenstrual syndrome, 192–193, 192t
Primaquine, 69
Probenecid, 12, 154b
Probiotics, 76, 179
Procainamide, 142–145, 143f, 143t
Procarbazine, 81–83
Prochlorperazine, 213–214, 215t
Progestins
    in contraceptives, 190–192, 191t
    in hormonal replacement therapy, 192–193, 193b

Prokinetic drugs, 175–176
Prolactin disorders, 188
Promethazine, 162
Propafenone, 142–145, 143f, 143t
Propofol, 204–205, 204t
Propranolol, 93–94, 106t, 107f, 108, 128–130, 129t, 145
Propylthiouracil, 186–187
Prostaglandins, 163t, 164f
Protamine, 34–35, 35t
Protease inhibitors, 75
Protein synthesis, prokaryotic, 53b, 54f
Protein synthesis inhibitors, 53–60, 54f
Protein-bound drugs, 7–8, 8b
Proton pump inhibitors (PPIs), 175, 175b, 175t
Psoriasis, 167
Psychomotor stimulants, 224
Psychoses. See Antipsychotics
Psyllium, 150–151
PTH. See Parathyroid hormone
Pulmonary arterial hypertension, 135–136, 136t
Pyrazinamide, 64
Pyridostigmine, 101

Q
QT interval, prolonged, 58–59, 62, 63b
Quantal dose-response curves, 18, 19b, 19f
Quetiapine, 213–214, 215t
Quinapril, 130–131
Quinidine, 142–145, 143f, 143t
Quinine, 69
Quinupristin, 60

R
RAA pathway. See Renin-angiotensin-aldosterone pathway
Rabeprazole, 175, 175t
Radioactive iodide, 186–187
Raloxifene, 193–195
Raltegravir, 76
Ramipril, 130–131
Ranitidine, 163, 174–175, 175t
Ranolazine, 137
Rasagiline, 216–218, 217t
Recreational drugs. See Drug abuse
Rectal administration, 5–6
5α-Reductase inhibitors, 196
Regional anesthesia. See Local anesthetics
Renal clearance, 155, 155b, 155f
Renal system, 153–160, 154f, 160t
    carbonic anhydrase inhibitors in, 156–157, 156f
    complementary and alternative medicine and, 159–160, 160b
    elimination and, 154–155, 155b, 155f
    hyponatremia and, 159
    loop diuretics in, 157, 157f
    osmotic diuretics in, 155–156

Renal system (Continued)
    potassium-sparing agents in, 158–159, 158f
    thiazides in, 157–158, 158f
Renin, 183b, 183f
Renin inhibitors, 127f, 132
Renin-angiotensin-aldosterone (RAA) pathway, 159b
Reproductive disorders. See Men's reproductive disorders; Women's reproductive disorders
Retapamulin, 59
Reteplase, 119, 120t
Retinoids, 167
Reye syndrome, 118b
Rheumatoid arthritis, 170–172, 171t
Ribavirin, 72–73, 73t
Rifampin, 64
Rifaximin, 63
Rimantadine, 71f, 72
Risperidone, 213–214, 215t
Ritodrine, 108
Ritonavir, 75
Rituximab, 85–86, 86t
Rivastigmine, 101, 218, 218t
Rizatriptan, 221
RNA synthesis inhibitors, 62–63
Rocuronium, 98–100
Romiplostim, 123
Ropinirole, 216–218, 217t
Rosiglitazone, 198, 198f
Rosuvastatin, 147–148
Rotigotine, 216–218, 217t
Routes of administration, 3–7, 4b
    inhalation, 6
    mucous membranes, 6
    parenteral, 6, 6b, 6t
    rectal, 5–6
    sublingual and oral, 4–5, 4f, 5b, 5t, 6b
    topical, 7
Rufinamide, 206–207, 206f, 208t

S
Salicylates, 117–118, 117f, 118f
Salicylic acid, 2b, 29–30, 30t
Salmeterol, 108
Saquinavir, 75
Sargramostim, 122
Sarin, 101
Saxagliptin, 198–199
Schizophrenia, 212–213, 213t, 214f, 215t
Scopolamine, 100–101
Secobarbital, 222, 222t
Sedative-hypnotics, 221–223
    alcohol, 222t, 223
    barbiturates, 222, 222f, 222t
    benzodiazepines, 221, 222b, 222f, 222t
    GABA receptor modulators, 221, 222t
    nonbenzodiazepine GABA$_A$ receptor modulators, 221–222, 222t
Seizure disorders, 206–207, 206f, 207b, 208t
β$_2$-Selective agonists, 167–169

Selective distribution, 8, 8b, 8f
Selective estrogen receptor modulators, 193–195
Selective norepinephrine reuptake inhibitors (SNRIs), 209f, 210t, 211, 211b
Selective serotonin reuptake inhibitors (SSRIs), 209f, 210t, 211, 211b
Selegiline, 216–218, 217t
Sermorelin, 187–188
Seropterin, 123
Serotonin, 202t, 209, 209f
Serotonin receptor (5HT3) antagonists, 178t
Serotonin syndrome, 32–33, 33b, 33t, 34t, 212b
Sertraline, 210t, 211
Sevoflurane, 203–204, 203t
Shock, 167b
Signal transduction, 20–24, 21f, 22f, 23f, 24b, 24f, 25f, 26f
Signal transduction inhibitors, 86–87
Sildenafil, 195, 195t
Silodosin, 106–107, 196
Silver sulfadiazine, 60–61, 60f, 61b, 61t
Simvastatin, 147–148
Sinecatechins, 74
Sirolimus, 88–89
Sitagliptin, 198–199
Skin disorders, 167, 168t, 169b
SLUD syndrome, 30
SNRIs. See Selective norepinephrine reuptake inhibitors
Sodium, water retention and, 131b
Sodium channel blockers, 142–145, 143f, 143t
Sodium nitrate, 38
Sodium nitroprusside, 134–135
Sodium thiosulfate, 38
Solifenacin, 100–101
Soman, 101
Somatostatin analogs, 179t
Somatropin, 187–188
Sorafenib, 86–87
Sotalol, 128–130, 129t, 145–146
Spare receptor, 20
Spasmolytics, 206
Spironolactone, 132
  as diuretic, 158–159, 158f
  for heart failure, 138, 140b
  for hirsutism and PCOS, 159b
SSRIs. See Selective serotonin reuptake inhibitors
St. John's wort, 39, 199, 225
Stable angina, 136–137, 136b, 137b, 137t
  nitrates for, 136–137, 137b
  partial fatty acid oxidation inhibitor, 137
Statins, 147–148, 147f, 148b
Stavudine, 74, 74b
Steroids. See Adrenal gland
Steroidal antiinflammatory drugs, 163–167, 163t, 164f
Steroid-mediated signal transduction, 185b, 185f
Stevens-Johnson syndrome, 61b

Stimulants, 209f, 224
Stomach, acid release in, 173b, 174f
Streptogramins, 60
Streptokinase, 119
Streptomycin, 53–55
Streptozocin, 81–84
Sublingual administration, 4–5, 4f, 5b, 5t
Substance P/neurokinin-1 receptor antagonists, 178t
Substrate reduction therapy, 26
Succimer, 37t, 38
Succinylcholine, 98–100, 205, 205t
Sucralfate, 176
Sulfacetamide, 60–61, 60f, 61b, 61t
Sulfadiazine, 60–61, 60f, 61b, 61t
Sulfamethoxazole, 60–61, 60f, 61b, 61t
Sulfasalazine, 60–61, 60f, 61b, 61t, 176, 176t
Sulfisoxazole, 60–61, 60f, 61b, 61t
Sulfonamides, 60–61, 60f, 61b, 61t
Sulfonylureas, 197, 198f
Sulindac, 165
Sumatriptan, 221
Sunitinib, 86–87
Susceptibility testing, 41–42, 44f
Sympathetic nervous system, 91, 92b, 92f, 92t. See also Adrenergic systems
  neurotransmitters of, 91–92, 93f
  physiologic responses of, 93–94, 94t
  receptors of, 92–93, 93t
Synthetic reactions. See Phase II reactions
Synthetic thyroxine, 187, 187b

T

T$_4$. See Thyroxine
Tabun, 101
Tachyphylaxis, 137
Tacrine, 101, 218, 218t
Tacrolimus, 88–89
Tadalafil, 195, 195t
Tamoxifen, 87
Tamsulosin, 106–107, 196
T-cell immunomodulators, 167
Tegafur, 83
Telavancin, 52
Telbivudine, 72–73, 73t
Telmisartan, 131–132
Telomerase, 81b
Temazepam, 221
Temozolomide, 81–83
Temsirolimus, 88–89
Tenecteplase, 119, 120t
Tenofovir, 74, 74b
Terazosin, 106–107, 132, 196
Terbinafine, 65f, 68
Terbutaline, 106t, 107f, 108
Testosterone replacement therapy, 195
Tetrabenazine, 218–219
Tetracyclines, 55–56, 55f, 55t, 56t
Thiazides, 128, 157–158, 158f, 160t
Thiazolidinediones, 198, 198f
Thioguanine, 83
Thionamides, 186–187

Thiopental, 204–205, 204t
Thioridazine, 213–214, 215t
Thiotepa, 81–83
Thrombin inhibitors, direct, 114
Thrombolytic drugs, 119
  first-generation, 119
  second-generation, 119, 120t
Thromboxanes, 163t
Thyroid disorders, 185–187, 186f, 187t
  Graves disease, 186–187
  hypothyroidism, 187, 187b, 187t
Thyroxine (T$_4$), 185–186, 187, 187b
Tiagabine, 206–207, 206f, 208t
Ticarcillin, 47t, 48
Ticlopidine, 118–119
Tigecycline, 55–56
Time-response relationships, 19, 19f
Timolol, 107f, 108, 128–130, 129t
Tinidazole, 63
Tinzaparin, 112–113, 112b
Tiotropium, 100–101
Tipranavir, 75
Tirofiban, 119
Tissue plasminogen activators (t-PA), 119, 120t
Tobramycin, 53–55
Tocainide, 142–145, 143f, 143t
Tocilizumab, 171t, 172
Tolcapone, 216–218, 217t
Tolerance, 224b
Tolterodine, 100–101
Tolvaptan, 159
Topical administration, 7
Topiramate, 206–207, 206f, 208t
Topoisomerase, 84b
Torsemide, 157
Tositumomab, 85–86, 86t
Total peripheral resistance, 125
Toxicology, 29–39
  approaches to patient, 29–30
  cardiovascular drugs/poisons, 34–35
    carbon monoxide, 34, 35t
    hematologic and cardiovascular toxidromes, 34–35, 35t
  complementary and alternative medicines, 39
  cyanide poisoning, 38
  heavy metal poisons, 36–38
  hepatic, 36
  neurologic, 30–34
    anticholinergics, 31, 32t
    benzodiazepines, 31, 32t
    methanol, 33–34, 34b, 34f, 35t
    opioids, 31–32, 32t
    organophosphates, 30–31, 31f, 31t
    serotonin syndrome, 32–33, 33b, 33t, 34t
  specific antidotes for, 30–38
t-PA. See Tissue plasminogen activators
Tranquilizers. See Antipsychotics
Transdermal formulations, 7
Transient protein C deficiency, 112b
Trans-uranium elements, 38

Tranylcypromine, 211–212
Trastuzumab, 85–86, 86*t*
Trazodone, 209–210, 210*t*
Triamcinolone, 166–167
Triamterene, 158–159, 158*f*
Triazolam, 221, 222*t*
Tricyclic antidepressants, 209–210, 209*f*, 210*t*
Trihexyphenidyl, 216–218, 217*t*
Trimethaphan, 98–100
Trimethoprim, 60*f*, 61–62
Trimetrexate, 83
Triptans, 221
Trospium, 100–101
Tubocurarine, 205
Tubulin, 85*b*
Type 2 diabetes, 196–198, 196*b*, 198*f*
Tyramine, 211–212, 211*b*

U
Ulcerative colitis, 176–177, 176*t*
Unfractionated heparins, 111*b*, 112–114
Uracil mustard, 81–83
Urea, 155–156
Uricosurics, 169
Urokinase, 119
Uterine fibroids, 192–193

V
Vaccine, for HPV, 73*b*
Valacyclovir, 72–73, 73*t*
Valganciclovir, 72–73, 73*t*

Valproic acid, 206–207, 206*f*, 208*t*
Valrubicin, 83–84
Valsartan, 131–132
Vancomycin, 52, 53*t*
Vardenafil, 195, 195*t*
Vasodilators, 134–135, 134*f*, 135*b*
Vasopressin analogs, 188–189, 189*b*, 189*f*
Vecuronium, 98–100, 205, 205*t*
Venlafaxine, 210*t*, 211
Ventricular membrane depolarization, 144*b*
Verapamil, 132–133, 146
Very-low-density lipoproteins (VLDLs), 148*b*
Vigabatrin, 206–207, 206*f*, 208*t*
Vinblastine, 84–85
Vincristine, 84–85
Vinorelbine, 84–85
Viral infection, mechanics of, 72*b*
Viral neuraminidase inhibition, 72
Viral uncoating inhibition, 71*f*, 72
Vitamin B$_{12}$, 120–122, 123*b*
Vitamin D, 193, 193*b*, 194, 194*t*
Vitamin K, 34–35, 35*t*, 120
Vitamin K antagonists, 114–116, 114*t*, 115*b*, 115*t*
VLDLs. *See* Very-low-density lipoproteins
Vomiting, 177, 178*t*
Voriconazole, 66
Vorinostat, 86–87

W
Warfarin, 114–116, 114*t*, 115*b*, 115*t*, 116*t*
Water retention, sodium and, 131*b*

Weak acids, detoxification of, 156*b*
Weak bases, detoxification of, 156*b*
Women's reproductive disorders, 189–195
   contraception, 190–192, 191*t*
   menopause, 192–193, 193*b*
   menstrual disorders, endometriosis, and uterine fibroids, 192–193, 192*t*
   osteoporosis, 193–195, 193*b*, 194*t*
   pregnancy, 189–190, 190*b*, 190*t*

X
Xanthine oxidase inhibitors, 169, 170*f*

Y
Yeast infections, 76
Yohimbine, 106–107, 106*t*, 107*f*

Z
Zafirlukast, 164*f*, 168
Zalcitabine, 74, 74*b*
Zaleplon, 221–222
Zanamivir, 71*f*, 72
Zidovudine, 74, 74*b*
Zileuton, 164*f*
Ziprasidone, 213–214, 215*t*
Zolmitriptan, 221
Zolpidem, 221–222, 222*t*
Zonisamide, 206–207, 206*f*, 208*t*